Orthodontics & Paediatric Dentistry

Commissioning Editor: *Alison Taylor*
Senior Development Editor: *Ailsa Laing*
Project Manager: *Frances Affleck*
Designer: *Stewart Larking*
Illustration Manager: *Bruce Hogarth*

CLINICAL **PROBLEM SOLVING** IN DENTISTRY
SERIES

SECOND EDITION

Orthodontics & Paediatric Dentistry

Declan Millett

BDSc DDS FDSRCPS (Glasg) DOrthRCSEng MOrthRCSEng
Professor of Orthodontics
Cork University Dental School and Hospital
University College Cork
Ireland

Richard Welbury

MBBS BDS PhD FDSRCS FDSRCPS FRCPCH
Director of Postgraduate Education
Professor of Paediatric Dentistry
Glasgow Dental Hospital and School
University of Glasgow
UK

with a contribution from

Caroline Campbell

MSc BDS MFDS RCPS(Glasg) MPaedDent(Ed) FDSPaedDent(Glasg)
Consultant in Paediatric Dentistry
Department of Paediatric Dentistry
Glasgow Dental Hospital and School
University of Glasgow
UK

CHURCHILL LIVINGSTONE

ELSEVIER

Edinburgh London New York Oxford Philadelphia St Louis Sydney Toronto 2010

CHURCHILL
LIVINGSTONE
ELSEVIER

© 2010 Elsevier Ltd. All rights reserved.

First edition 2005
Second edition 2010
    Reprinted 2011 (twice), 2013

ISBN 978-0-7020-3124-3

British Library Cataloguing in Publication Data
A catalogue record for this book is available from the British Library

Library of Congress Cataloging in Publication Data
A catalog record for this book is available from the Library of Congress

Notices

Knowledge and best practice in this field are constantly changing. As new research and experience broaden our understanding, changes in research methods, professional practices, or medical treatment may become necessary.

Practitioners and researchers must always rely on their own experience and knowledge in evaluating and using any information, methods, compounds, or experiments described herein. In using such information or methods they should be mindful of their own safety and the safety of others, including parties for whom they have a professional responsibility.

With respect to any drug or pharmaceutical products identified, readers are advised to check the most current information provided (i) on procedures featured or (ii) by the manufacturer of each product to be administered, to verify the recommended dose or formula, the method and duration of administration, and contraindications. It is the responsibility of practitioners, relying on their own experience and knowledge of their patients, to make diagnoses, to determine dosages and the best treatment for each individual patient, and to take all appropriate safety precautions.

To the fullest extent of the law, neither the Publisher nor the authors, contributors, or editors, assume any liability for any injury and/or damage to persons or property as a matter of products liability, negligence or otherwise, or from any use or operation of any methods, products, instructions, or ideas contained in the material herein.

ELSEVIER your source for books, journals and multimedia in the health sciences
www.elsevierhealth.com

Working together to grow
libraries in developing countries

www.elsevier.com | www.bookaid.org | www.sabre.org

ELSEVIER . BOOK AID International Sabre Foundation

The
publisher's
policy is to use
paper manufactured
from sustainable forests

Printed in China

Contents

1 Median diastema   1

2 Unerupted upper central incisor   5

3 Absent upper lateral incisors   10

4 Crowding and buccal upper canines   15

5 Severe crowding   20

6 Palatal canines   26

7 More canine problems   32

8 Infra occluded primary molars   37

9 Increased overjet   41

10 Incisor crossbite   47

11 Reverse overjet   50

12 Increased overbite   54

13 Anterior open bite   58

14 Posterior crossbite   62

15 Bilateral crossbite   66

16 Late lower incisor crowding   74

17 Prominent chin and TMJDS   77

18 Drifting incisors   83

19 Appliance related problems   87

20 Tooth movement and related problems   91

21 Cleft lip and palate   96

22 Nursing and early childhood caries   100

23 High caries risk adolescents   103
by Caroline Campbell

24 The uncooperative child   107

25 Disorders of eruption and exfoliation   110

26 Pain control and carious primary teeth   113

27 Facial swelling and dental abscess   116

28 The displaced primary incisor   119

29 The fractured immature permanent incisor crown   122

30 The fractured permanent incisor root   125

31 The avulsed incisor   128

32 Poor quality first permanent molars   131

33 Tooth discoloration, hypomineralization and hypoplasia   135

34 Mottled teeth   139

35 Dental erosion   143

36 Multiple missing and abnormally shaped teeth   146

37 Amelogenesis imperfecta   150

38 Dentinogenesis imperfecta   153

39 Gingival bleeding and enlargement   156

40 Oral ulceration   159

41 Mind Maps®   162

Appendices:

A1 The index of orthodontic treatment need: dental health component   203

A2 Lateral cephalometric analysis   204

Index   206

Preface to the second edition

In view of the favourable response from students who used the first edition, we were pleased when the publishers asked us to do a second edition. The problem-solving approach, with question and answer format, has proved popular, as have the Mind Maps®.

The philosophy of the book remains the same as that of the first edition, in that the reader is presented with a clinical problem and then taken logically through sequential steps of case assessment, diagnosis and treatment planning. All chapters have been updated where relevant. Four new chapters (with Mind Maps®) are included, dealing with severe crowding, more canine problems, bilateral crossbite and high caries risk adolescents. The reference list in each chapter incorporates the best of current evidence for self-directed learning and reflection. As several medical conditions affect dental and orthodontic management of the child and adolescent patient, the reader is referred, where appropriate, to Scully C, Cawson RA 2005 Medical Problems in Dentistry, 5th edn, Edinburgh, Churchill Livingstone.

We hope that the second edition will continue to prove useful to undergraduates and postgraduates in the early years of specialty training.

DTM
RRW
Cork and Glasgow 2010

Preface to the first edition

Problem solving is a core skill which the dental undergraduate must develop and refine for examinations and everyday clinical practice. As orthodontics and paediatric dentistry interface broadly, combined clinical teaching and examinations in these disciplines are linked increasingly to encourage holistic problem solving of dental and occlusal problems in the child and adolescent patient.

This book aims, therefore, to address a range of common clinical problems encountered in orthodontic and paediatric dental practice. The format promotes a logical approach to problem solving through history taking, clinical examination and diagnosis, which underpin the principles of treatment planning for both disciplines. A short reference list is provided with each chapter to facilitate further directed learning.

Mind Maps® are also given for each topic to provide a focused framework for learning and revision. Each Mind Map® links key words, or key points, which are highlighted throughout the text, to create an overview of the subject and is designed to trigger information recall.

Intended primarily for the undergraduate, we hope this book will be of value also to the junior postgraduate and to those preparing for membership examinations.

DTM
RRW
Cork and Glasgow 2004

Acknowledgements

We are particularly grateful to Mrs K Shepherd and Mrs G Drake for their help and support in the preparation of photographic material. We would also like to thank especially Dr G McIntyre, Ms R Bryan, Mr J C Aird, Dr A Shaw, Miss D Fung, Dr T Ubaya, Dr C Campbell, Dr K O'Rourke, Dr P Murray and Mr S A Fayle for provision of some of the illustrations. Mr J Brown also kindly assisted with the drawings of appliances and editing of photographic material along with Ms J Howard. We are also grateful to Buzan Centres Ltd for the style for the Mind Maps®. Our gratitude is extended to the staff of Elsevier who have been very helpful throughout.

1

Median diastema

SUMMARY

Brian is almost 8 years of age. He presents with a gap between his upper front teeth and crooked lower front teeth (Fig. 1.1). What are the causes of these problems and what treatment would you recommend?

History

Complaint

Brian's mother noticed the gap between his upper front teeth and the irregularity of his lower front teeth. She is anxious about his appearance and is keen for treatment to be provided.

History of complaint

Brian's primary front teeth had a pleasing appearance with a small midline space in the upper arch; the lower primary front teeth were not spaced. There is no history of trauma. The permanent incisors erupted in their present positions.

- no trauma
- ?p

Medical history

Brian is fit and well.

Dental history

Brian attends his general dental practitioner every 6 months but has not required any treatment.

Family history

Brian's father had an upper midline space that was closed with a fixed appliance.

Examination

Extraoral examination

Brian has a Class I skeletal pattern with average FMPA and no facial asymmetry. Lips are competent with the lower lip resting at the incisal third of the upper central incisors. There are no temporomandibular joint signs or symptoms.

Intraoral examination

Soft tissues are healthy and the dentition is caries-free. The intraoral views are shown in **Figures 1.1** and **1.2**.

■ *What do you observe?*

✱ Low-lying maxillary labial frenum.

The following teeth are clearly visible: $\dfrac{6\,e\,d\,c\,b\,|\,|\,|\,b\,c\,d}{6\,e\,d\,c\,2\,|\,|\,|\,2\,c\,d\,e\,6}$

(note $\underline{|e6}$ present but $\underline{|6}$ erupting into $\underline{|e}$).

Mild lower labial segment crowding with distolabial rotations of $\overline{1|1}$; slight spacing distal of $\overline{2|2}$.

Upper median diastema with the crowns of $\underline{1|1}$ flared distally.

- Class III incisor relationship.

- Crossbites $\dfrac{b\,|\,b}{c\,|\,c}$.

■ *What is the aetiology of the $\overline{1|1}$ rotations?*

Incisor rotations are usually a manifestation of inherent crowding in the arch, which is genetic in origin. The lack of primary lower incisor spacing reported by the child's mother is predictive of likely crowding of the permanent successors. Incisor rotations may also result from ectopic position of the tooth germs or from the presence of a supernumerary tooth.

- lack of spacing 1°
low lying frenum

Fig. 1.1 Anterior occlusion at presentation.

Fig. 1.2 Lower occlusal view (note $\overline{6|6}$ erupted but not shown).

■ **What are the possible causes of the upper median diastema?**

These are listed in **Table 1.1**.

Table 1.1 Causes of an upper median diastema

Causes	Comments
Developmental	Due to pressure of $2\mid2$ on $1\mid1$ roots (formerly referred to as 'ugly duckling' stage); tends to resolve by the time $3\mid3$ erupt
Dentoalveolar disproportion	Small teeth in a large arch
Absent or peg-shaped 2's	
Supernumerary tooth/teeth in midline	
Proclination of $21\mid12$	May be due to digit sucking habit
Prominent labial frenum	Implicated where there is blanching of the incisive papilla on stretching the frenum and notching between $1\mid1$ is seen in radiograph
Pathological	Cyst/tumour
	Juvenile periodontitis

■ **Is the dental and occlusal development normal?**

Dental development is normal. Eruption dates of the primary and permanent dentition are given in **Table 1.2**.

Table 1.2 Eruption dates for primary and permanent teeth

Primary	Months	Permanent	Years
Upper		**Upper**	
Central incisor	6–7	Central incisor	7–8
Lateral incisor	7–8	Lateral incisor	8–9
Canine	18–20	Canine	11–12
First molar	12–15	First premolar	10–11
Second molar	24–36	Second premolar	10–12
		First molar	6–7
		Second molar	12–13
		Third molar	17–21
Lower		**Lower**	
Central incisor	6–7	Central incisor	6–7
Lateral incisor	7–8	Lateral incisor	7–8
Canine	18–20	Canine	9–10
First molar	12–15	First premolar	10–12
Second molar	24–36	Second premolar	11–12
		First molar	5–6
		Second molar	12–13
		Third molar	17–21

It is common for some crowding to be present as the lower incisors erupt, which usually manifests itself as slight lingual placement and/or rotation of the teeth, but the slight distal tilt and rotations of $1\overline{\mid}1$ may indicate inherent crowding. Also, there is no lower primate (anthropoid) space between the primary canines and first primary molars.

Spacing between the upper permanent central incisors (flared distally and formerly described as the 'ugly duck-ling' stage, terms best avoided with concerned parents) is also normal at this stage, but generalized spacing of the upper primary teeth including the upper primate spaces (located between the upper primary lateral incisors and the upper primary canines) should exist.

Although the primary incisor relationship is commonly edge-to-edge at 5–6 years with incisor attrition, it is not usual for the permanent incisor relationship to be similar. Rather a Class I incisor relationship should be present.

A crossbite should not exist on $\dfrac{b\mid b}{c\mid c}$.

The first permanent molars should normally be in half-unit Class II relationship due to the 'flush terminal planes' relationship of the second primary molars.

Key point

On eruption:

- Some crowding of $\overline{21\mid12}$ is usual.
- A median diastema between $1\mid1$ is normal.

■ **In the developing dentition, how is space created for the upper permanent incisor teeth?**

Space is obtained from three sources: the spacing which should exist between the primary incisors; an increase in intercanine width; and by the permanent upper incisors erupting more labially and proclined compared with their predecessors.

Investigations

■ **What investigations would you undertake? Explain why.**

Clinical

Gently pull the upper lip upwards and observe if there is blanching of the incisive papilla from the frenal attachment. This may implicate the frenum in the possible aetiology of the upper median diastema. In Brian, slight blanching of the incisive papilla was detected.

Check if there is a mandibular displacement associated with the crossbites on $\dfrac{b\mid b}{c\mid c}$. If a displacement is detected, early crossbite correction is indicated. Brian, however, did not have a mandibular displacement, which was confirmed by the absence of a lower centreline shift.

Radiographic

A left bitewing radiograph could be taken to assess $\lfloor6$ position/status of any root resorption of $\lfloor e$ and an upper anterior occlusal radiograph to assess presence/absence of an upper midline supernumerary. Alternatively a dental panoramic tomogram, which is easier for the child to cooperate with, could be taken initially, which will also allow you to ascertain the presence, position and form of all unerupted teeth.

If a supernumerary tooth/teeth or other pathology is observed or suspected on the dental panoramic tomogram in the anterior premaxilla, an upper anterior occlusal radiograph should be taken.

Fig. 1.3 Dental panoramic tomogram.

■ *The dental panoramic tomogram is shown in* Figure 1.3. *What do you notice?*

Normal alveolar bone levels.

A normally developing dentition, which is consistent with the patient's chronological age.

Resorption of the distal root of e|e .

Impaction of |6.

Diagnosis

■ *What is the diagnosis?*

Mild Class III malocclusion in the early mixed dentition on a Class I skeletal base with average FMPA. Mild lower labial segment crowding; upper median diastema.

Crossbites $\frac{b|b}{c|c}$ with no mandibular displacement.

Impacted |6.

■ *What is the IOTN DHC grade (see p. 203)? Explain why.*

4t – due to partially erupted and impacted |6.

■ *What treatment would you advise for the labial segment problems? Explain why.*

No treatment is indicated at present. The mild lower labial segment crowding may reduce slightly by drift of $\overline{2|2}$ into the small existing spaces distal to them (**Fig. 1.4**). There is also likely to be some increase in lower intercanine width until about 9 years of age, which may reduce the lower incisor crowding further.

The upper median diastema is likely to reduce as the maxillary permanent lateral incisors and canines erupt. Brian's mother should be reassured about this. The attachment of the maxillary labial frenum, although initially to the incisive papilla during the primary dentition, moves to the labial attached mucosa as the permanent lateral incisors erupt and approximate the permanent central incisors (**Fig. 1.5**). In a spaced arch, this migration of the frenum is less likely. In contrast, where the upper arch is potentially crowded and the diastema is less than 4 mm, recession of the frenum and closure of the median diastema may be forthcoming eventually. However, in the present case, as Brian's father had an upper median diastema, there may be a tendency for the space to persist.

Fig. 1.4 Lower occlusal view 1 year after presentation.

Fig. 1.5 Anterior occlusion following eruption of 2's.

■ *How common is impaction of 6?*

This anomaly of eruption occurs in about 2–6% of children but has been reported in 20–25% of children with cleft lip and/or palate.

■ *What are the causes of impaction of 6?*

Impaction of 6 is indicative of crowding.

Both local and hereditary factors have been implicated (**Table 1.3**). A multifactorial mode of inheritance has been identified where both genetic and local factors can act in combination.

Table 1.3 Causes of impaction (ectopic eruption) of 6

Factor	Cause
Local	Significantly larger 6 and more pronounced mesial angle of eruption of 6
Hereditary	Familial tendency
	Small maxilla

■ *Describe the clinical features of ectopic eruption of 6 and classification of this anomaly.*

Ectopic eruption of 6 is manifested by eruption mesial of its normal path. Complete eruption of 6 is initially blocked by the distal surface of e, which then, in response to tooth contact, undergoes resorption.

Ectopic eruption of 6 is described as 'reversible' if disimpaction and full eruption ensue spontaneously. After 8 years of age, this occurs rarely. If 6 remains impacted until treated or premature loss of e happens spontaneously, ectopic eruption of 6 is described as 'irreversible'.

Treatment

■ *What treatment options are there for irreversible ectopic eruption of 6?*

Without extraction of e

A brass wire separator may be tightened around the contact area of e and 6 over several visits. Discing the distal surface of e and the use of a separating spring have also been proposed.

If 6 exhibits marked mesial tipping, more active distal movement is required. This may be achieved by a spring soldered to a transpalatal bar uniting the d's. The spring acts against a composite stop bonded to the occlusal surface of 6.

With extraction of e

If there is marked resorption or abscess formation of e, or if 6 cannot be disimpacted with a separating spring, or if 6 is carious and poor access impedes restoration, extraction of e is unavoidable. As 6 erupts with a mesial inclination, space loss occurs rapidly following loss of e. Consideration should be given to regaining space by distalizing 6 with a spring on an upper removable appliance in cases of unilateral loss of e. Where bilateral loss of e occurs, distal movement of 6's may be achieved by springs soldered to a transpalatal arch connecting both d's or by cervical traction to bands on 6's. Alternatively, management of the space loss resulting from extraction of e's can be deferred until the permanent dentition.

Key point

For impacted 6 consider:

- Brass wire separator.
- Discing distal surface of e.
- Move 6 distally.
- Extract e.

■ *How will the orthodontist manage impaction of |6 in this case?*

The various options regarding disimpaction of |6 should be discussed with Brian and his parents.

Fig. 1.6 Upper occlusal view following extraction of |e.

It should then be explained that if |e becomes abscessed, or attempts to disimpact |6 are unsuccessful, extraction of |e will be required. Treatment to deal with the resultant space loss will be required thereafter.

Brian was not keen for any orthodontic treatment and, therefore, it was decided to extract |e in view of the caries risk to |6. The consequent upper buccal segment crowding (**Fig. 1.6**) will be dealt with in the permanent dentition.

Impressions and a wax registration for study models should be recorded of the developing Class III malocclusion, which should then be monitored until the permanent dentition is fully established, when treatment planning can be completed.

Recommended reading

Bjerklin K, Kurol J, Valentin J 1992 Ectopic eruption of maxillary first permanent molars and association with other tooth and developmental disturbances. Eur J Orthod 14:369–375.

Foster TD, Grundy MC 1986 Occlusal changes from primary to permanent dentitions. Br J Orthod 13:187–193.

Huang WJ, Creath CJ 1995 The midline diastema: a review of its aetiology and treatment. Pediatr Dent 17:171–179.

Kurol J, Bjerklin K 1986 Ectopic eruption of maxillary first permanent molars: a review. ASDC J Dent Child 53:209–214.

For revision, see Mind Maps 1a and 1b, pages 162–3.

2

Unerupted upper central incisor

SUMMARY

Neil, a 9-year-old boy, presents with 1| unerupted (Fig. 2.1). What are the possible causes and how would you manage the problem?

History

Complaint

Neil's mother is very concerned about the unerupted 1| as he is 9 years old and the tooth has not yet appeared; 2| is also erupting over b| and she dislikes the appearance.

History of complaint

|a was lost at about 6 years and |1 erupted normally at 6.5 years. Unfortunately, Neil fell over while playing soccer with his class team 4 months ago and fractured |1, exposing the pulp, which was treated by a coronal pulpotomy and placement of calcium hydroxide.

■ *Is there anything else you would wish to elicit from the history?*

Neil's mother should be asked about any history of trauma to the primary incisors, particularly intrusion of ba|.

There is no history of trauma to the primary dentition.

Medical history

Neil is fit and well.

Examination

Extraoral examination

Neil has a mild Class II skeletal pattern with slightly increased FMPA. His lips are competent. No facial asymmetry or abnormal temporomandibular joint signs or symptoms were detected.

Intraoral examination

■ *The appearance of the mouth is shown in Figures 2.1 and 2.2. What do you notice?*

Oral hygiene is fair – calculus is visible on the buccal aspect of 6|.

Fig. 2.1 Upper labial segment at presentation.

Fig. 2.2 (A) Right buccal occlusion.

Fig. 2.2 (B) Anterior occlusion.

Fig. 2.2 (C) Left buccal occlusion.

Mild plaque deposits on most teeth associated with marginal gingival erythema.

Early mixed dentition with $\dfrac{6\,e\,d\,c\,2\,b\,a\,|\,1\,2\,c\,d\,e\,6}{6\,e\,d\,c\,2\,|\ \ |\,2\,c\,e\,6}$ present.

Restored incisal edge of $\underline{1}$, which also appears to be darker than the other incisors.

Class I malocclusion with mild lower and moderate upper labial segment crowding.

Upper centreline to the right; lower centreline to the left.

Potential crowding lower left quadrant.

Buccal segment relationship Class I bilaterally.

■ *Why are the centrelines displaced?*

An imbalance of upper anterior tooth size (the retained $a|$ is considerably smaller than an $1|$) has promoted the upper centreline shift, but this has been aggravated by inherent upper arch crowding.

The lower centreline shift is due to early unbalanced loss of $\overline{d}$ in a potentially crowded arch.

■ *Could the lower centreline shift have been prevented?*

Following removal of $\overline{d}$, the lower centreline should have been monitored at review visits. $\overline{d|}$ should have been extracted to balance for loss of $\overline{d}$ when the centreline appeared to be migrating.

■ *What are the possible causes of the unerupted $1|$?*

These are listed in **Box 2.1**.

Box 2.1 Causes of unerupted or missing upper permanent central incisor

Missing
- Congenitally absent.
- Avulsed.
- Extracted.

Present but unerupted
- Ectopic position of the tooth germ.
- Dilaceration and/or displacement due to trauma.
- Scar tissue.
- Supernumerary tooth.
- Crowding.
- Pathology, e.g. cyst, odontogenic tumour.

■ *How would you rate the likelihood in this case of each of the potential causes of unerupted $1|$ listed in **Box 2.1**?*

Congenital absence of $1|$ is highly unlikely. It would be very rare for $1|$ to be absent without other congenitally missing teeth.

Avulsion of $1|$ can be excluded as there is no history of $1|$ having erupted or of incisor trauma.

Extraction of $1|$ can be excluded also.

Ectopic position of the tooth germ is a possibility but is more likely to be secondary to some pathological cause or the presence of a supernumerary tooth.

Dilaceration and/or displacement due to trauma can be excluded due to the absence of a relevant history.

Scar tissue can be excluded also as this would result from trauma.

A supernumerary tooth (**Box 2.2**) is the most likely cause of unerupted $1|$. With an incidence of 1–3% in the premaxilla, supernumerary teeth (particularly the late-forming tuberculate type) are associated with delay or non-eruption of an upper permanent central incisor.

Box 2.2 Classification of supernumerary teeth by morphology
- Conical or peg-shaped – most often lies between $\underline{1}|\underline{1}$ and may produce no effect, a median diastema, incisor rotation or failure of $\underline{1}$ eruption.
- Tuberculate or barrel-shaped – most usually associated with unerupted $\underline{1}$.
- Supplemental – resembles and lies adjacent to the last tooth of a series (2's, 5's, 8's).
- Odontome – may either be compound or complex.

Crowding is an unlikely cause. Although the upper labial segment is crowded, only very severe crowding would prevent $1|$ erupting 2 years following its expected eruption time.

Pathology is also an unlikely cause. There is no evidence of alveolar expansion in the premaxilla, which would most likely be due to cyst formation possibly arising from $1|$, a supernumerary or odontome. Other rarer lesions would need to be excluded.

Key point

A supernumerary tooth is the most common cause of failure of eruption of $\underline{1}$.

Investigation

■ *What investigations are required? Explain why.*

Clinical

Palpation of the labial and palatal mucosae in the $1|$ area to detect if the unerupted $1|$ is present.

Sensibility testing of $|1$ to assess pulp status. $|1$ was vital on sensibility testing to all stimuli but as $1|$ was unerupted, it was not possible to compare responses to that tooth. Comparison with the 2's indicated that $|1$ had a diminished response to electric pulp testing.

Radiographic

The following views are required to determine the presence/absence of $1|$, and/or possible supernumerary teeth:

- *Dental panoramic tomogram* gives a general screen of the developing dentition allowing detection of the presence/absence of unerupted teeth.
- *Upper anterior occlusal or periapical views* provide greater detail of the anterior maxilla. In particular, the following can be assessed: the crown and root morphology of unerupted $1|$, the presence of supernumerary teeth and/or other pathology and their relation to the incisor roots, the root and periapical status of traumatized $|1$. On a panoramic radiograph these structures may be poorly defined due to superimposition of other anatomical features or by lying outside the focal trough of the tomogram. Periapical radiographs should include the

roots of adjacent teeth to determine if they were damaged during previous trauma to $\underline{1}$.

Used in combination and employing the principle of vertical parallax, the dental panoramic tomogram and the upper anterior occlusal or periapical views can be used to localize the position of any unerupted tooth and/or supernumerary relative to the dental arch.

■ *How would you determine the position of an unerupted tooth in the anterior premaxilla using vertical parallax?*

If the tooth moves in the <u>same</u> direction as the <u>tube</u> shift, it lies <u>palatal</u> to the arch; if it moves in the opposite direction to the tube shift, it lies buccal to the arch. Where there is no apparent shift in its position between the films, it lies in the line of the arch.

■ *Neil's radiographs are shown in* Figure 2.3*. What do these show?*

The panoramic tomograph shows all permanent teeth to be present including third molars. Dental development appears

Fig. 2.3 (A) Dental panoramic tomogram.

Fig. 2.3 (B) Upper anterior occlusal radiograph.

reasonably aligned with chronological age. There is a supernumerary tooth overlying $1\rfloor$. Root resorption of the remaining first primary molars is advanced and caries is evident in $\dfrac{d\mid}{ed\mid e}$. Bitewing radiographs would be required for more accurate assessment of the extent of carious involvement of the primary molars.

The upper anterior occlusal view shows that root resorption of $\underline{ba}\rfloor$ is advanced. $1\rfloor$ has a normal crown and root form, the root canal appears wide with an apical calcific bridge. A tuberculate supernumerary overlies the crown of $1\rfloor$. The composite tip repair to $\lfloor 1$ is visible and root formation is incomplete with apical narrowing.

Application of vertical parallax to these radiographs indicates that $1\rfloor$ and the supernumerary tooth are palatally positioned.

Diagnosis

■ *What is your diagnosis?*

Class I malocclusion on a mild Class II skeletal base with slightly increased FMPA.

Generalized mild marginal gingivitis.

Caries in $\dfrac{d\mid}{ed\mid e}$; trauma to $\lfloor 1$ involving the pulp.

Upper and lower arch crowding.

$\underline{ba}\rfloor$ retained; $2\rfloor$ erupting labially; $1\rfloor$ unerupted with associated tuberculate supernumerary.

Upper centreline shift to the right; lower centreline shift to the left.

Buccal segment relationship Class I bilaterally.

■ *What is the IOTN DHC grade (see p. 203)? Explain why.*

5i – due to impeded eruption of $1\rfloor$ caused by the presence of a supernumerary tooth.

Treatment

■ *What are your aims of treatment?*

- Restore gingival and dental health.
- Relief of crowding.
- Correction of centrelines.
- Alignment of $1\rfloor$. Definitive restoration of $\lfloor 1$.

■ *What is your treatment plan?*

For treatment planning, you should make arrangements for Neil to be referred for joint consultation by an orthodontist, oral surgeon and paediatric dentistry colleague regarding management of unerupted $1\rfloor$, associated supernumerary, the prognosis of $\lfloor 1$ and the carious molars. The plan agreed was:

1. Oral hygiene instruction.
2. Dietary advice with the aid of a diet diary.
3. Provide a custom-made mouthguard for soccer practice. The fit may need to be modified with regard to some aspects of treatment given below.
4. Determine the prognosis of $\lfloor 1$. The likelihood of apical closure was deemed to be good and $\lfloor 1$ was to be monitored radiographically at 3-month intervals.

5. Determine the prognosis of the second primary molars from bitewing radiographs. e̲'s were deemed to be of reasonable prognosis but e̅'s require formocresol pulpotomy and stainless steel crowns or extraction in view of the pulpal carious involvement. More than half the root length of e̅|e̅ remains and in view of the space loss that already exists in the lower arch, it would be wise to minimize any further extractions except in an attempt to correct the centreline shift.

6. Fit an upper removable appliance to open space for 1| and correct the upper centreline.

7. Taking the poor prognosis of $\dfrac{d|}{d|}$ into account, and to allow relief of upper arch crowding at this stage, to create space for centreline correction and for 1| to be accommodated, the following extractions are indicated $\dfrac{d c b a \mid c d}{d \quad \mid}$.

   Removal of |d is required to balance the extraction of d|. Extraction of d̅| will balance the loss of |d̅ and tend to encourage correction of the lower centreline shift.

8. The supernumerary tooth will also need to be surgically removed and an attachment with a length of gold chain should be bonded to 1| followed by flap replacement (closed technique). 1| should not be surgically exposed with an open technique.

9. In this case it will be necessary to await further eruption of 2| following removal of ba̲|, before moving 2| and |12 distally to create space for 1|.

■ What design of upper removable appliance would you use to achieve the desired tooth movements?

The appliance should be designed with the aid of the acronym ARAB (activation, retention, anchorage, baseplate) while the patient is still in the dental chair, so that nothing is overlooked.

- *Activation:* Palatal finger springs (0.5 mm stainless steel wire) to 2|12 .
- *Retention:* Adams clasps (0.7 mm stainless steel wire) to 6|6 . Recurved labial bow (0.7 mm stainless steel wire) for mesial of each e̲.
- *Anchorage:* From baseplate.
- *Baseplate:* Full palatal acrylic coverage (**Fig. 2.4**).

Fig. 2.4 Upper removable appliance to open space for 1|.

When space for 1| has been created, a hook may be soldered to the labial bow to allow attachment of the gold chain for 1| extrusion or the bow may be modified to create a buccal arm for this purpose.

Key point

Sequence in design of an upper removable appliance: ARAB acronym

- Activation.
- Retention.
- Anchorage.
- Baseplate.

■ Will an upper removable appliance achieve all the treatment objectives?

An upper removable appliance will achieve the simple tooth movements (tipping and extrusion) required in this case at this stage. It is likely that further treatment, probably loss of a premolar unit from each quadrant and fixed appliance therapy, will be required at a later date and detailing of 1| position can be undertaken at that stage (**Fig. 2.5**).

■ What is the recommended root filling material for |1 during orthodontic tooth movement?

When apical closure is evident on |1, no root canal treatment is required as the tooth has vital pulp tissue.

■ Does orthodontic tooth movement pose any risk to |1?

There is an increased risk of root resorption. Neil and his mother should be warned about this during the informed consent process. |1 may also become non-vital and require endodontic treatment.

■ Are there any precautions you would take during orthodontic treatment to minimize this risk?

As with all orthodontic tooth movement, excessive forces should be avoided. Sensibility testing and a periapical radiograph should be taken prior to starting treatment and then, for monitoring, at 6 months after the commencement of treatment. Neil and his mother should be informed of this also during the consent process. Neil should be advised to wear the mouthguard provided during contact sport to minimize the risk of repeat trauma.

|1 became non-vital nearing completion of 1| alignment and required endodontic treatment with gutta percha. This was completed uneventfully.

Fig. 2.5 Following extraction of four first premolars, fixed appliance therapy and further restorative treatment to |1.

■ *How would you ensure long-term stability of* 1⌋ *following alignment?*

Bonded palatal retention will be required to guarantee long-term alignment of 1⌋.

Labial gingivoplasty may be required at a later stage in relation to 1⌋ to obtain coincidence of the gingival margins of 1|1.

Key point
Sequence in management of unerupted 1.
• Obtain oral surgical/orthodontic opinion (and possibly paediatric dental opinion); if prognosis for 1 alignment judged satisfactory then,
• Open space for unerupted 1 (may involve primary tooth extractions).
• Remove supernumerary.
• Bond attachment to 1.
• Do not surgically expose 1.
• Align 1 with appropriate appliance.
• Maintain 1 correction with bonded retainer.
• Reassess malocclusion regarding further treatment needs.

Recommended reading

Becker A, Brin I, Ben-Bassat Y et al 2002 Closed-eruption surgical technique for impacted maxillary incisors: a postorthodontic periodontal evaluation. Am J Orthod Dentofacial Orthop 122:9–14.

Yaqoob O, O'Neill J, Gregg T et al 2010 Management of unerupted maxillary incisors. Faculty of Dental Surgery of the Royal College of Surgeons of England. Available at: **http://www.rcseng.ac.uk/fds/publications-clinical-guidelines/clinical_guidelines/index.html**

Kindelan SA, Day PF, Kindelan JD et al 2008 Dental trauma: an overview of its influence on the management of orthodontic treatment. Part 1. J Orthod 35:68–78.

Mason C, Azam N, Holt RD, Rule DC 2000 A retrospective study of unerupted maxillary incisors associated with supernumerary teeth. Br J Oral Maxillofac Surg 38:62–65.

For revision, see Mind Map 2, page 164.

Absent upper lateral incisors

SUMMARY

Sarah, aged 12 years, presents with spacing of her upper anterior teeth** (Fig. 3.1). **What are the possible causes and how may it be treated?

History

Complaint

Sarah does not like the gaps between her upper front teeth. She has just moved to a new school and feels self-conscious about the appearance of her teeth.

History of complaint

All primary teeth were present and were lost normally. When her upper permanent front teeth erupted, there was considerable spacing between them and this has not altered much since then. The permanent teeth erupted at a normal age and none have been extracted or avulsed.

Medical history

Sarah is fit and well.

Dental history

Sarah attends her general dental practitioner regularly but has had no intervention other than placement of fissure sealants to her first permanent molars.

Fig. 3.1 Anterior occlusion at presentation.

Family history

Sarah's mother also has a small space between her upper front teeth due to one missing tooth (2|).

Social history

Sarah is a keen clarinet player and not motivated to wearing a fixed appliance.

■ ***How will her instrument playing impact on orthodontic treatment?***

Wearing an orthodontic appliance will temporarily affect her musical performance but with practice and motivation, most wind instrument players adjust. With a woodwind instrument such as a clarinet, it is likely that Sarah will adjust very quickly to wearing an orthodontic appliance and for playing to return to normal within a few weeks. It would, however, be advisable to avoid fitting an appliance close to dates of music exams, auditions or performances. Any orthodontic appliance, particularly fixed appliances, may rub the inside of the lips and cheeks when fitted but wax may be applied to minimize this. As Sarah is not keen for a fixed appliance and provided treatment is possible with a removable appliance, this could be removed while playing. In advance of any orthodontic treatment, it would be useful for the orthodontist to ascertain how many hours Sarah practises per day as leaving the appliance out for long periods is likely to influence treatment outcome.

Examination

Extraoral

Sarah has a Class I skeletal pattern with average FMPA; there is no facial asymmetry. Her lips are competent with the lower lip covering the incisal third of the upper incisors. The temporomandibular joints are symptom-free.

■ ***What else should you check for?***

- Thinning of the hair.
- Absence of palmar sweat glands.

These signs are present in anhidrotic ectodermal dysplasia, which is associated with marked hypodontia (see Chapter 36). Neither was evident in Sarah's case.

Intraoral

■ ***The intraoral views are shown in** Figures 3.1 **and** 3.2**. What do these show?***

The soft tissues appear healthy and overall oral hygiene seems good, although there are small plaque deposits labially on the lower incisors. All teeth are of good quality and no caries is evident.

The following teeth are present:

```
7 6 5 4 3 1 | 1 3 c 4 5 6 7
7 6 5 4 3 2 1 | 1 2 3 4 5 6 7
```

There is a retained fragment of e͞|.

There is mild imbrication of the lower incisors; the upper arch is spaced.

The incisor relationship is Class I with a complete overbite.

The lower centreline is shifted slightly to the left.

Fig. 3.2 (A) Lower occlusal view.

Fig. 3.2 (B) Upper occlusal view.

Fig. 3.2 (C) Right buccal occlusion.

The buccal segment relationship is half unit Class II bilaterally.

■ *What other clinic assessment would you undertake?*

The labial and palatal mucosae in the 2 area should be palpated for the presence of an unerupted tooth or any pathology.

Fig. 3.2 (D) Left buccal occlusion.

■ *What are the possible causes of the upper labial segment spacing?*

These are listed in **Table 3.1**.

Table 3.1 Possible causes of the upper labial segment spacing

Cause	Aetiology
Absence of 2|2	Hypodontia (affects ~2% of Caucasians) — also associated with cleft lip and palate, Down syndrome and ectodermal dysplasia
	Avulsion
	Extraction
Failure of/delayed eruption of 2's	Crowding
	Ectopic position
	Supernumerary tooth
	Scar tissue
	Dilaceration
	Cyst/tumour

■ *What is the most likely cause in this case?*

Congenital absence of 2\|2 is most likely. This is more common in females than males. The genetic linkage is indicated by Sarah's mother, who has absence of 2\|.

Key point

Congenital absence of 2's is more common in females.

■ *What further investigations would you undertake?*

Clinical

- Mobility testing of the retained upper primary canine (|c) is required. Grade 1 mobility was detected.

Radiographic

- A dental panoramic tomogram is required to determine the presence/absence of 2's, 8's, supernumerary teeth or any pathology.

Sarah's dental panoramic tomogram showed:

- Normal alveolar bone height.
- Absence of 2\|2 and third molars; short root on |c.

• No pathology associated with any erupted or unerupted teeth.

Occlusal

• Impressions and a wax registration should be taken for study models to allow further assessment of the occlusion.

■ *What is your diagnosis?*

Class I malocclusion on a Class I skeletal base with average FMPA. Well cared for mouth. Mildly imbricated lower incisors but otherwise uncrowded lower arch; spaced upper arch with absent 2|2 and retained |c. Buccal segment relationship is half-unit Class II bilaterally.

■ *What is the IOTN DHC grade (see p. 203)?*

4h – due to absence of 2|2.

■ *What are the treatment options?*

These are:

1. Accept the spacing – not a realistic option as Sarah is concerned by it.
2. Build up the mesiodistal width of 1's and 3's with composite or by veneering to reduce the spacing but not to close it completely. The median diastema is too large for restorative build up of 1|1 to look aesthetic. Some recontouring of the cusp tips of 3's would also be required to improve the final appearance.
3. Orthodontic space closure. This would require a considerable amount of tooth movement along with |c extraction, the wearing of a fixed appliance and reverse headgear or alternative anchorage support.
4. Orthodontic space opening (this would require extraction of |c) for replacement of 2's on resin-retained bridges, by fixed bridgework or by implants in late teenage years. Replacement of 2's by autotransplantation of lower premolars is not a viable consideration as: (i) the lower arch does not warrant premolar extractions; and (ii) root formation on lower premolars is in advance of the ideal stage (two-thirds to three-quarters complete).

As option 2 will only partly address Sarah's concerns it has to be ruled out. The choice then is between the two orthodontic options.

Key point

Management options with absent 2's are to:
• Maintain or close 2 space.
• Open space for 2 replacement.

■ *What factors would you consider in deciding between space closure or space opening?*

Sarah should be seen with a restorative colleague who will provide input regarding the restorative implications of each treatment option. Then, it is often wise to undertake a trial set-up of the optimal treatment option using duplicate study models and to show this to the patient, to allow a fuller appreciation of what will be the likely outcome.

The following factors should be considered:

The patient's attitude to orthodontic treatment. If the patient is not keen on wearing fixed appliances, this may necessitate a change in treatment plan.

The anteroposterior and vertical skeletal relationships. In Class II cases with an increased overjet, space closure is desirable as it will eliminate the overjet, whereas in Class III cases this would tend to worsen the incisor relationship. Space opening is optimal in Class III cases where proclination of the incisors is likely to correct an anterior crossbite. Where the FMPA is reduced, space opening is preferable to space closure and the converse is true where an increased FMPA exists.

The colour, size, shape and angulation of the canine and incisor teeth. Where the maxillary canine is considerably darker than the incisors and/or it has a marked canine form, space closure is not advisable as considerable recontouring of 3's will be required to enable them to resemble 2's. Where the canine and incisor teeth are so angulated that it is possible to reposition them into their desired locations by tipping movements, a removable rather than a fixed appliance may be used.

Whether the arches are spaced or crowded, and the buccal segment occlusion. In uncrowded or mildly crowded arches, where the buccal segment occlusion is Class I or at most half-unit Class II, space opening is best. Space closure is preferable where crowding exists and the buccal segment relationship is a full-unit Class II.

In this case, it was decided to proceed with space opening for replacement of 2|2, ultimately on resin-retained bridges. This required an initial phase of distal movement of the upper buccal segments to achieve a Class I molar relationship, extraction of |c, followed by retraction of 3's to a Class I relationship with 3‾'s and space opening for 2's replacement. Importantly, overbite reduction was also undertaken in conjunction with these tooth movements to provide space for the metal framework of the resin-retained bridges.

Ideally, a fixed appliance would be indicated to achieve these objectives, but as Sarah was not keen for this form of treatment, an acceptable though not optimal outcome was deemed achievable by upper removable appliance therapy.

Key point

With absent 2's consider:
• Patient's attitude to orthodontic treatment.
• Skeletal relationships.
• Colour, size, shape and angulation of 3 and 1.
• Crowding/spacing.
• Buccal segment occlusion.

■ *How could the upper buccal segments be moved distally using a removable appliance to achieve a Class I molar relationship?*

An upper removable appliance with bilateral screws to move 6 5 4| and |4 5 6 distally is an option. Anchorage needs to be reinforced by allowing provision for headgear to be attached to the appliance. The appliance should also incorporate:

- Adams clasps (0.7 mm stainless steel wire) with headgear tubes soldered to 6's clasp bridges; Adams clasps (0.7 mm stainless steel wire) to 4's also.
- Short labial bow 3| to |3 (0.7 mm stainless steel wire).
- Flat anterior biteplane to half the crown height of 1|1 and extended 3 mm further palatally than the maximum overjet measurement.

When there is evidence of full-time appliance wear, headgear should be fitted for anchorage with an upward direction of pull to prevent the appliance becoming dislodged when the headgear is being worn.

■ What force and duration of headgear wear is required for anchorage?

A force of 200–250 g per side for 10–12 hours per day is required.

■ What precautions must be adhered to when prescribing headgear?

Two safety mechanisms must be fitted to the headgear assembly, preferably a safety release spring mechanism attached to the headcap and a facebow with locking device. Verbal and written safety instructions must be issued to both patient and parent(s)/guardian. The headgear should be checked at each visit.

When compliance with headgear wear is evident, then Sarah should be instructed to turn each screw once per week. |c should be extracted to allow for potential distal drift of |3 as the buccal segments are retracted to Class I. Some over-retraction is advisable to allow for any slight anchorage slip during the next phase of treatment when 3̲'s will be retracted to a Class I relationship with 3̄'s, 1̲'s will be approximated and overbite reduction will be maintained.

■ What design of upper removable appliance would you consider for these tooth movements?

Palatal finger springs to 31|13 (0.5 mm stainless steel wire). Adams clasps 6|6 (0.7 mm stainless steel wire) with headgear tubes soldered to the clasp bridges.
Long labial bow with 'U' loops (0.7 mm stainless steel wire) from 4| to |4.
Flat anterior biteplane to half the crown height of 1|1 and extended 3 mm further palatally than the maximum overjet measurement. This is an important component of the appliance to ensure that overbite reduction is maintained, creating sufficient interocclusal clearance for placement of the metal framework on the resin-bonded bridges.

■ When space has been created for 2|2, what should be done?

The patient should be seen again with a restorative colleague to ensure that the tooth movements achieved will allow restorative treatment to proceed as planned. Then a removable retainer should be fitted for 6 months carrying replacement 2|2 and ensuring that space for them is maintained by placing wire spurs in contact with the adjoining teeth (**Fig. 3.3**).

Fig. 3.3 Upper removable appliance retainer with replacement 2̲'s.

Fig. 3.4 Final restorations.

Key point

- Always place wire spurs on the removable retainer, to the teeth adjoining the 2 space after space opening.

■ What design of resin-retained bridge is required?

Maintenance of closure of the median diastema requires permanent retention. A bonded palatal retainer framework linking 1|1 together is indicated along with resin-retained bridges with single wing, off 3|3. It is better that 1|1 are retained as a separate unit rather than risk the retention integrity and success of the bridges by incorporating 1|1 retention in the bridge design.

Implant replacement of 2|2 later is unlikely as the roots of 31|13 are tipped toward the 2|2 space, compromising access for implant positioning. The final result with 2|2 replaced on adhesive bridgework is shown in **Figure 3.4**.

Recommended reading

British Orthodontic Society: Advice for Musicians 2007. Available at:
www.bos.org.uk/orthodonticsandyou/ orthodonticsforschools/adviceformusicians.htm.

Carter NE, Gillgrass TJ, Hobson RS et al 2003 The interdisciplinary management of hypodontia: orthodontics. Br Dent J 194:361–366.

Harrison JE, Bowden DE 1992 The orthodontic/restorative interface. Restorative procedures to aid orthodontic treatment. Br J Orthod 19:143–152.

Mossey PA 1999 The heritability of malocclusion: part 2. The influence of genetics in malocclusion. Br J Orthod 26:195–203.

Robertsson S, Mohlin B 2000 The congenitally missing upper lateral incisor. A retrospective study of orthodontic space closure versus restorative treatment. Eur J Orthod 22:697–710.

For revision, see Mind Map 3, page 165.

Crowding and buccal upper canines

SUMMARY

Gemma, an 11-year-old girl, attends for a 6-month dental assessment at your practice with both upper permanent canines erupting buccally (Fig. 4.1). What is the cause and how may it be treated?

History

Complaint

Gemma does not like the 'squint' appearance of her top and bottom teeth, in particular the position of the upper eye teeth, which she says 'look like fangs'.

History of complaint

The crookedness of Gemma's teeth has been getting worse for the past year. The appearance of her upper teeth has become of more concern to her in recent months when both upper eye teeth started to erupt. She is now teased at school and called 'Fangs', which annoys her.

Gemma's mother reports that her daughter's baby teeth were also slightly crooked. Both she and Gemma are very keen for treatment.

Medical history

Gemma has had asthma since she was 5 years of age and uses a salbutamol (Ventolin) inhaler; otherwise she is fit and well.

Fig. 4.1 Anterior occlusion at presentation.

Dental history

Gemma has attended for routine dental examinations since she was 3 years, but has not undergone any active dental treatment.

Examination

Extraoral

Gemma has a Class I skeletal pattern with average FMPA. There appears to be slight facial asymmetry with the chin point deviated mildly to the right. The lips are competent.

No temporomandibular signs or symptoms were detected or reported.

Gemma and her mother were unaware of Gemma's slight facial asymmetry and have noticed no change in her facial appearance over recent years.

■ *Would you be concerned by the mild facial asymmetry?*

A mild degree of facial asymmetry is normal and as facial appearance is reportedly unaltered for several years there is no cause for concern.

Intraoral

■ *Gemma's intraoral views are shown in* Figures 4.1 *and* 4.2. *What do you notice?*

Generalized marginal gingival erythema.

Plaque deposits visible on several teeth, notably both 3's.

Fig. 4.2 (A) Lower occlusal view.

Fig. 4.2 (B) Upper occlusal view.

Fig. 4.2 (C) Right buccal occlusion.

Fig. 4.2 (D) Left buccal occlusion.

Fig. 4.3 Dental panoramic tomogram.

There are no restorations and there is no obvious caries. Gemma is in the late mixed dentition stage with the following teeth present: $\dfrac{6\,5\,4\,c\,3\,2\,1 \,|\, 1\,2\,3\,4\,5\,6}{7\,6\,5\,4\,3\,2\,1 \,|\, 1\,2\,3\,4\,e\,6\,7}$ (note 5| and 7|7 are partially erupted).

- The lower labial segment is moderately crowded with 2|2 bodily displaced lingually and 1|1 slightly mesiolabially rotated.

  3| is distally inclined; |3 is mesially inclined.

  The lower right buccal segment is also crowded with insufficient space for 5|; the lower left buccal segment is uncrowded with |e present.

  The upper labial segment is moderately crowded, with 1|1 slightly mesiolabially rotated and 3|3 erupting buccally; c| is present. 3| is upright and |3 is slightly distally inclined. The upper buccal segments are aligned.

  In occlusion, there is a Class I incisor relationship.

  The overbite is average and complete.

  The lower centreline is slightly to the right.

  The right molar relationship is Class III and the left molar relationship is Class I.

■ **What are the possible reasons for 3's erupting buccally?**

- *Crowding* – buccal displacement of 3's is often a manifestation of inherent crowding in the upper arch. A contributory factor is 3 being the last tooth to erupt anterior to the first permanent molars.
- *Retention of the primary canine* – this usually leads to slight buccal displacement of 3.

Key point

Buccal displacement of 3 is more usual in a crowded arch.

Investigations

■ *What investigations would you request and why?*

A dental panoramic tomogram is required to provide a general view of the developing dentition and confirm the presence and position of all unerupted permanent teeth.

■ *Gemma's dental panoramic tomogram is shown in Figure 4.3. What do you notice?*

  Alveolar bone level is normal.

  Presence of a full complement of developing permanent teeth including third molars.

  All teeth appear caries-free.

■ *What is your diagnosis?*

  Class I malocclusion on a Class I skeletal base with average FMPA, with the chin point displaced slightly to the right.

  Generalized marginal gingivitis.

  Moderate upper and lower arch crowding with the lower centreline displaced slightly to the right.

  Right molar relationship is Class III; left molar relationship is Class I.

■ *What is the IOTN DHC grade and why (see p. 203)?*

4d – due to severe displacements of teeth, greater than 4 mm.

Treatment

■ *What treatment is likely to be required in this case? Explain why.*

Extractions are required to relieve the moderate crowding. Fixed appliance therapy is indicated in view of the distal inclination of most canines, the rotations of the central incisors, the bodily lingual displacement of 2's and the centreline shift.

■ *What would you do now?*

  Explain to the patient the likely plan for correction of her malocclusion.

  Arrange for several visits of oral hygiene instruction by the practice hygienist, and assuming that oral hygiene improves

Expansion of the lower intercanine width is unstable as is forward movement of the lower labial segment (with a few exceptions which will be dealt with elsewhere); distal movement of the lower first permanent molars is difficult without extraction of lower second permanent molars and is undertaken rarely. Enamel stripping is usually only considered in adults to gain 1–2 mm of space in total. In view of these considerations, extractions are the only realistic option of gaining space in Gemma's case.

Key point

Always consider the lower arch first in treatment planning.

▪ **What factors govern the choice of extraction?**

The prognosis of teeth.

The site of crowding.

The degree of crowding.

Individual tooth position, e.g. grossly displaced or ectopic teeth.

In this case, there are no lower teeth of poor prognosis and in view of the site and degree of crowding, the lower first premolars would be the teeth of choice for extraction.

▪ **Why are first premolars a common choice of extraction?**

They are in the middle of the arch and, therefore, provide space for relief of moderate labial and buccal segment crowding.

The contact point between the canine and second premolar is as good as between the canine and the first premolar.

If a canine is mesially inclined, considerable scope exists for spontaneous alignment of the labial segment as the canine uprights into the extraction space. For maximum spontaneous improvement, it is best to extract the first premolars as the permanent canines are erupting.

Any residual space is not at the front of the mouth and is likely to close further with mesial drift of the buccal segments.

2. *Imagine the corrected position of* $\overline{3}$. $\overline{3|}$ is mesially inclined and will upright spontaneously following removal of $\overline{|4}$, thereby providing space for labial segment alignment; $\overline{3|}$, however, is distally inclined and will require bodily retraction with a fixed appliance.

3. *Mentally reposition* $\underline{3}$ *to be in a Class I relationship with the corrected position of* $\overline{3}$. Space is required in Gemma's case for this. Extraction of both upper first premolars should provide adequate space for retraction of $\underline{3}$'s. As $3|$ is upright and $|3$ is distally inclined, fixed appliance therapy is indicated to effect this movement.

4. *Plan the upper labial segment.* The incisors are mildly crowded and slightly rotated, so fixed appliance therapy is required to produce ideal alignment.

5. *Decide on the final molar relationship.* As upper and lower first premolar extractions are planned, the final molar relationship should be Class I. Closure of residual buccal segment spacing following the extractions will require fixed appliance therapy.

6. *Assess the anchorage needs.* As almost all of the upper first premolar extraction spaces will be required for relief of upper arch crowding, and retraction of the upright/

Practice address

Date

Dear

Re [patient's name, address, date of birth]

I would be grateful if you could see Gemma for orthodontic assessment and treatment.

Gemma is very concerned about the crowding of her teeth. Apart from using a salbutamol (Ventolin) inhaler for asthma, she is in good health.

Gemma's oral hygiene is improving following several visits to our hygenist. She has a caries-free dentition. She is very keen for treatment and is prepared to wear fixed appliances.

She has a Class I malocclusion on a Class I skeletal base with average FMPA and the chin point slightly to the right. The upper and lower arches are moderately crowded and the lower centreline is slightly to the right. The right molar relationship is Class III; the left molar relationship is Class I.

I enclose current study models and a recent dental panoramic tomogram.

Yours sincerely

Fig. 4.4 Example of a referral letter.

satisfactorily, take upper and lower impressions and a wax registration for study models.

Arrange referral to an orthodontist and enclose the study models and dental panoramic tomogram.

Write a referral letter to the orthodontist (**Fig. 4.4**).

▪ **What aims of treatment do you think will be proposed by the orthodontist?**

Relief of crowding.

Upper and lower arch alignment.

Correction of lower centreline.

Correction of right molar relationship.

Closure of any residual spacing.

▪ **Describe how you would approach treatment planning.**

1. *Consider the lower arch first and plan the lower labial segment.* As the latter is in a narrow zone of soft tissue balance between the lips and the tongue, it is best to consider this sacrosanct. First the alignment of the labial segment must be assessed and if it is crowded, as in Gemma's case, the degree of crowding must be assessed to ascertain if this is sufficient to warrant extractions.

As Gemma has moderate lower labial segment crowding, space will be required to achieve alignment.

▪ **What possible means are there of creating space?**

Extractions.

Arch expansion (laterally and/or anteroposteriorly).

Distal movement of the molars.

Enamel stripping.

Any combination of the above.

distally inclined <u>3</u>'s is needed, anchorage would be best reinforced with a palatal arch attached to bands on <u>6</u>'s or temporary anchorage devices (TADs).

7. *Plan retention*. The prognosis is favourable, but bonded retention to the lower labial segment would be wise in view of the bodily lingual displacement of $\overline{2|2}$. Upper removable retention for at least 12 months (6 months full-time except meals, followed by 6 months at night only) should be planned.

Key point

- Always plan anchorage at the treatment planning stage.
- The amount of space and type of intended tooth movement influence anchorage demands.
- Always consider retention in the treatment plan.

■ What is the final orthodontic treatment plan likely to be?

No appliance therapy would be considered until Gemma has demonstrated that she is capable of maintaining a high standard of oral hygiene. Then the orthodontic plan would be:

- Fit palatal arch for anchorage or TADs (see below).
- Extraction of four first premolars (provided there is satisfactory cooperation with wear of the palatal arch). TADs (see Chapter 5) could be placed, instead of the palatal arch, at the time of the upper arch extractions.
- Upper and lower fixed appliance therapy.
- Upper removable retainer and lower canine to canine bonded retainer.

■ What risks should the patient be warned of regarding fixed appliance orthodontic treatment?

The patient should be warned of the risk of:
Decalcification.
Root resorption.
Loss of tooth vitality.
Relapse.

■ Gemma's final occlusion is shown in *Figure 4.5*. What undesirable sequelae of treatment are visible?

Several teeth are affected by white spot lesions or decalcification, indicating early carious involvement.

■ How common is this with fixed appliance therapy and which teeth are affected mostly?

The reported incidence is 2–96%. Upper lateral incisors and lower canines are affected most commonly.

■ How may the problem be prevented or minimized?

Careful patient selection. Ensure a high standard of oral hygiene pre-treatment.
Advise the patient that fizzy drinks and sugary foods should not be consumed between meals.
The teeth should be brushed with a fluoridated dentifrice after each meal.
Regular surveillance of oral hygiene and oral hygiene instruction should be undertaken by a hygienist throughout treatment.

Fig. 4.5 (A) Post-treatment. Right buccal occlusion.

Fig. 4.5 (B) Post-treatment. Anterior occlusion.

Evidence exists that regular application of a fluoride varnish around the brackets during treatment is effective.
Daily use of a fluoride mouthrinse (0.05% sodium fluoride) is recommended during treatment.

■ How may these 'white spots' be managed?

Usually, following removal of the appliances, the white spots regress slightly as maintenance of an improved standard of oral hygiene is facilitated.

Application of high concentration fluoride varnish is inadvisable as this leads to hypermineralization of the white spot, which makes it more visible and less likely to regress.

Where the white spot lesions are extensive and pose an obvious aesthetic insult, acid-pumice abrasion with 0.2% hydrofluoric acid may be carried out. In severe cases, veneers or composite restorations are likely to be required.

Key point

Decalcification with fixed appliances:
- Is common (2–96% incidence).
- Mostly affects <u>2</u>'s and $\overline{3}$'s.
- Is best prevented by careful patient selection, dietary advice and use of a fluoride mouthrinse.

Recommended reading

Benson PE, Shah AA, Millett DT et al 2005 Fluorides, orthodontics and demineralization: a systematic review. J Orthod 32:102–114.

Little RM, Wallen TR, Reidel RA 1981 Stability and relapse of mandibular anterior alignment-first premolar extraction cases treated by traditional edgewise orthodontics. Am J Orthod 80:349–365.

Mitchell L 1992 Decalcification during orthodontic treatment with fixed appliances – an overview. Br J Orthod 19:199–205.

Stecksen-Blicks C, Renfors G, Oscarson ND et al 2007 Caries-preventive effectiveness of a fluoride varnish: a randomized controlled trial in adolescents with fixed orthodontic appliances. Caries Res 41:455–459.

Stephens CD 1989 The use of natural spontaneous tooth movement in the treatment of malocclusion. Dent Update 16:337–338, 340–342.

For revision, see Mind Map 4, page 166.

Severe crowding

SUMMARY

Amy, an almost 11-year-old girl, presents with marked space shortage for both unerupted 3's (Fig. 5.1). What has caused this problem and how may it be treated?

History

Complaint

Amy does not like the appearance of the upper 'side teeth' being beside her upper front teeth; the 'side teeth' she thinks 'look like two rows of teeth'. She also does not like the crookedness of her lower front teeth.

History of complaint

Amy has become aware of the worsening appearance of her teeth over the past year. In that time, she has lost some baby teeth and the new teeth have come through crooked.

Amy's mother reports that her daughter's baby teeth looked good with only mild irregularity of the lower front teeth. Both she and Amy are keen for treatment.

Medical history

Amy's mother reports that her daughter had a heart murmur as a baby and attended a cardiologist at the local hospital. She fractured her right wrist in a fall from her mountain bike 4 months ago and has been attending for physiotherapy at the local hospital since the cast was removed. Mobility is almost back to normal now but she has difficulty with some procedures such as toothbrushing. Otherwise she is fit and well.

■ *What implications does the medical history have for any proposed orthodontic treatment?*

Amy's cardiologist should be consulted regarding the cardiac status and the possible need for antibiotic prophylaxis for procedures likely to produce bacteraemia because of the potential risk of infective endocarditis. The National Institute for Health and Clinical Excellence (NICE, which governs clinical practice in England and Wales) guidelines (2008) recommend no antibiotic prophylaxis for any cardiac defect whereas the American Heart Association (AHA) recommends antibiotic cover only for those at high risk.

Amy's cardiologist confirmed that her cardiac murmur had fully resolved and that antibiotic prophylaxis was not required prior to any dental or orthodontic (separator placement, fitting / removal of bands) procedures.

As excellent oral hygiene is essential with any orthodontic treatment, the impact of lack of optimal wrist mobility on oral hygiene should be assessed. Assistance with toothbrushing by a parent may be required until wrist mobility is fully restored; compared with manual brushes, powered brushes with a rotation oscillation action provide protection against gingivitis in the long and short term as well as better plaque removal in the short term.

Amy's mother is already assisting with her daughter's toothbrushing using a powered toothbrush.

Dental history

Amy is a regular attender at her general dental practitioner. She had several of the baby back teeth extracted a few years ago and has some fissure sealants placed in the first permanent molars. She brushes her teeth twice per day but her mother says that she needs reminding about toothbrushing; currently her mother assists with toothbrushing (see above).

Examination

Extraoral

Amy has a Class I skeletal pattern with average FMPA, average lower facial height and no facial asymmetry. Her lips are competent with the lower lip resting in the mid-labial third of the upper central incisors.
↝ No abnormal temporomandibular joint signs or symptoms were detected.

Intraoral

■ *The intraoral views are shown in Figures 5.1 and 5.2. Describe what you see.*

Poor oral hygiene with plaque deposits visible on several teeth and associated generalized gingival marginal erythema.

Fig. 5.1 Anterior occlusion at presentation

Fig. 5.2 (A) Lower occlusal view.

Fig. 5.2 (B) Upper occlusal view.

Fig. 5.2 (C) Right buccal occlusion.

Fig. 5.2 (D) Left buccal occlusion.

Stained occlusal fissures in $\overline{6|}$, brown staining on the mesial of $\overline{|6}$ and decalcification at the gingival margin level on the buccal aspects of $\overline{6|6}$; fissure sealants are visible in the occlusal surface of the first permanent molars. $5|$ has a mildly hypoplastic palatal cusp (this was non-carious).

All permanent teeth present from second permanent molar to second permanent molar in the lower arch ($\overline{5}$'s are partially erupted); in the upper arch, all permanent teeth (except 3's) erupted from second permanent molar to second permanent molar.

Mild lower labial segment crowding with $\overline{|1}$ mesiolabially rotated; $\overline{3|}$ slightly mesially inclined and $\overline{|3}$ upright. Lower right and left buccal segments exhibit mild crowding.

Overall, summing the labial and buccal segments, the lower arch is moderate to severely crowded.

Severe upper labial segment crowding; 2's very slightly mesiolabially rotated; both 3's are about to erupt buccal to the line of the arch; $3|$ is more buccally positioned than $|3$.

Upper buccal segments are not crowded; there is mesiopalatal rotation of $5|$ and distopalatal rotation of $4|$; small amount of space on either side between the premolar teeth and between the first premolars and lateral incisors.

Class I incisor relationship; overbite is average and complete; lower centreline shifted slightly to the right.

Class I molar relationship on right and left.

■ *What is the likely cause of the enamel hypoplasia on $5|$?*

This is most likely due to pulpal pathology in the overlying $e|$ affecting amelogenesis, often referred to as a Turner's tooth or Turner's hypoplasia.

■ *What are the likely causes of the severe upper arch crowding?*

- Inherent dentoalveolar disproportion manifesting as crowding – this is genetically determined and represents a mismatch in tooth and alveolus size. Added to this, the maxillary canines are the last permanent teeth to erupt anterior to the first permanent molars and are often squeezed buccally in a crowded arch.
- Early loss of primary teeth – this leads to mesial drift of the buccal segments and aggravates crowding.
- Supernumerary teeth and megadont teeth are other causes of crowding but not relevant in this case.
- Any combination of the above causes.

■ *What factors influence the rate of space loss following early loss of a primary molar? What are the effects of early loss of a primary molar?*

These are given in **Table 5.1**.

Table 5.1 Factors affecting the rate of space loss following early loss of a primary molar

Factor	Effect*
Age at loss	The younger the age at loss, the greater the potential for space loss
Degree of crowding	The more crowded the arch, the more space that will be lost
Tooth extracted	Early loss of an e, rather than of a d, is likely to lead to more space loss (see below regarding arch). 5's may erupt and be excluded palatally/lingually or be impacted; 5 may be in crossbite; centreline shift if asymmetrical extraction and in case of e, if early loss before age 7
Arch from which tooth is lost	Greater loss is likely in the upper, rather than in the lower arch, as mesial drift tendency is greater in the former
Type of occlusion	Less space loss will occur where good buccal interdigitation exists

*The effects listed above are those that are, in general, likely to result from each of the factors given. Individual variation with regard to outcome is, however, possible.

Key point

On average, space loss is greater following extraction of a primary molar:

- The younger the age at extraction.
- In the upper, rather than the lower arch.
- In a crowded arch.
- Where the second rather than the first primary molar is extracted.
- Where there is poor occlusal interdigitation.

■ *What are the likely causes of the upper premolar rotations?*

Developmental – where the tooth germ is rotated in its crypt which could be a manifestation of inherent crowding.

Acquired – due to early loss of the primary predecessor, most likely due to caries, which removes its main guidance into occlusion and allows the premolar to initially rotate in the tooth crypt, and become characteristically mesiopalatally rotated later due to mesial drift pressure of the first permanent molars.

A retained primary molar or its root fragment may also induce rotation of the successor if it fails to erupt in the correct position.

Investigations

■ *What investigations would you request and why?*

A dental panoramic tomogram is required to determine the presence and position of all unerupted teeth. Bitewing radiographs would be advisable in view of the fissure and mesial surface staining observed related to 6⌋ and ⌊6, respectively. These will also allow the status of 5⌋ to be assessed.

The presence of all permanent teeth including third molars was confirmed; enamel caries was detected in 6⌋ and ⌊6 (this had not penetrated through to dentin).

■ *What is your diagnosis?*

- Class I malocclusion on a Class I skeletal base with average FMPA.
- Generalized marginal gingivitis; enamel caries in 6⌋⌊6.

- Moderate to severe lower arch crowding; severe upper arch crowding with 3's unerupted but positioned buccally; lower centreline displaced slightly to the right.
- Class I molar relationship on right and left.

■ *What is the IOTN DHC grade (see p. 203)? Explain why.*

5i – due to the impacted maxillary canines.

Treatment

■ *What are the aims of treatment?*

To improve oral hygiene and restore dental health.
To relieve crowding.
To align upper and lower arches.
To correct the lower centreline.
To close residual buccal segment spacing, maintaining Class I incisor and molar relationships.

■ *What is your treatment plan?*

1. Provide oral hygiene instruction and dietary advice.
2. Topical fluoride (Duraphat) application to early enamel lesions on lower first permanent molars.
3. Composite restoration of the palatal aspect of 5⌋.
4. Referral, with the recently taken radiographs, to an orthodontist for further assessment and management of the severe crowding.

■ *Explain the treatment options for Amy's severe upper arch crowding and moderate to severe lower arch crowding. What are the implications of each option?*

Although Amy's principal concern relates to her upper arch crowding, it is essential that treatment planning begins in the lower arch. (See p. 17 for an explanation of this and options for relief of crowding.) Based on the assessment of the overall severity of the lower arch crowding, extraction of first premolars will be required. This will relieve impaction of the second premolars and provide space for the canines to move distally to facilitate labial segment alignment. The latter is more likely to occur spontaneously on the right side due to the uprighting of the slightly mesially inclined 3⌋. Provided oral hygiene has improved sufficiently, fixed appliances will then be required because of the inclination of ⌊3, rotation of ⌊1, the need for centreline correction and space closure.

Following on the same scheme given on pages 17–18 for treatment planning, after you:

Imagine the corrected position of 3̄ (in this case taking the need to move the lower centreline to the left), the next step is to

Mentally reposition 3 to be in a Class I relationship with the corrected position of 3̄. For Amy, space is required to achieve this.

■ *How would you assess the space required in the upper arch?*

As space is at a premium, the distance from the distal of the lateral incisor to the mesial of the first permanent molar should be measured with fine pointed stainless steel dividers.

This measured 16 mm on the right and left sides.

■ Is this sufficient to achieve the treatment objectives?

Removal of both upper first premolars will provide space for alignment of 3's but it will be insufficient to achieve this completely and obtain a Class I canine relationship with the 3⎮3 positions corrected unless *all* the space from the upper arch extractions is maintained. No space loss is permissible. Anchorage reinforcement is required. It is important to realize that removal of an upper first premolar creates usually 7 mm of space but the average mesiodistal width of the permanent maxillary canine is 8 mm – so generally, on average, 15 mm of space is required to accommodate 3 and 5. Fortunately, in Amy's case, there is a small amount of space present in the upper premolar areas which will assist correct positioning of 3's with the aligned 3's.

Removal of both upper canines is another possibility; if they erupt buccal to the line of the arch in a few months time, they could be extracted or if not, surgical removal could be undertaken. Upper fixed appliance therapy would then be required to rotate the first premolars slightly mesio-palatally to hide the palatal cusp and occupy a greater mesiodistal width akin to that of the extracted canine; the palatal cusp of 4's should also be ground to avoid interferences in lateral excursions. Bonded retention would also be needed to maintain the final position of 4's.

Removal of upper 4's addresses Amy's concern and is likely to give the better final appearance.

Key point

An upper first premolar extraction space will not accommodate an upper permanent canine.

■ Finalize your treatment planning.

The next steps are:

Plan the upper labial segment. The mild rotation of 2's is best dealt with by fixed appliance therapy.

Decide on the final molar relationship. With four first premolar extractions, this should be Class 1; residual space closure in the lower arch will necessitate fixed appliance therapy.

Assess the anchorage needs. The high anchorage demands in the upper arch have already been identified. A space maintainer with anchorage support via headgear must be fitted in the upper arch and good cooperation with wear of each appliance demonstrated before any extractions are requested. Anchorage demands in the lower arch are modest; there is no need for anchorage reinforcement.

Plan retention. Upper and lower vacuum-formed retainers (Essix retainers) should be adequate with full-time wear for the first 2 days (except mealtimes), then night-time only for 1 year followed by a second year of every second night wear.

■ What is the final orthodontic treatment plan?

Assuming that Amy's oral hygiene improves and is maintained at a high standard following instruction, then the plan would be as follows:

Fit an upper removable appliance space maintainer with headgear support to be worn at night (the headgear would only be added when wear of the upper removable appliance is judged satisfactory; headgear wear would then need to be as required before proceeding to the next stage – see below).
Extraction of four first premolars.
Upper and lower fixed appliances.
Upper and lower Essix retainers.

Key point

Where anchorage is at a premium, always reinforce anchorage before any extractions for relief of crowding.

■ Design the upper removable appliance space maintainer.

Activation: there are no active components.
Retention: Adams clasps 6⎮6 (0.7 mm stainless steel wire) with headgear tubes soldered to the 6's clasp bridges; flat stops distal of 2⎮2.
Anchorage: full palatal acrylic coverage; also headgear to be added to fit into molar clasp tubes.
Baseplate: full palatal acrylic coverage.

The upper removable appliance should be worn full-time except for contact sports and after meals when it should be removed for cleaning. Details regarding headgear force and wear for anchorage reinforcement as well as safety precautions necessary are given on page 13.

■ Are there any alternatives to this appliance?

Space could be maintained with headgear alone fitted to bands on the upper first permanent molars, with a force of 200–250 g per side, worn 10–12 hours per day. Should the headgear not be worn as required in this case, then mesial drift of the second premolar and first permanent molar will compromise space required for 3's.

A transpalatal arch soldered to bands on the upper first permanent molars is an alternative but as space is critical in this case, soldering a Nance button in addition to the transpalatal arch to the molar bands would be advisable; alternatively a transpalatal arch could be connected to an implant in the anterior vault of the palate. The transpalatal arch confers anchorage by maintaining the intermolar distance thereby preventing mesial drift and molar tipping whereas the resistance of mucosal contact with the anterior vault of the palate is the means of anchorage reinforcement by the Nance extension.

A temporary anchorage device (TAD) or bone screw could be inserted distal to 6's and used to keep the 6's and second premolars from moving mesially.

■ If all the space from lower premolar extractions had been required for lower labial segment alignment, how could anchorage have been reinforced there?

A lower removable appliance is not well tolerated due to encroachment on tongue space, interference with speech and difficulty with achieving good appliance retention due to the lingual inclination of the molars. A lower lingual arch, soldered to bands on the first permanent molars is a better option (**Fig. 5.3**). Alternatively, a TAD could be inserted into the retromolar area and used to keep the first permanent molars and second premolars from moving mesially while providing anchorage for canine retraction.

Fig. 5.3 Lingual arch.

Fig. 5.4 (A) Post-treatment. Right buccal occlusion.

Fig. 5.4 (B) Post-treatment. Anterior occlusion.

Key point

Options for reinforcing anchorage in upper arch:

- Upper removable appliance space maintainer with headgear support.
- Headgear to molar bands.
- Transpalatal arch (with/without Nance button or palatal implant).
- TAD.

Options for reinforcing anchorage in lower arch:

- Lingual arch.
- TAD.

Fig. 5.4 (C) Post-treatment. Left buccal occlusion.

■ How effective are TADs at reinforcing anchorage?

From the limited evidence available, TADs appear to be an effective, non-compliant, means of reinforcing anchorage or of moving upper first permanent molars distally. More quality research evidence is required in this area of clinical practice.

■ Are there any risks with TADs?

Risks include:

- Screw breakage during insertion (5%).
- Root contact during placement (should heal uneventfully).
- Early failure necessitating TAD replacement/removal (15–20%).
- Infection (unlikely if area around screw is brushed gently with a small headed toothbrush and fluoride toothpaste and chlorhexidine mouthrinse (0.2%) is used for first 5 days after insertion).
- Screw loosening (may be replaced in original or different position).

Greater than 80% success rates have been reported.

■ At review, 2 weeks after fitting the upper removable appliance, how will you know if it is being worn as instructed?

Amy should be speaking normally with the appliance in place; she should also be able to remove and insert the appliance unaided by a mirror. The appliance should have lost its shine; there should be evidence of mild gingival erythema along the palatal margins of the baseplate and at the posterior extension of the baseplate (if the appliance had a bite platform, there would be marks from the occlusion also).

The occlusion following appliance wear with headgear support is shown in **Figure 5.4**. The lower centreline shift corrected without appliance treatment. At this stage, Amy indicated that she was sufficiently pleased with the improvement in her dental appearance that she did not wish to proceed to further fixed appliance therapy. This was fortunate as she was not keen on assisted tooth brushing by her mother and had struggled, due to continuing problems with right wrist mobility, to maintain a high standard of oral hygiene during removable appliance treatment, despite the use of a powered toothbrush.

An Essix retainer was fitted in the upper arch only; Amy was instructed to wear this for 2 days full-time, with the exception of mealtimes, and then to proceed to night-time wear for 6 months initially.

■ *What is an Essix retainer and what are its potential advantages over a Hawley retainer in the upper arch? Aside from the usual advice regarding retainers, what specific advice should the patient be given regarding this retainer?*

An Essix retainer is a clear vacuum-formed thermoplastic retainer. Some of its potential advantages over a Hawley retainer are:

- Better aesthetics.
- Less difficulty with speaking.
- Cheaper.
- Easier to make.

Vacuum-formed retainers are more effective than Hawley retainers at maintaining correction of the upper and lower labial segments, with greater effectiveness in the upper than the lower arch.

The retainer must not be worn while eating and must never be worn while consuming beverages, especially carbonated drinks, as with these there is a high risk of decalcification.

Recommended reading

Benson PE, Tinsley D, O'Dwyer JJ et al 2007 Midpalatal implants vs headgear for orthodontic anchorage – a randomized clinical trial: cephalometric results. Am J Orthod Dentofacial Orthop 132:606–615.

National Institute for Health and Clinical Excellence 2008 Prophylaxis against infective endocarditis. Clinical Guideline No. 64. London: NICE.

British Orthodontic Society 2009 Patient Information Leaflet: Orthodontic Mini-screws. London: British Orthodontic Society.

Prabhu J, Cousley RR 2006 Current products and practice: bone anchorage devices in orthodontics. J Orthod 33:288–307.

Reynders R, Ronchi L, Bipat S 2009 Mini-implants in orthodontics: a systematic review of the literature. Am J Orthod Dentofacial Orthop 135:564e1–564e19.

Robinson P, Deacon SA, Deery C et al 2005 Manual versus powered toothbrushing for oral health. Cochrane Database Syst Rev Issue 2: CD002281.

Rowland H, Hitchens L, Williams A et al 2007 The effectiveness of Hawley and vacuum-formed retainers: a single-center randomized controlled trial. Am J Orthod Dentofacial Orthop 132:730–737.

For revision, see Mind Map 5, page 167.

Palatal canines

SUMMARY

Diane, a 15-year-old girl, presents with both upper primary canines retained (*Fig. 6.1*). What is the cause and what treatment possibilities are there?

History

Diane is concerned about the size of the baby upper 'eye' teeth that are present and by the spaces on either side of her upper two front teeth. She is not bothered by the small space between the upper front teeth. c| is also slightly loose and she is worried in case it is lost, producing a big space.

History of complaint

Diane has been aware that the baby 'eye' teeth should have been lost a few years ago. Her previous general dental practitioner, who retired last year, advised her that these teeth would eventually fall out by themselves and that when the new 'eye' teeth came through, she would then need a brace to close the spaces between her top teeth. There is no history of trauma to c|c areas and all other primary teeth were lost naturally. All permanent teeth have erupted on schedule.

She has noticed that c| has been loose intermittently for the past 18 months. It does not appear to have got looser in recent months. Diane is very keen to improve the appearance of her upper teeth.

Medical history

Diane is fit and well.

Fig. 6.1 Anterior occlusion at presentation.

Dental history

Diane is a regular attender at her general dental practitioner but has never had any dental treatment.

Examination

Extraoral

Diane has a Class I skeletal pattern with average FMPA and lower facial height and no facial asymmetry. Her lips are competent with the lower lip at the level of the incisal third of the upper incisors.

There is a slight lateral mandibular displacement to the left on closure on $\frac{4|}{4|}$.

Intraoral

■ ***The intraoral views are shown in*** *Figures 6.1* ***and*** *6.2.* ***Describe what you see.***

Oral hygiene is fair with mild marginal gingival erythema related to 2|2 and the upper left buccal segment teeth.

No obvious buccal swellings in the c areas but there seem to be mucosal swellings palatal to c2|2c, perhaps indicating the position of unerupted 3's.

Fig. 6.2 (A) Lower occlusal view.

Fig. 6.2 (B) Upper occlusal view.

Fig. 6.2 (C) Right buccal occlusion.

Fig. 6.2 (D) Left buccal occlusion.

Slight enamel decalcification buccally on 6|6.

$$\frac{7\ 6\ 5\ 4\ c\ 2\ 1\,|\,1\ 2\ c\ 4\ 5\ 6\ 7}{7\ 6\ 5\ 4\ 3\ 2\ 1\,|\,1\ 2\ 3\ 4\ 5\ 6\ 7}$$ erupted.

Mild lower labial segment crowding; 1|1 very slightly mesiolingually rotated; lower buccal segments spaced.

Upper arch uncrowded; spacing in the upper labial segment.

Class I incisor relationship with a centreline shift (clinically the lower centreline was 1.5 mm to the left).

Buccal segment relationship Class I bilaterally; lingual crossbite of 4| with |4; buccal crossbite of |6 with |6.

■ *What are the potential causes of c's being retained?*

Absence of 3's. This is highly unlikely (0.3% of Caucasians).

Ectopic position of 3's – this is the most likely cause (1–2% in Caucasians with 8% of these bilateral).

■ *What factors are implicated in maxillary canine ectopia?*

The aetiology of maxillary canine ectopia is obscure but most probably multifactorial. Possible causative factors are:

1. Genetic – palatally displaced 3 appears to result from a polygenic multifactorial mode of inheritance, with associated anomalies including incisor-premolar hypodontia and peg-shaped 2 (see below). Class II division 2 malocclusion is also associated with an increased incidence of palatal 3.
2. Crypt displacement – where the position of 3 is grossly displaced, this may be an aetiological factor.
3. 3 has the longest path of eruption of any permanent tooth.
4. Arch length discrepancy – palatal displacement of 3's has been mostly associated with an uncrowded or spaced arch. Note the spacing present in Diane's upper arch.

5. Trauma to the maxillary anterior area at an early stage of development – this has been suggested but there is no history of trauma in this case.
6. Peg-shaped, short-rooted 2's or absent 2's – guidance for 3 is reduced where these features are evident, doubling the incidence of palatal impaction of 3.

Key point

Palatal displacement of 3 is more common in an uncrowded arch and is associated with small, absent or abnormal formation of 2's and Class II division 2 malocclusion.

Note in Diane's case, the mesiodistal width of 2's were the same as those of $\overline{2}$'s, indicating that 2's are smaller than average and that a tooth-size discrepancy (TSD) or Bolton discrepancy exists between the upper and lower labial segment teeth.

■ *What is the prevalence of TSD and which teeth are most commonly affected?*

Between 5–14% of the population have a significant overall TSD, whereas 20–30% have a significant anterior TSD (see below). Although a TSD is most commonly due to a size anomaly of the upper lateral incisor, premolars or other teeth may also be responsible.

■ *How would you assess for a TSD?*

Quick-check method

- For anterior TSD: compare the width of the upper and lower lateral incisors; if the upper lateral incisor is not wider than the lower, a TSD exists.
- For posterior TSD: compare the width of the upper and lower second premolars; these should be about equal size.

Computational method

A tooth-size analysis, often referred to as a Bolton analysis after its developer, may also be performed. The mesiodistal width of each permanent tooth, excluding second and third molars, is measured and then the summed widths of the maxillary to mandibular teeth are compared with a standard table. This allows calculation of Bolton anterior (canine to canine) and overall (first molar to first molar) ratios as follows:

(Sum mandibular anteriors)/(sum maxillary anteriors) × 100 = anterior ratio (%).

(Sum mandibular 6–6)/(sum maxillary 6–6) × 100 = overall ratio (%).

Bolton obtained an anterior ratio of 77.2 ± 1.65% and an overall ratio of 91.3 ± 1.91%. Discrepancies greater than 2SD beyond these mean values have been regarded as clinically relevant to treatment planning. Tooth-size analysis may also be undertaken using digital models; the measurements are as accurate and reliable as those obtained from plaster models.

■ *What are the implications of a TSD?*

The teeth must be proportional in size to ensure good occlusion. Rarely is a TSD of less than 1.5 mm of significance with regard to treatment planning, but where larger discrepancies exist, adjustment of the mesiodistal tooth width through either addition to the enamel (e.g. composite build-ups or porcelain veneers) or enamel removal (e.g. interdental enamel stripping/reproximation) may be required to close or open spaces in the opposing arch.

Key point

TSD:

- May be assessed comprehensively by a Bolton analysis: mean anterior ratio is 77.2 ± 1.65%; mean overall ratio is 91.3 ± 1.91%.
- Is rarely significant if < 1.5 mm.
- Clinically significant for treatment planning if >2SD beyond Bolton mean values.

Investigations

■ *What investigations would you undertake regarding the retained c's? Explain why.*

It would be essential to determine if 3's are present and to localize their position. Initial assessment should be clinical, and where suspicion of 3 displacement exists, radiographic examination should follow.

Clinical

Palpation of the buccal sulci and palatal mucosae in the upper canine regions, as well as observation of the 2 inclination, usually provides a reasonable guide to the probable position of an unerupted 3. Labial displacement of 2 crown indicates 3 to be lying high and buccal over 2 root or low and palatal.

Radiographic

Two films taken with either a vertical or a horizontal tube shift are required to assess accurately the location of unerupted 3's. Alternatively, cone beam computed tomography (CBCT) may be used. A dental panoramic tomogram (DPT) gives a general good assessment of 3 position, although its potential for alignment is presented more favourably. The root length of c, vertical and mesiodistal position of 3 relative to the incisor roots, the axial angulation and apex location should be assessed. An upper anterior occlusal radiograph or a periapical film of each 3 is useful for detecting incisor resorption and determining the prognosis of the c's. Either of these views, used in combination with the panoramic view and application of parallax (a palatal 3 moves with the tube shift), can be used to locate 3's. Localization of a palatally impacted canine, however, has been shown to be best undertaken using the combination of an occlusal and a periapical radiograph allowing horizontal parallax. A lateral cephalometric radiograph is not indicated in Diane's case, but where it is justified on clinical grounds it provides valuable information about the position of 3's, when used in combination with the panoramic view.

Three-dimensional evaluation of the canine position and any suspected resorption to the roots of other teeth is provided by CBCT, which could in time, to replace the radiographic views given above for canine localization. Using CBCT, the incidence of incisor root resorption from an impacted maxillary canine has been estimated to be as high as 68%, more than five times higher than that reported from conventional radiographs. A more robust research base for orthodontic application of this technique, however, is required before it can be advocated more widely.

Key point

Using CBCT:

- Incidence of incisor root resorption associated with an ectopic maxillary canine may be five times higher than with conventional radiographs.

■ *How does the radiation dose from CBCT compare with that of a DPT?*

Although the effective radiation dose is less than that of a conventional CT, one exposure equates to about 2–8 conventional panoramic radiographs.

■ *Are there any disadvantages to CBCT in orthodontics?*

Currently, CBCT units are costly and considerable time must be allocated to view, and report on, all the data obtained, in line with medicolegal requirements.

■ *Diane's DPT and upper anterior occlusal radiograph are shown in Figure 6.3. What are the features of note?*

- Four developing third molars.
- Presence of 3|3, which are palatal.
- Resorption of the roots of c|c.

■ *Is there any way in which ectopia of 3's may be intercepted?*

Early detection of an abnormal eruption path of 3 is essential in order to provide, if appropriate, an opportunity for interceptive measures to be undertaken. From 9 years, palpation for unerupted 3's should be carried out routinely. Importantly, the position of 3 must be localized before considering any interceptive extractions. Radiographic investigation is required when a difference is detected on clinical palpation of the upper buccal sulcus between opposite sides of the arch.

Where 3 is displaced palatally in an uncrowded arch, in a child aged 10–13 years old, removal of c may lead to 3 reverting to a normal path of eruption. The amount of improvement depends on the degree of overlap of 3 over 2 root, with a better prognosis when 3 overlies the distal rather than the mesial half of 2 root. Although improvement in 3 position may occur even where 3 is markedly displaced, specialist advice must be obtained before removal of c. Consideration must be given to balancing the extraction of c with removal of the opposite c to prevent a centreline shift. Normally, following extraction of c, clinical and radio-

Fig. 6.3 (A) Dental panoramic tomogram.

Fig. 6.3 (B) Upper anterior occlusal radiograph.

graphic re-evaluation should be undertaken at 6-monthly intervals. If no improvement in 3 position is observed on a DPT within 12 months, alternative treatment is required.

> **Key point**
>
> Removal of c's between 10 and 13 years may encourage improvement in the position of a palatally ectopic canine.

When 3 displacement is associated with crowding, elimination of crowding and space maintenance, if required, may stimulate 3 position to improve.

> **Key point**
>
> In planning treatment for a palatally ectopic canine, assess the following on radiograph:
> • The root length of c and not root status of incisors.
> • The vertical and mesiodistal position relative to the incisor roots.
> • The axial angulation.
> • The apex location.

What is your diagnosis?

Class I malocclusion on a Class I skeletal base with average FMPA.

Lateral mandibular displacement on closure on $\frac{4}{4}$.

Marginal gingivitis related to 2's and upper left buccal segment teeth; enamel decalcification buccally on 6's. Mild lower labial segment crowding but spaced buccal segments; uncrowded upper arch with c's retained (3's unerupted and displayed palatally); lower centreline shift to the left.

Class I molar relationship bilaterally; lingual crossbite 4 with 4; buccal crossbite 6 with 6.

What is the IOTN DHC grade (see p. 203)? Explain why.

5i – due to impeded eruption (owing to palatal ectopia) of 3's.

Treatment

What management options are there for Diane's unerupted 3's? What are the indications for each option?

These are summarized in **Table 6.1**.

> **Key point**
>
> Surgical exposure and orthodontic alignment of a palatal 3 requires a well-disposed patient with good oral hygiene and dentition.

Which option would you favour?

As Diane is a highly motivated patient with a high standard of general dental care and the roots of c's are resorbing with 3's in reasonably favourable positions for orthodontic alignment, surgical exposure of 3's and orthodontic alignment would be optimal.

What are the ideal aims of treatment?

Alignment of 3's.
Build up 2's to increase mesiodistal width.
Correction of crossbite of 4|6.
Correction of lower centreline shift.

For treatment planning, Diane should be seen by an orthodontist, oral surgeon and restorative colleague to discuss management of 3's and 2's. Orthodontic alignment of 3's, following their surgical exposure, was agreed. Build-up of 2's mesially was to precede this. Mid-treatment, after 3's were across the occlusion, build-up of 2's distally was planned. Diane, however, decided not to have 2 mesial build-ups and the likely affect of this on the final result was explained to her.

The need for lower centreline correction should be reassessed following crossbite correction on $\frac{4}{4}$.

How would you proceed with treatment?

Create space for 3's alignment. This will be obtained by moving 2|2 slightly mesially. As they are distally inclined, mesial tipping only is required. These movements as well as palatal

Table 6.1 Management options, with indications, for palatally displaced unerupted 3's*

Option	Indications	Comments
Early removal of c's	See comments in the text in relation to interceptive treatment	Not a viable option in this case as Diane is 15 years old
Retain 3 and observe	Patient not keen for treatment	Need to monitor radiographically the unerupted 3 for cystic degeneration and/or root resorption of incisors
	Pathology or resorption of adjacent teeth not evident	
	Good aesthetics/prognosis of c's or 2 and 4 in good contact	
	3 severely displaced with no associated pathology evident	
Surgical exposure of 3's and orthodontic alignment	Highly motivated patient with excellent general dental health	Prognosis is good: the nearer 3 is to the occlusal plane, 3 overlaps at most the distal half of 1 root, when 3 long axis is ≥30° to the midsagittal plane, when root of 3 is not dilacerated or ankylosed or 3 apex is not more distal than 5. Bond gold chain, bracket or magnet to 3 at surgery; alignment of 3 may commence with removable appliance but fixed appliance required to align 3 apex
	Spaced arch or possible to create space; vertical, anteroposterior and transverse position of 3 crown and root favourable	
Remove 3	Patient not keen for alignment of 3 and radiographic evidence of associated cystic degeneration	Prosthetic replacement of c required when lost
	Hopeless prognosis for alignment of 3, 2 and 4 in good contact, or good root length on c with good aesthetics or patient willing to undergo fixed appliance therapy to substitute 4 for 3	
	Early resorption of adjacent teeth	
Transplant 3	Adequate space in arch for 3	Prognosis best if root of 3 is 50–75% formed, minimal handling of 3 root at surgery, and rigid splinting is avoided
	Intact removal of 3 possible	
	Adequate buccal/palatal bone	

*May need to address any associated TSD.

movement of 4| and buccal movement of |6, could be accomplished easily by upper removable appliance therapy.

■ *Detail the design of a suitable removable appliance.*

Activation
Palatal finger springs (0.5 mm stainless steel wire to move 2's mesially).
Buccally approaching spring (0.7 mm stainless steel wire) with 'u' loop to 4|.
Screw section to move |6 buccally.

Retention
Adams clasps 6|6 (0.7 mm stainless steel wire).
Southend clasp 1|1 (0.7 mm stainless steel wire).

Anchorage
From baseplate.

Baseplate
Full palatal acrylic coverage.
Posterior bite platforms ~2 mm in thickness to facilitate crossbite correction on 4|6. The acrylic needs to be relieved palatal and occlusal to 4|.

■ *What instructions would you give the patient regarding turning of the screw?*

It should be turned one quarter turn once per week (this is ~0.25 mm).

■ *When the crossbites on 4|6 have been corrected what would you do?*

Reduce the posterior capping to half its height at one visit and then remove it completely at the following visit to allow the posterior occlusion to settle. It would then be advisable to place an upper fixed appliance. A transpalatal arch, attached to bands on 6's, should be cemented for anchorage. Brackets should be bonded to all other upper teeth except 7c|c7 and alignment continued until a rectangular stain-

less steel stabilizing archwire (019 × 025 stainless steel in an 022 slot) can be placed.

Then arrange for surgical exposure of 3's. If TADs, rather than a palatal arch, are used for anchorage, these could be placed at the same time as surgical exposure of 3's.

■ *What methods of surgical exposure are there?*

Three methods exist:
1. Open surgical exposure followed by spontaneous eruption. 3 needs to be of correct angulation for this to succeed.
2. Open surgical exposure of 3 with packing. About 1 week postoperatively the pack is removed and an attachment is bonded to 3 to facilitate alignment with a fixed appliance.
3. Closed surgical exposure of 3 with attachment bonded during surgery. An eyelet or gold chain bonded to the mid-buccal aspect of 3 crown has the best prospect of bond survival.

■ *How may the 3's be aligned?*

Elastic traction may be applied from the attachment bonded to 3's to the archwire (**Fig. 6.4**) or to a temporary anchorage

Fig. 6.4 Mid-treatment view.

device. Light forces (20–60 g) should be used. When movement of 3's is evident, c's should be extracted. Once 3's are close to the line of the arch, a bracket should be bonded to the mid-buccal aspect of each tooth. It is essential that the roots of 3's are adequately torqued to finalize their positioning.

■ *What factors may you consider for retaining 3's in their corrected positions?*

Aside from full correction of torque, early correction of rotations should be undertaken followed by circumferential fibreotomy to 3's and then the provision of a bonded retainer.

Recommended reading

Husain J, Burden D, McSherry P 2010 Management of the palatally ectopic maxillary canine. Faculty of Dental Surgery of the Royal College of Surgeons of England. Available at:
http://www.rcseng.ac.uk/fds/publications-clinical-guidelines/clinical_guidelines/index.html

Kokich VG, Spear FM 1997 Guidelines for managing the orthodontic-restorative patient. Semin Orthod 3:3–20.

McSherry PF 1998 The ectopic maxillary canine: a review. Br J Orthod 25:209–216.

Othman SA, Harradine NW 2006 Tooth-size discrepancy and Bolton's ratios: a literature review. J Orthod 33:45–51.

Parkin N, Benson PE, Shah A et al 2009 Extraction of primary (baby) teeth for unerupted palatally displaced permanent canine teeth in children. Cochrane Database Syst Rev Issue 2: CD004621.

For revision, see Mind Map 6, page 168.

More canine problems

Cases 1 and 2

SUMMARY

Two similar canine-related problems are shown. What is the cause of each and how may they be managed?

■ *What do you notice in* *Figure 7.1?*

Fair oral hygiene with marginal gingival erythema related to several teeth.

Fig. 7.1 (A) Case 1 at presentation: right buccal occlusion.

Fig. 7.1 (B) Case 1 at presentation: lower sectional occlusal view.

$\dfrac{654321|1}{7654321|12}$ visible with $\overline{3|}$ erupting mesial of $\overline{2|}$.

Uncrowded upper and lower arches: space mesial to $\overline{3|}$; $\overline{2|}$ bodily displaced lingually and tilted distally; $\overline{3|}$ rotated distobuccally; space between $\overline{1|1}$. Class I incisor relationship. Molar relationship slightly Class III; $\overline{3|}$ in crossbite with $\underline{2|}$.

■ *What do you notice in* *Figure 7.2?*

Mild marginal gingival erythema related to most teeth, more marked interproximally.

$\dfrac{654c21 \mid 12}{654321 \mid 123}$ visible with $\underline{4|}$ erupted forward of $\underline{3|}$ and displaced palatally.

Moderate lower and upper arch crowding; mesiopalatal rotation of $\underline{3|}$; distopalatal rotation of $\underline{2|}$; mesiolabial rotation of $\underline{1}$. Class I incisor relationship.

Molar relationship Class I ($\underline{4|}$ was in buccal crossbite with $\overline{4|}$).

■ *What is the term used to describe the anomaly in position of the canine teeth? How common is this?*

The term used is transposition (positional interchange of two adjacent teeth or tooth development/eruption in a position normally occupied by a non-adjacent tooth). In the general population, prevalence remains under 1% but varies according to the sample investigated.

■ *Which arch and which teeth are affected mostly? Is there a gender difference in incidence?*

Fig. 7.2 (A) Case 2 at presentation: right buccal occlusion.

Fig. 7.2 (B) Case 2 at presentation; upper sectional occlusal view.

Transposition is more common in the upper arch, where it most commonly affects the canine and first premolar, followed by the canine and lateral incisor. In the lower arch, it seems to affect exclusively the canine and lateral incisor. The left side seems to be favoured in the upper arch and the right side in the lower arch.

A female predilection has been highlighted in some studies whereas others have indicated either no difference in gender prevalence or male predilection.

■ *What is the aetiology of this anomaly?*

Although several theories have been proposed – interchange of developing tooth buds, altered eruption paths, presence of retained primary teeth, trauma – the aetiology is now suggested to be multifactorial with involvement of complex relationships between genetic and environmental factors. There is evidence of associated gender predilection, hypodontia, peg-shaped maxillary lateral incisors and retained primary teeth.

Key point

Transposition:
- In maxilla: more commonly affects $\underline{3}$ and $\underline{4}$ than $\underline{3}$ and $\underline{2}$.
- In mandible: affects $\overline{3}$ and $\overline{2}$ almost exclusively.
- Prevalence: less than 1%.
- Aetiology: genetic and environmental.

■ *Could you classify this anomaly?*

The transposition may be partial or complete, the apices of the affected teeth being transposed in the latter.

■ *What factors would you consider in treatment?*

These are given in **Table 7.1**.

Table 7.1 Factors to consider in treatment planning for transposition

Factor(s)	Reason(s)
Underlying malocclusion, facial aesthetics, degree of crowding	These will influence need for extraction(s)
Stage of dental development and position of root apices	When root development is complete, interception (by extraction of primary teeth) is unlikely to lead to spontaneous improvement in tooth position
	With complete transposition and root apices closed, acceptance of transposition may be best due to the root resorption and periodontal (e.g. gingival recession, alveolar dehiscence) risks involved in correction
Dental morphology	If transposition is to be maintained, re-shaping is necessary to disguise for incorrect tooth position
Occlusal considerations	Judicious grinding of the palatal cusp of a maxillary first premolar will be required where it is aligned in the canine position

■ *What are the treatment options?*

These are as follows:

Interceptive treatment: if detected early (on average, between 6 and 8 years), extraction of primary teeth may be undertaken in an attempt to guide the transposed teeth to their normal positions while ensuring that space is maintained either by an upper removable appliance/palatal bar or lingual arch. This approach is only possible where the teeth affected are tilted so their roots are near the desired positions (sometimes called pseudotransposition).

Acceptance: especially if transposition and root formation are complete, followed by reshaping of incisal/occlusal surfaces and/or composite additions to camouflage for tooth position.

Extraction of the most displaced tooth: this strategy has been recommended where the arch is crowded or for caries; appliance therapy may be required thereafter.

Orthodontic alignment: whether the affected teeth are aligned in their transposed positions or whether these are corrected, depends on the relative position of the root apices.

Key point

Management options for transposition:
- Intercept.
- Accept/tooth reshaping.
- Extract most displaced tooth.
- Align orthodontically: consider relative position of root apices.

■ *How would you manage Case 1 and Case 2?*

Request a periapical radiograph of transposed teeth to determine position of root apices.
- Case 1: This indicated that the apex of $\overline{2}|$ was slightly ahead of the long axis of $\overline{3}|$; root formation was nearing completion. No root resorption was observed.
- Case 2: this indicated half the root length of $\underline{c}|$ remaining; root apices of $\underline{4}|$ were marginally ahead of $\overline{3}|$ root; no root resorption was visible.

Treatment options are to align the transposed teeth in their transposed position or to correct the transpositions.
- Case 1: In view of the relation of the $\overline{2}|$ apex to $\overline{3}|$ root, it was decided to proceed with orthodontic alignment, correcting the transposition.
- Case 2: a periodontal specialist opinion, deemed that as $\underline{4}|$ was quite markedly palatal (almost in line with palatal cusp of $\underline{5}|$), there was adequate alveolar bone to align $\underline{3}|$ in its correct position without risk of gingival recession/ alveolar dehiscence. To encourage $\underline{3}|$ to move mesially, $\underline{c}|$ was removed initially and an upper removable space maintainer was fitted. It was decided to commence treatment on a non-extraction basis and to review need for extractions based on further cephalometric evaluation of profile and incisor angulations when the arches were aligned.

■ *What appliance type will be required? Explain why.*

Fixed appliance therapy is indicated in both cases in view of the need for bodily movement. These are: Case 1 the positions of $\overline{3}|$ and $\overline{2}|$ to be corrected; rotational correction of $\overline{3}|$; space closure. Case 2: positions of $\underline{43}|$ to be corrected; rotational correction of $\underline{321}|$; correction of incisor relationship; space closure.

In Case 1, the upper arch also required fixed appliance therapy to close the median diastema. In Case 2, the lower arch required fixed appliance alignment.

Fig. 7.3 (A) Case 1 following fixed appliance alignment.

Fig. 7.3 (B) Case 2 following fixed appliance alignment.

■ *How would you check that the positions of the corrected transposed teeth are optimal?*

Palpate the labial/buccal sulci for root position of the corrected teeth (case 1: 3̄| and 2̄|; additional labial crown torque may be required in a rectangular steel or TMA archwire to maximize root positions; case 2: 4| and 3|; additional buccal root torque may be required to 4| and palatal root torque to 3| in rectangular steel or TMA wires for maximum correction).

Take a *periapical radiograph* to check root alignment and any root resorption of the corrected teeth.

Check *functional occlusion*, lateral and protrusive movements, to ensure no occlusal interferences.

The occlusion following fixed appliance alignment for Case 1 and Case 2 is shown in **Figure 7.3 (A)** and **(B)**, respectively. An example of a case where the transposition of 3̄| and 2̄| was accepted is shown in **Figure 7.4**.

Recommended reading

Ciarlantini R, Melsen B 2007 Maxillary tooth transposition: correct or accept? Am J Orthod Dentofacial Orthop 132:385–394.

Ely NJ, Sherriff M, Cobourne MT 2006 Dental transposition as a disorder of genetic origin. Eur J Orthod 28:145–151.

Peck S, Peck L 1995 Classification of maxillary tooth transpositions. Am J Orthod Dentofacial Orthop 107:505–517.

Fig. 7.4 (A) Pre-treatment following surgical exposure of |3̄ .

Fig. 7.4 (B) Following fixed appliance alignment accepting the transposed positions of |3̄ and |2̄.

Fig. 7.5 (A) Case 3 at presentation: right buccal occlusion.

Fig. 7.5 (B) Case 3 at presentation: left buccal occlusion.

Case 3

Adrienne, an 11.5 year-old girl, presents with mobile 2's and c's with 3's unerupted and not palpable buccally (**Fig. 7.5**). You order a dental panoramic tomogram and upper anterior occlusal radiograph.

Fig. 7.6 (A) Case 3 at presentation: dental panoramic tomogram.

Fig. 7.6 (B) Case 3 at presentation: upper anterior occlusal radiograph.

■ *What do you notice in Figure 7.5?*

Mild marginal gingival erythema.

654c21|12c456 visible.

654321|123456

Attrition of c̲'s.

Uncrowded upper and lower arches.

Class I (tending toward Class III) incisor relationship.

Molar relationship Class 1 bilaterally.

■ *Why are radiographs requested?*

To localize the position of the unerupted 3̲'s and to determine the cause of mobility of 2̲'s.

■ *What do you notice on the radiographs (Fig. 7.6)?*

Normal alveolar bone height.

All permanent teeth present except for third molars; all erupted permanent teeth appear to be caries free with possible exception of |6̲.

Root resorption of c21|2c with less than half the root length of 2| remaining; slight pipette root morphology of |1 and apical curvatures developing on 5|45.

3̲'s palatally positioned (3| much more so than |3 by parallax; see p. 28).

■ *What is the most likely cause of the root resorption to 2̲'s?*

Much debate and conflicting evidence exists with regard to the trigger for this resorption and potential aetiological factors involved (see p. 93). It is, however, probably caused by a combination of inherent pressure due to migration of the displaced, erupting canine and its physical contact with the incisor root.

■ *What is the incidence of root resorption of 2̲'s by ectopic 3̲'s? What sites are most commonly affected? Is it more common in females?*

Depending on the modality of diagnosis and population sampled, an incidence of between 12% and 68% has been reported, with the apical and middle thirds of the incisor roots most commonly affected. It is more common in females.

■ *How accurate is the information regarding resorption of 2̲'s from the radiographs?*

Due to superimposition of the malpositioned canine, especially when it is buccal or palatal to the incisor root, the true extent of the injury may be obscured. If, however, the angulation of 3̲ to the midline is greater than 25°, the risk of incisor resorption increases by 50%.

Even without overlapping teeth, intraoral radiographs make it difficult to detect resorption on the palatal side.

> ### Key point
>
> Incisor resorption by an ectopic maxillary canine:
> - Has an incidence of 12–68%.
> - Is more common in females.
> - Risk increases by 50%, if angulation of 3̲ to the midline is greater than 25°.

■ *How may more detailed information regarding 2̲'s resorption be obtained?*

Cone beam computed tomography (CBCT; see p. 28) has proved useful.

> ### Key point
>
> Detection of incisor root resorption may be:
> - Difficult on conventional radiographs.
> - Facilitated by CBCT.

■ *What other investigations would you do in relation to 2̲'s?*

Sensibility tests and periodontal assessment (pocket depths/bleeding on probing/attachment loss) should be undertaken. It would also be wise to enquire regarding bruxing habits.

Both 2̲'s were vital on electric pulp testing; aside from mild bleeding on probing consistent with slight marginal gingivitis, no periodontal pocketing of >2 mm or loss of attachment was noted; no bruxing habits were reported.

■ *What are the treatment options in relation to 2̲'s?*

Accept and monitor: this is not advisable as the resorption of 2̲'s is likely to worsen due to presence of 3̲'s impinging on their roots. Swift intervention is required as the progression of incisor resorption can be rapid.

Extraction of c2|2c: both 3̲'s may erupt spontaneously or |3 may erupt and 3| may require surgical exposure. In view of the lack of upper arch crowding, it would be difficult to then close the upper labial segment spacing by fixed appliance therapy without creating a reverse overjet; opening space for the lateral incisors, to be replaced with resin-retained bridges or by implants at a later stage would likely be a better option.

Extraction of c's and surgical exposure of 3's: orthodontic alignment by fixed appliance therapy would then be required; lower arch fixed appliance therapy may also be required to detail the occlusion.

There is a risk of further root resorption to 2's by aligning 3's; however if this occurs and prognosis of 2's is deemed hopeless, retaining 2's for as long as possible will preserve alveolar bone for possible implant placement later. Otherwise 2's may be replaced on resin-retained bridges.

After discussion with Adrienne and her mother, they decided to proceed with the last option. They were both warned in relation to the possible resorption risk to several other teeth due to their root morphology.

Key point

Swift intervention is required for incisor resorption by an ectopic 3.

■ *How would you monitor resorption of the upper incisors during orthodontic treatment?*

This is dealt with on page 93.

■ *What is the short–medium term prognosis of 2| with the markedly resorbed root?*

From the limited evidence available in the literature, this should be reasonable. In a Swedish study, even in cases of severe resorption, the incisor roots showed good healing when assessed at a mean time of 3.5 years (range 2–10 years) after treatment with fixed appliances. Such healing was observed in most cases after management of the ectopic canine either by surgical exposure and orthodontic alignment or by surgical removal. The resorbed incisors were incorporated in the orthodontic appliance system and endodontic treatment was not indicated to arrest further root resorption.

Key point

Severely resorbed maxillary incisors:
- May heal following management of the associated ectopic canine.
- May be incorporated in an orthodontic appliance.
- Do not require endodontic treatment to arrest further root resorption.

Radiographic follow-up during treatment (**Fig. 7.7**) showed minimal change in 2| root resorption after surgical exposure and fixed appliance alignment of 3's (**Fig. 7.8**). There was minor further resorption of the other upper incisors.

Fig. 7.7 Case 3: upper anterior occlusal radiograph mid-treatment.

Fig. 7.8 Case 3: occlusal view following surgical exposure of 3's and during fixed appliance alignment.

Recommended reading

Alqerban A, Jacobs R, Lambrechts P et al 2009 Root resorption of the maxillary lateral incisor caused by impacted canine: a literature review. Clin Oral Investig 13:247–255.

Bjerklin J, Bondemark L 2008 Ectopic maxillary canines and root resorption of adjacent incisors. Does computed tomography (CT) influence decision-making by orthodontists? Swed Dent J 32:179–185.

Falahat B, Ericson S, Mak D'Amico R, Bjerklin K 2008 Incisor root resorption due to ectopic maxillary canines: a long-term radiographic follow-up. Angle Orthod 78:778–785.

For revision, see Mind Map 7, page 169.

Infraoccluded primary molars

SUMMARY

Aileen is 11 years old. She is referred by her general dental practitioner for infraoccluded lower primary molars (Fig. 8.1). What is the cause and how would you treat it?

History

Complaint

Aileen is unconcerned by the position of her back teeth.

History of complaint

Aileen and her mother were unaware of any problem with her molars until this was brought to their attention recently by their general dental practitioner. There is no discomfort associated with these teeth and they are not loose.

Medical history

Aileen is fit and well.

Dental history

She is a regular attender at the family's general dental practitioner. No dental treatment has been required to date.

Family history

Aileen's mother has several permanent teeth missing and these have been replaced by bridgework.

Examination

Extraoral examination

Aileen has a mild Class II skeletal pattern with average FMPA and no facial asymmetry. The lips are incompetent with the lower lip lying at the incisal edges of the upper incisors. There are no temporomandibular joint signs or symptoms.

Intraoral examination

Soft tissues of the tongue, floor of mouth, palate/oropharynx and the oral mucosa are healthy. The intraoral views are shown in **Figures 8.1** and **8.2**.

Fig. 8.2 (A) Upper occlusal view.

Fig. 8.2 (B) Right buccal occlusion.

Fig. 8.2 (C) Anterior occlusion.

Fig. 8.1 Lower occlusal view at presentation.

Fig. 8.2 (D) Left buccal occlusion.

■ *What do you see?*

Plaque deposits on many teeth with associated marginal gingival erythema.

Dentition appears caries-free; fissure sealants are present occlusally in the first permanent molars.

6e4321|1234e6 erupted.
6e4321|1234e6

Uncrowded lower labial segment; e͞le infraoccluded; uncrowded upper arch.

Mild Class II division 1 incisor relationship (overjet is 4.5 mm measured clinically); overbite slightly increased and complete.

Lower centreline to the right.

First molar relationship: right half unit Class II with 6e| in crossbite; left Class I.

■ *What is the prevalence of infraocclusion of primary molars?*

It is between 8% and 14%.

■ *Why does infraocclusion of primary molars occur?*

Separate phases of resorption and repair occur in the exfoliation of primary teeth. Although resorption predominates in most cases, sometimes repair prevails temporarily leading to ankylosis of a primary molar. As alveolar growth and eruption of the adjacent teeth continue, the tooth infraoccludes.

Key point

Infraocclusion of a primary molar is due to ankylosis of the tooth while alveolar growth and eruption of the adjacent teeth continues.

Investigations

■ *What investigations would you undertake? Explain why.*

Clinical
Assess:

1. Mobility of e͞'s – if these are mobile this tends to indicate that they are close to exfoliation and that the permanent successors are present.
2. Extent of infraocclusion of e͞'s – if these teeth are in danger of submerging below gingival level, their removal is indicated. (For grading of infraocclusion, see p. 112.)
3. If e͞'s ankylosed – typically a 'tin-can' sound is audible when the occlusal surface is percussed with the handle

Fig. 8.3 Dental panoramic tomogram.

end of a dental mirror and the sound compared with that obtained from percussion of adjacent fully erupted teeth.

4. Overeruption of opposing teeth – this could lead to interferences in functional occlusion and present difficulties if prosthetic replacement of e͞'s spaces is required in the absence of 5͞'s.

Key point

With infraoccluded e͞'s, assess:
- Mobility of e͞'s.
- Extent of infraocclusion.
- If e͞'s are ankylosed.
- Overeruption of opposing teeth.
- If 5͞'s are present.

Radiographic

1. A dental panoramic tomogram – to determine if unerupted teeth are present, in normal developmental position and of normal form and size.
2. A lateral cephalometric radiograph may be required later if fixed appliance therapy is planned and the patient is keen to proceed. It would allow more accurate determination of the skeletal pattern in the anteroposterior and vertical dimensions and for the incisor angulations to be assessed.

Both e͞'s were found to be non-mobile and were not infraoccluded below gingival level, but clinically both were ankylosed.

■ *The dental panoramic tomogram is shown in* Figure 8.3. *What are the findings of note?*

- Dental development corresponds with chronological age.
- Extensive resorption of the roots of e's; short roots on e͞'s.
- Absent 5͞'s and all third molars.
- Absence of periodontal ligament space related to e͞le.

■ *Which teeth does hypodontia affect most commonly?*

The prevalence of hypodontia in the permanent dentition is 3.5–6.5%. The most distal tooth of any tooth type is usually affected, i.e. the lateral incisor, the second premolar, the third molar. In Caucasians, third molars are most commonly affected (25–35%) followed by $\overline{5}$ (3%) and then $\underline{2}$ (2%). Females are affected more than males and tooth size in the remainder of the dentition tends to be reduced.

Key point

Hypodontia:

- Prevalence: 3.5–6.5% in permanent dentition.
- Frequency: 8's, then $\overline{5}$, $\underline{2}$.
- Females more than males.

Following perusal of the panoramic tomogram and preliminary discussion of treatment options with Aileen and her mother, a lateral cephalometric radiograph was taken. Analysis revealed the following:

SNA = 82°; SNB = 76.5°; ANB° = 5.5°; $\underline{1}$ to maxillary plane = 112°; $\overline{1}$ to mandibular plane = 92°; MMPA = 26°; facial % = 55%.

■ *What do these values tell you (see p. 204)?*

They confirm the clinical impression of a mild Class II skeletal pattern with average FMPA. Incisor angulations to their underlying dental bases are also within the normal range.

Diagnosis

■ *What is your diagnosis?*

Class II division I malocclusion on a mild Class II skeletal base with average FMPA. Generalized marginal gingivitis, uncrowded lower arch with infraoccluded ē's. Uncrowded upper arch. First molar relationship right half unit Class II with $\underline{6e}$| in crossbite; left Class I. Hypodontia of $\overline{5}$'s and third molars.

■ *What is the IOTN DHC grade (see p. 203)?*

4h – due to absent $\overline{5}$'s.

Treatment

■ *What treatment options are there for the lower arch? Explain why.*

In view of the lack of crowding:

1. Accept the position and status of $\overline{e|e}$, realizing their poor long-term prognosis due to the short root length, but build up $\overline{e|e}$ with occlusal onlays to bring them into occlusion. This procedure has been shown to improve longevity of infraoccluded molars. When eventually they are lost, resin-bonded or conventional bridgework or implants may be used to replace the missing units. Aileen and her mother would need to be aware of the implications of this treatment proposal over the lifetime of the dentition including the need for replacement of any prosthesis as required.

2. Extract $\overline{e|e}$ in view of their poor long-term prognosis and as infraocclusion is likely to progress with absence of $\overline{5}$'s. Then, close the extraction spaces with a lower fixed appliance. This has the advantage of removing the need

for a prosthesis but a retainer would need to be worn post-treatment for several years at night to minimize the likelihood of space opening. Alternatively bonded retainers could be placed on the buccal aspects of $\overline{6\,4|4\,6}$ to maintain space closure.

■ *What implications do these options have for the upper arch?*

If ē's are retained, the slight overjet increase could be accepted as the teeth are aligned and provided the patient is in agreement.

If ē's are to be extracted and a lower fixed appliance planned, it would be sensible to resort to an upper premolar extraction on either side in the upper arch (probably $\underline{5}$'s in view of the small overjet and absence of crowding, although it will be necessary to await their eruption) and proceed to fixed appliance therapy to achieve Class I molar and incisor relationships.

Following discussion, Aileen and her mother decided to proceed with fixed appliance therapy (**Fig. 8.4**) after Aileen's oral hygiene improved following several visits to the hygienist. The occlusion following removal of $e|e$, then $\underline{5|5}$ and ē's and fixed appliance therapy is shown in **Figure 8.5**.

■ *If $\overline{5}$'s had been present radiographically, what would have been your treatment plan?*

Ankylosis of ē's is likely to be temporary when permanent successors exist, and ē's should exfoliate within a normal time frame. The position of ē's should be monitored until then, and if the infraocclusion progresses extraction is recommended, particularly if the crown of ē moves to lie below gingival level (reinclusion) and/or apical closure is almost complete on $\overline{5}$.

Fig. 8.4 Fixed appliances.

Fig. 8.5 (A) Post-treatment: right buccal occlusion.

Fig. 8.5 (B) Post-treatment: anterior occlusion.

Fig. 8.5 (C) Post-treatment: left buccal occlusion.

Key point

Management options for infraoccluded $\bar{e}$:

- $\bar{5}$ present, no reinclusion: allow $\bar{e}$ to exfoliate.
- $\bar{5}$ present, and reinclusion: extract or surgically remove $\bar{e}$.
- $\bar{5}$ absent: retain and place onlay:
  - extract and space close.
  - extract and prosthetic replacement.

Recommended reading

Bjerklin K, Al-Najjar M, Karestedt H, Andren A 2008 Agenesis of mandibular second premolars with retained primary molars: a longitudinal radiographic study of 99 subjects from 12 years of age to adulthood. Eur J Orthod 30:254–261.

Hudson AP, Harris AM, Morkel JA, Amra I 2007 Infraocclusion of primary molars: a review of the literature. SADJ 62:114,116,118–122.

Kurol J, Koch G 1985 The effect of extraction of infraoccluded deciduous molars: a longitudinal study. Am J Orthod 87:46–55.

For revision, see Mind Map 8, page 170.

9

Increased overjet

SUMMARY

Emma, aged 11, is teased at school about her prominent upper front teeth (Fig. 9.1). What are the possible causes and how may it be treated?

History

Complaint

Emma's upper front teeth stick out. Her mother is very concerned about her daughter's appearance and is anxious for her to be treated.

History of complaint

The upper front teeth have always been prominent, even when the primary incisors were present. Emma is teased about her teeth at school and the teasing is upsetting her. She recently fell in the school yard and hit her two upper front teeth on the ground. Fortunately there was only minimal incisal enamel damage to 1|1.

■ *Medical history.*

Emma has had asthma since she was 4 years old. This is managed with a salbutamol inhaler (Ventolin).

Key point

Increased overjet may predispose to teasing and upper incisor trauma.

Fig. 9.1 Right buccal occlusion at presentation.

Examination

Extraoral

Emma's full facial and profile views are shown in **Figure 9.2**.

■ *How would you assess Emma's skeletal pattern?*

The skeletal pattern is the relationship of the mandibular to the maxillary dental base in all three planes of space – anteroposterior, vertical and lateral. With the patient seated upright with the Frankfort plane (superior aspect of the external auditory meatus to the inferior aspect of the orbital margin) horizontal, the lips in repose and the teeth in maximum interdigitation, assessment should be as follows:

1. *Anteroposterior.* Viewing the soft tissue facial profile in most cases allows the following classification to be made:
    Class I: the mandible lies 2–3 mm behind the maxilla.

Fig. 9.2 (A) Full face view.

Fig. 9.2 (B) Profile.

Class II: the mandible lies more than 2–3 mm behind the maxilla.

Class III: the mandible lies less than 2–3 mm behind the maxilla.

Due to variation in lip thickness, this method is not always reliable and palpation of the alveolar bases over the apices of the upper and lower incisors in the midline has been claimed to give a better estimate of skeletal pattern.

Emma has a Class II skeletal pattern.

2. *Vertical.*

   Lower facial height. The distance from the mid eyebrow level to the base of the nose (upper facial height) should equal that from the base of the nose to the inferior aspect of the chin (lower facial height). The lower facial height is reduced when the latter measurement is reduced and the converse is true when this distance is increased.

   Frankfort-mandibular planes angle (FMPA). With a finger along the lower border of the mandible and a ruler placed along the Frankfort plane, project both of these lines backwards in the imagination to estimate the FMPA. The FMPA is then classified as average (both lines intersect at the back of the skull, occiput), reduced (both lines meet beyond occiput) or increased (both lines meet anterior to occiput).

   Emma has a slightly reduced lower facial height and FMPA.

3. *Transverse.* Stand directly behind the patient and look down across the face, checking the coincidence of the midlines of the nose, upper and lower lips and midpoint of the chin. Alternatively assess the face from the front. It is important to note that slight facial asymmetry is common. The location (upper, middle or lower facial third) and extent of any asymmetry should be recorded. Emma's chin point is marginally to the right. As this is very mild and has not been noticed by her or her mother before now, and as a slight degree of facial asymmetry is regarded as normal, there is no cause for concern.

   No mandibular deviation on closure or temporomandibular signs/symptoms were detected.

The lips are habitually competent with the lower lip tending to lie under the upper incisors at rest (**Fig. 9.2B**).

Intraoral

■ *The intraoral views are shown in Figures 9.1 and 9.3. What do these show?*

There are plaque deposits on several teeth and overall mild marginal gingival erythema.

All teeth appear to be good quality.

Emma is in the permanent dentition with

$$\frac{6\,5\,4\,3\,2\,1\,|\,1\,2\,3\,4\,5\,6}{6\,5\,4\,3\,2\,1\,|\,1\,2\,3\,4\,5\,6}$$ present. (Note $\overline{7|7}$ are erupting.)

The upper and lower arches are uncrowded.

There is a Class II division 1 incisor relationship with increased overjet (measured 7 mm clinically); the overbite is increased and complete. The buccal segment relationship is

Fig. 9.3 (A) Anterior occlusion.

Fig. 9.3 (B) Left buccal occlusion.

a half-unit Class II bilaterally. There is a lingual crossbite (scissors bite) affecting $\left|\frac{4}{4}\right.$.

■ *What are the causes of an increased overjet?*

These are given in **Table 9.1**.

Table 9.1 Causes of an increased overjet

Cause	Aetiology
Skeletal pattern	May be Class I, II or III
	If Class II, mandibular deficiency is almost entirely the primary cause but may be excessive horizontal maxillary growth or a combination of the two factors
Soft tissues*	Lower lip lying under the upper incisors to create an anterior oral seal will procline the upper incisors and retrocline the lower incisors (likely if there is a Class II skeletal pattern, reduced lower facial height and lip incompetence)
	Hyperactive lower lip will retrocline the lower incisors
	Primary atypical swallowing pattern (endogenous tongue thrust) will tend to procline upper (but also lower) incisors
Digit sucking habit	If present for more than 6 hours out of 24, it will procline upper incisors, retrocline lower incisors, create an anterior open bite and a tendency to buccal segment crossbite
	Overjet increase is often asymmetrical due to digit positioning
Crowding	Labial displacement of upper incisors and/or lingual displacement of lower incisors
Any combination of above	

*Effects determined principally by the skeletal pattern, and thereafter by the manner in which an anterior oral seal is produced.

Investigations

What radiographs are indicated?

A dental panoramic tomogram is required to check the presence, position, developmental stage and abnormalities of crown and root of any unerupted teeth. Untreated caries should also be noted and bitewing radiographs requested, if necessary. In view of the history of trauma to the upper incisor area, a periapical view or an upper anterior occlusal radiograph should be taken and examined for possible apical pathology.

A lateral cephalometric radiograph is indicated as there is an anteroposterior and a vertical skeletal discrepancy. In addition, anteroposterior movement of the incisors is planned.

The findings of the cephalometric analysis are:

SNA = 82°; SNB = 76°; SN to maxillary plane = 9°; MMPA = 22°; $\underline{1}$ to maxillary plane = 114°; $\overline{1}$ to mandibular plane = 92°; facial % = 52%.

What do these indicate (see p. 204)?

ANB value of 6° (SNA minus SNB) indicates a Class II skeletal pattern.
Reduced MMPA and Facial %.

Relative to mean Caucasian values, the upper incisors are proclined (but within the normal range) and the lower incisors are slightly retroclined. Although within the normal range the $\overline{1}$ to mand. plane must be considered with the MMPA as there is an inverse relationship between the two values. $\overline{1}$ to mand. plane (93°) and MMPA (27°) should total 120° or, alternatively, $\overline{1}$ to mand. plane angle should be 120° − MMPA. Hence in this case, the $\overline{1}$ to mand. plane angle should be 120° − 22° = 98°. At 92°, it is retroclined.

Would you consider any other investigations?

It would be wise to do sensibility tests of 1|1. These proved positive for all tests, with no marked difference in recordings between teeth.

Diagnosis

What is the diagnosis?

Emma has a Class II division 1 malocclusion on a mild Class II skeletal base with reduced FMPA. There is generalized marginal gingivitis. 1|1 have suffered recent trauma. There is no crowding of the upper and lower arches. The buccal segment relationship is a half-unit Class II bilaterally with a lingual crossbite of $\overline{4}$.

What is the IOTN DHC grade (see p. 203)?

4a – due to overjet >6 mm but ≤9 mm.

What factors predispose to upper incisor trauma?

The overjet increase – the risk is doubled where the overjet exceeds 9 mm.
Lip incompetence – this places the incisors at greater risk of trauma.

Gender of the patient – boys experience more upper incisor trauma than girls.

What are the aims of treatment?

To reduce the overbite and overjet to establish a Class I incisor relationship.
To correct the buccal segment relationship to Class I.
To correct the crossbite on $\left|\dfrac{4}{4}\right.$.

What treatment would you advise? Explain why.

Emma's malocclusion should be amenable to correction by growth modification with functional appliance therapy. Favourable features are the patient is likely to be growing and is approaching the pubertal growth spurt. The skeletal pattern is mildly Class II, due to mandibular retrusion rather than maxillary protrusion. The arches are uncrowded and aligned; the lower incisors are slightly retroclined; the buccal segment relationship is a half-unit Class II so a modest shift of the arch relationship is required for it to be corrected to Class I.

Functional appliances are usually contraindicated where the lower incisors are proclined, as they induce further proclination through generation of Class II intermaxillary traction. Following functional appliance therapy, fixed appliances may be required to detail the occlusion. It would be advisable then to retain the result by night-only wear of a functional appliance until growth is complete.

Key point

A functional appliance:
- Aims to 'modify' growth.
- Is only effective in growing children, preferably just pre-pubertal.

Describe the records you would take to allow fabrication of the functional appliance?

The records required are upper and lower impressions as well as a wax registration taken with the mandible postured forward to an edge-to-edge incisor relationship, the bite open about 4–6 mm and with no appreciable shift in the upper and lower dental midlines. This 'working bite' may be recorded by softening several layers of wax in warm water, forming this to a horseshoe shape indexed firmly over the upper teeth and finally guiding the mandible to the correct anteroposterior and vertical position by checking the relationship of the centrelines and the incisal opening. Alternatively, layers of wax may be adapted to a proprietary bite registration fork, which has graduated markings to facilitate assessment of the postured mandibular position. The wax registration should then be chilled, examined for adequate dental registration and re-checked for accuracy in the mouth before forwarding with the impressions to the laboratory.

■ *On issuing the functional appliance, what instructions would you give Emma?*

Assuming that this is a Twin-Block appliance, which is now the most universally adopted type of functional appliance, the instructions would be as follows:

- The appliance should be worn full-time, including at mealtimes, from insertion. The only time it is removed is after meals for cleaning and also for contact sports, during which time it should be stored in a hard plastic tub provided.

- Speaking and eating will be difficult for the first few days but will improve if you persevere.

- You must avoid eating hard or sticky foods or consuming fizzy drinks while wearing the appliance as these are likely to damage the appliance and/or your teeth. The appliance and the teeth should be cleaned thoroughly after every meal.

- Mild jaw discomfort and muscle tenderness are common for the first few days but reduce after that. It may be necessary to take a mild analgesic, as required, during this 'settling-in' period.

- Should a sore spot develop or there be any breakage of the appliance, you should return immediately to have any adjustments carried out.

■ *How does a Twin-Block work and what effects does it produce?*

The Twin-Block appliance consists of upper and lower appliances incorporating buccal blocks with interfacing inclined planes (at about 70°), which posture the mandible forward on closure (**Fig. 9.4**). This appliance works by using the forces generated by the orofacial musculature, tooth eruption and dentofacial growth. The upper midline expansion screw is usually adjusted once per week by the patient until the arch widths are coordinated with the mandible postured forward in a Class I incisor relationship. In this case no expansion was required in view of the scissors bite on $\frac{4}{4}$. The effects are usually as follows:

Skeletal

Forward growth of the mandible.
Lower anterior facial height increase.

Dental

Retroclination of upper incisors/proclination of lower incisors.
Promotion of mesial and upward eruption of lower posterior teeth (see below).
Distal movement of the upper molars.
Upper arch expansion.

Key point

A functional appliance for Class II correction:

- Postures the mandible downward and forward.
- Generates intermaxillary traction.
- Uses, removes or modifies forces of the orofacial musculature, tooth eruption and dentofacial growth.

Fig. 9.4 Design of a Twin-Block appliance (from Heasman (2008), with permission).

■ *Following overjet correction by Twin-Block therapy, what occlusal anomaly is usually manifest posteriorly in the dental arches?*

A posterior open bite is usually present bilaterally due to the buccal blocks.

■ *How may this be corrected?*

There are three possible means available to allow correction of the posterior open bite by eruption of the buccal segment teeth:

The patient may be instructed to proceed to part-time wear of the appliance.

The buccal blocks may be trimmed progressively over a period of a few months until a posterior occlusion is established.

Wear of the Twin-Blocks may be ceased and the patient fitted with an upper Hawley retainer (Adams clasps 0.7 mm on 6|6, labial bow 0.7 mm 3| to |3) with a steep anterior inclined biteplane, which aims to maintain overjet correction by posturing the mandible forward while encouraging eruption of the lower buccal segment teeth. Full-time wear of the appliance is required, except for contact sports and tooth cleaning, until a well-interdigitating posterior occlusion is established. Then night-only wear of the appliance, until growth has ceased or until a second phase of treatment commences, is permissible.

■ If there is no progress at 6 months, what action would you take?

Lack of overjet correction could be due to poor patient response to the appliance, improper design or poor compliance. Treatment should be discontinued and a re-evaluation made. The patient's standing height should be recorded and compared to the pre-treatment measurement. This will give an indication of growth over the intervening period. Provided Emma remains keen for orthodontic treatment, new records, including a progress cephalometric radiograph, should be taken and analysed to allow a new treatment plan to be devised.

■ What other treatment options are there?

- ❦ If a *design problem* with the appliance is identified as the cause of lack of treatment progress, then remaking the appliance incorporating appropriate design modifications could be undertaken and treatment recommenced.

- ↪ If *poor compliance* is to blame for no progress, then the reason(s) should be ascertained from discussion with the child. If lack of motivation or interest in treatment is the cause, it would be prudent to avoid any further appliance therapy until such time as the child has a change of heart regarding orthodontic treatment.

- ↪ *Orthodontic camouflage* – by retraction of the upper incisors into first premolar extraction spaces, accepting the Class II skeletal pattern. Importantly, this treatment should not be detrimental to facial aesthetics. Although some amount of tipping movement of the upper incisors is permissible, fixed appliances would be required to ensure an optimal interincisal angle is created. A useful rule of thumb with tipping movement is that each millimetre of incisor retraction approximates to a 2.5° change in angulation. With an original overjet of 8 mm and a target overjet of 3 mm (representing a 5 mm reduction), this would equate to a 12.5° change producing a final incisor angulation of 101.5°. This value is outside the normal range (109° ± 6°) and the incisors would be quite upright. An upper incisor angulation of 95° to the maxillary plane is regarded as the limit for acceptable retraction by tipping movements.

■ What factors govern stability of the corrected overjet?

For the best prospects of stability the interincisal angle should be within normal limits (135° ± 10°) and the overjet completely reduced with the incisors in soft tissue balance, i.e. no tongue thrust and the lower lip covering at least one-third of the labial surface of the upper incisors. A period of retention will nonetheless be required and this should extend until growth is complete following functional appliance therapy.

Key point

After functional appliance therapy:
- Ensure the upper incisors are in soft tissue balance and controlled by the lower lip.
- Retain until growth is complete.

Fig. 9.5 (A) After functional appliance therapy: profile.

Fig. 9.5 (B) After functional appliance therapy: left buccal occlusion.

Fig. 9.5 (C) After functional appliance therapy: anterior occlusion.

The profile and occlusion following functional appliance therapy are shown in **Figure 9.5**.

Recommended reading

DiBiase AT, Sandler PJ 2001 Malocclusion, orthodontics and bullying. Dent Update 28:464–466.

Harrison JE, O'Brien KD, Worthington HV 2007 Orthodontic treatment for prominent upper front teeth in children. Cochrane Database Syst Rev Issue 3: CD003452.

Heasman P 2008 Master Dentistry, vol. 2. Restorative Dentistry, Paediatric Dentistry and Orthodontics, 2nd edn. Churchill Livingstone, Edinburgh.

King GJ, Keeling SD, Hocevar RA, Wheeler TT 1990 The timing of treatment for Class II malocclusions in children: a literature review. Angle Orthod 60:87–97.

O'Brien K, Wright J, Conboy F et al 2003 Effectiveness of treatment for Class II malocclusion with the Herbst or twin-block appliances: a randomized, controlled trial. Am J Orthod Dentofacial Orthop 124:128–137.

O'Brien K, Wright J, Conboy F et al 2009 Early treatment for Class II Division 1 malocclusion with the Twin-Block appliance: a multi-centre, randomized, controlled trial. Am J Orthod Dentofacial Orthop 135:573–579.

Tulloch JFC, Phillips C, Proffit WR 1998 Benefit of early Class II treatment. Progress report of a two-phase randomized clinical trial. Am J Orthod Dentofacial Orthop 113:62–72.

For revision, see Mind Map 9, page 171.

10

Incisor crossbite

SUMMARY

Matthew is 8 years old. He presents with an upper incisor in crossbite (Fig. 10.1). What is the cause and how would you manage it?

History

Complaint

Matthew's mother is concerned that her son's upper front teeth are not straight and is anxious for treatment to be undertaken soon.

History of complaint

1| erupted inside the lower teeth. There is no history of a fall or other trauma to the primary predecessor or to 1|. a| was lost over a year ago, a little later than |a.

Medical history

Matthew is in good health.

Dental history

d| was extracted uneventfully under local anaesthesia 8 months ago.

Fig. 10.1 Anterior occlusion at presentation.

Examination

Extraoral

The skeletal pattern is Class I with an average FMPA. There is no facial asymmetry. The lips are competent.

There are no abnormal temporomandibular joint signs or symptoms.

Intraoral

■ *What features are visible on the intraoral views (Figs 10.1 and 10.2)?*

Oral hygiene is fair. Marginal gingival erythema is evident related to the incisor teeth. There is marked attrition of c|c with carious involvement of |c mesially and d|d distally. With the exception of the lower right quadrant where d| has been lost, 6edc 21 are present in each quadrant.

Gingival recession appears to be evident on the labial aspect of 1|. 1| is displaced labially; the lower arch appears uncrowded. 2|2 are rotated mesiolabially; 1| is displaced slightly palatally and there is a small median diastema.

Fig. 10.2 (A) Upper occlusal view.

Fig. 10.2 (B) Right buccal occlusion.

Fig. 10.2 (C) Left buccal occlusion.

Otherwise the upper arch appears uncrowded. The incisor relationship is Class I and $\underline{1|}$ is in crossbite; $\underline{|2}$ is partially erupted with the distoincisal aspect in crossbite with $\overline{|c}$.

■ *What specific features would you check? Explain why.*

1. *The periodontal status of $\overline{1|}$* – degree of mobility and pocket probing depth associated with $\overline{1|}$ should be assessed to determine its prognosis as it is being displaced labially by deflecting occlusal contact (see below) and gingival recession is present. $\overline{1|}$ exhibited grade 2 mobility but probing pocket depth was less than 2 mm, indicating good periodontal prognosis in the event the crossbite relationship is corrected.

2. *Can the patient achieve an edge-to-edge relationship on $\frac{1|}{1|}$?*

   If so, this indicates that only a small amount of labial movement of $1|$ is required to correct the crossbite relationship. An edge-to-edge relationship of $\frac{1|}{1|}$ was easily achievable by the patient.

3. *Is there a mandibular displacement on closure?* If the mandible is shifted anteriorly or laterally on closure from initial tooth contact, on $\frac{1|}{1|}$ or $\frac{|2}{|c}$, into maximum interdigitation, early treatment to eliminate the displacement is indicated on dental health grounds.

   → The rationale for this approach is that in susceptible individuals, mandibular displacement on closure due to premature tooth contact(s) may lead eventually to temporomandibular joint dysfunction syndrome. A 3 mm anterior mandibular displacement on closure was detected from initial contact on $\frac{1|}{1|}$; there was no lateral mandibular displacement associated with the crossbite affecting $\frac{|2}{|c}$.

4. *The amount of overbite on $1|$* – as the amount of overbite post-treatment is a major factor governing stability of incisor crossbite correction and as overbite reduces when the incisor edge is moved upwards and forward during incisor proclination, a deep overbite pre-treatment is a favourable feature. In this case the overbite was 3.5 mm on $1|$ and there is a good prospect of adequate overbite following crossbite correction.

5. *The inclination of $1|$* – an upper incisor that is upright or retroclined ($1|$) is better for proclination than one that is already labially inclined. Further proclination of the latter may not be possible or could result in unfavourable occlusal loading.

6. *The amount of space required to procline $1|$* – space already exists in the upper incisor area and there is no need for any extractions.

Key point

Where an incisor crossbite is present, check:
- Periodontal status of lower incisors.
- If an edge-to-edge incisor occlusion is achievable.
- If mandibular displacement is present.
- Amount of overbite.
- Incisor inclination.
- Amount of space required for correction.

Investigations

■ *What special investigations would you request? Why?*

As a dental panoramic tomogram taken 6 months prior to this visit by a previous general dental practitioner (see below), was available for inspection, a repeat film of this nature was not indicated on clinical grounds. From this radiograph it was possible to check the presence/absence of permanent teeth and whether there is a supernumerary tooth present in the upper midline. Should there have been any suspicion of the latter, a maxillary anterior occlusal view would be indicated to note the relation of the supernumerary tooth to the roots of the upper incisors. No supernumerary tooth was evident in the upper midline. A periapical radiograph of the lower central incisors is not required as the clinical examination does not lend significant cause for concern to the prognosis of these teeth.

Bitewing radiographs should be taken to diagnose accurately the extent of carious involvement of the primary molars.

■ *The dental panoramic tomogram taken 6 months prior to this visit is shown in* Figure 10.3*. What does it show?*

Normal alveolar bone height except for apparent angular bone defects related to the mesial aspects of $\overline{6|6}$. (Both teeth, however, were not mobile and pocket depths were <2 mm on the mesial and distal aspects of $\overline{6|6}$.)
$\overline{d|}$ absent; caries in $\frac{d|c\,d}{e|d\,e}$.
All permanent teeth (except 8's) present, of normal size and in normal developmental positions.

Diagnosis

■ *What is your diagnosis?*

Matthew has a Class I malocclusion on a Class I skeletal base with average FMPA.
Mild marginal gingivitis related to the incisor teeth.
Gingival recession related to $\overline{1|}$ labially.
Caries in $\frac{d|c\,d}{e|d\,e}$.
Crossbite on $1|$ with associated mandibular displacement.
Misalignment of upper and lower labial segments.

Fig. 10.3 Dental panoramic tomogram.

■ *What is the IOTN DHC grade (see p. 203)?*

4c – due to mandibular displacement >2 mm between the retruded contact position (RCP) and the intercuspal position (ICP).

■ *What would you deem to be the prognosis for the labial recession related to 1̅?*

For accurate assessment of the extent of the labial recession, the soft tissues should be healthy, and at present gingival inflammation is evident. There appears, however, to be some attached gingiva labially and the recession does not extend to the sulcus reflection. It is also not associated with a frenal pull. At this stage, provided oral hygiene improves and the crossbite is corrected, the gingival recession should not worsen, although the width of attached gingiva will not increase.

■ *Why is 1̲ in crossbite?*

This is most likely due to a slightly palatal ectopic position of 1̲ tooth bud.

Treatment

■ *What treatment would you provide and why?*

1. *Oral hygiene instruction* – this is required to improve gingival health and to remove the plaque insult to the gingival recession related to 1̅.

2. *Caries management* – a diet diary should be completed over 3 consecutive days (one of which should be a weekend day) and then appropriate dietary advice should be given based on the findings (see Chapter 22). Although several primary molars are carious, none have associated symptoms. Restorative management of carious primary teeth is dealt with in Chapters 22 and 26.

3. *Upper removable appliance therapy to procline 1̲*. Due to the mandibular displacement that is producing periodontal trauma to 1̅, correction of the crossbite on 1̲ is required urgently.

4. *Monitor the lower centreline*. Consider removal of d̅ if a centreline shift develops.

■ *Describe the appliance design you would use to align 1̲.*

The appliance would have the following design:
Activation: Z spring (0.5 mm stainless steel wire) to procline 1̲.
Retention: Adams clasps 6d|d6 (clasps on 6|6 in 0.7 mm stainless steel wire; clasps on d|d in 0.6 mm wire).
Anchorage: From baseplate.
Baseplate: Acrylic baseplate with full palatal coverage incorporating posterior capping (~2 mm in height).
The appliance is shown in **Figure 10.4**.

Fig. 10.4 Upper removable appliance to procline 1̲.

Fig. 10.5 Post-treatment.

■ *What will determine stability of crossbite correction on 1̲?*

Provided there is 2–3 mm of overbite on 1̲ following proclination, the prospect of stability is good. Subsequent mandibular growth must also be favourable.

The occlusion following crossbite correction on 1̲ is shown in **Figure 10.5**.

Key point

Early treatment of an incisor crossbite is advisable if there is associated mandibular displacement and/or periodontal trauma.

Recommended reading

Gravely JF 1984 A study of the mandibular closure path in Angle Class III relationship. Br J Orthod 11:85–91.

McComb JL 1994 Orthodontic treatment and isolated gingival recession: a review. Br J Orthod 21:151–159.

For revision, see Mind Map 10, page 172.

Reverse overjet

SUMMARY

Alistair, 8.5 years old, presents with a reverse overjet on all of his upper incisors (Fig. 11.1). What is the cause and how may it be treated?

History

Complaint

Alistair is not bothered about the way his teeth bite together and is not concerned about any aspect of his facial appearance. His father, however, feels that Alistair's chin is somewhat prominent and gives the boy an aggressive-looking appearance. Sometimes Alistair is teased about his chin at school.

History of complaint

Alistair's permanent upper front teeth erupted behind his lower teeth. His mother's recollection is that the bite of his 'milk' teeth was similar. Alistair is not bothered by the occasional teasing he gets about his chin.

Alistair's parents are keen for treatment, if possible, at this stage to correct his bite and reduce the prominence of his chin, which would remove the source of teasing at school.

Medical history

Alistair is fit and well.

Fig. 11.1 Right buccal occlusion at presentation.

Family history

Alistair's father reports that his own teeth meet in a manner similar to the boy's and he also has a slightly prominent chin but is unconcerned by it. His father had orthodontic treatment with extraction of two lower teeth and fixed appliances when he was a teenager to correct the bite of his front teeth. His bite changed a lot after he stopped wearing the retainers.

Examination

Extraoral

Alistair has a mild Class III skeletal pattern with average FMPA (**Fig. 11.2**) and no facial asymmetry.

■ *What other features would you check for?*

- The presence/absence of a mandibular displacement on closure.
- Temporomandibular joint signs/symptoms.

Alistair could just achieve an edge-to-edge incisor relationship.

A 3 mm anterior mandibular displacement on 1|1 was detected from RCP to ICP. No temporomandibular joint signs were noted and Alistair reported no temporomandibular joint symptoms. There was no masticatory muscle tenderness.

Intraoral

■ *What are your observations from the intraoral views (Figs 11.1 and 11.3)?*

The soft tissues appear healthy with the exception of mild marginal gingival erythema related to the incisor teeth. Oral hygiene is fair. The dentition appears caries free. 6 e d c 2 1 are present in each quadrant.

Upper and lower incisors are very mildly crowded and in crossbite. The overbite is average to slightly increased and complete. Upper and lower centrelines are displaced. The buccal segment relationship is Class III bilaterally.

Fig. 11.2 Profile.

Fig. 11.3 Left buccal occlusion.

■ *What are the possible causes of the reverse overjet?*

These are listed in **Table 11.1**.

Table 11.1 Causes of reverse overjet

Cause	Aetiology
Skeletal	Usually Class III due to any of the following: long mandible, forward placement of glenoid fossa positioning the mandible more anteriorly; short and/or retrognathic maxilla; short anterior cranial base
Anterior mandibular displacement on closure	A premature contact may displace the mandible forward on closure into maximum interdigitation
Retained primary upper incisors	These may deflect the eruption path of their successors palatally into crossbite
Pattern/excessive mandibular growth	Forward pattern of mandibular growth will exacerbate a Class III skeletal pattern
	Excessive mandibular growth may be due to excess growth hormone resulting from a pituitary adenoma
Restraint of maxillary growth	Found in repaired cleft lip and palate and attributed to the effect of post-surgical scar tissue

■ *What radiographic investigations would you request and why?*

A dental panoramic tomogram would be required to account for the presence and position of all the remaining permanent teeth.

A lateral cephalometric radiograph is indicated to assess more accurately the magnitude of the Class III skeletal pattern and the incisor angulations, which will facilitate treatment planning. It will also form a baseline from which treatment progress/growth changes can be evaluated by comparison with future cephalometric films.

The panoramic radiograph showed all permanent teeth to be developing.

■ *What is your interpretation of the following cephalometric findings?*

SNA = 80°; SNB = 82°; $\underline{1}$ to maxillary plane = 106°; $\overline{1}$ to mandibular plane = 97°; maxillary mandibular planes angle = 25°; facial % = 53%.

The skeletal pattern is Class III (SNA − SNB = ANB = −2°) due to mild maxillary retrognathism and mandibular prognathism. The upper incisors are slightly retroclined relative to the mean (109°) but within the normal range. Taking account of MMPA, $\overline{1}$ angulation should be 120° − 25° = 95°, but is 2° proclined at 97°. The MMPA and facial proportions are slightly reduced from average values but are within the normal range.

Diagnosis

■ *What is your orthodontic diagnosis?*

Alistair has a Class III malocclusion on a Class III skeletal pattern with slightly reduced facial proportions. There is an anterior mandibular displacement on closure on $\underline{1|1}$. Marginal gingivitis related to the upper and lower incisors. Upper and lower arches exhibit mild incisor crowding; the upper incisors are in crossbite. Upper and lower centrelines are slightly displaced. The buccal segment relationship is Class III bilaterally.

■ *What is the IOTN DHC grade (see p. 203)?*

4c – due to >2 mm mandibular displacement between the RCP and ICP.

■ *What dental health reasons are there for orthodontic treatment?*

Mandibular displacement on closure may increase the likelihood of temporomandibular joint dysfunction in susceptible individuals. In addition, displacing occlusal contacts may lead to lower incisor mobility and contribute to gingival recession.

■ *What factors would you assess in orthodontic treatment planning?*

These are given in **Table 11.2**.

Table 11.2 Factors to assess in treatment planning

Factor	
Degree of anteroposterior and vertical skeletal discrepancy	Most important factor
	Reflected directly in facial and dental appearance; patient's perception of these will influence complexity of treatment undertaken
Potential direction and extent of future facial growth	Assess relevant family history, age and gender of the patient and vertical facial proportions
	Reverse overjet is likely to worsen with a forward growth rotation and horizontal pattern of mandibular growth, usually observed when the anterior facial height is reduced or average
	The converse is likely where there is an increased vertical facial height
Incisor angulations	If dentoalveolar compensation is already marked, further orthodontic compensation is unlikely to be stable or to produce an aesthetic result
Amount of overbite	The deeper the overbite, the better the likelihood of stable correction of the reverse overjet
Ability to achieve edge-to-edge incisor contact	If this is not possible, correction of the incisor relationship by simple means is unlikely
Degree of upper and lower arch crowding	Delay upper arch extractions until the reverse overjet is corrected as this may provide space for relief of mild/moderate crowding
	If extractions are undertaken in the upper arch only, the reverse overjet may worsen by the upper labial segment moving palatally
	If mid upper arch extractions are necessary, extraction of $\overline{4|4}$ is usually advisable to allow correction of the incisor relationship

[Handwritten notes at bottom of page:]
Reverse Twin Block.
Encourage maxillary development
Reverse occlusal inclined planes at 70°
Drive 4 teeth forward by forces of occlu

Treatment

■ *What orthodontic treatment would you undertake and why?*

In view of the already apparent Class III skeletal pattern, the ability of the patient to just achieve an edge-to-edge incisor relationship, the inherent tendency for downward and forward mandibular growth and the family history, a sensible option would be to accept the malocclusion for the present and reassess in the light of further mandibular growth. Alistair has not yet entered the pubertal growth spurt, which is likely to exacerbate the Class III malocclusion and chin prominence as mandibular growth proceeds. On average, mandibular growth continues until 19 years in boys, but it may progress for longer.

Key point

Class III malocclusion in the mixed dentition is likely to worsen with mandibular growth, especially in boys.

As the parents are keen for treatment if possible, to try to reduce any further teasing at school, another option to consider would be growth modification by functional appliance therapy (Fränkel III [or FR III; FR stands for Function Regulator]; **Fig. 11.4**) to correct the incisor relationship because:

- The skeletal pattern is mildly Class III.
- There is an anterior mandibular displacement on closure, i.e. Alistair can achieve edge-to-edge incisor contact.
- The MMPA is slightly reduced.
- The upper incisors are not proclined.
- The lower incisors are very mildly proclined.
- The overbite is average to slightly increased.

It is essential, however, that Alistair and his parents are aware of the need for prolonged retention during continuing growth and of the need for reassessment in the light

Fig. 11.4 Fränkel III appliance.

of ensuing growth. This form of treatment should only be undertaken by a specialist and only when Alistair's oral hygiene has improved.

■ *How would you take a wax registration for this appliance?*

The mandible is rotated downward and backward until the incisors are brought to an end-to-end relationship or better, with the bite open about 2 mm. Alistair may be instructed to place the tip of his tongue at the back of the hard palate and to maintain it there while closing slowly into a horse-shoe of softened wax placed over the upper teeth until the desired position is reached. This wax registration should then be chilled in cold water and its accuracy rechecked in the mouth before forwarding to the laboratory with impressions of the dental arches to allow appliance construction.

■ *How much should Alistair wear this appliance?*

He should build up wear over the first week so that it is worn for at least 14 hours out of 24. Encouragement should be given to increasing wear to full-time with the exception of mealtimes and for sports, although this may prove difficult for some children. As its name implies, the Function Regulator was designed with the intention of altering function of the circumoral and masticatory musculature. For this reason, the patient should be instructed to 'exercise' these muscles, by gently opening and closing into the appliance. Alistair should be given a time sheet to allow him to record the number of hours wear per day. This should be inspected at each visit and used to encourage progress.

■ *What effects will this appliance have?*

The response is a downward and backward rotation of the mandible accompanied by an increase in facial height. There is no direct restraining force on the mandible and overall attempts to modify growth in Class III cases have proved disappointing. The lower incisors are uprighted and the upper incisors may be proclined slightly. The upper molars should erupt more than the lowers.

Key point

Attempts to 'modify' growth in Class III malocclusion:
- Tend to be disappointing.
- Are mostly limited to dentoalveolar changes.

■ *What other treatment options are there?*

An alternative approach to try to modify growth where mandibular excess exists is by chincup therapy. This requires specialist management. The line of force application should be oriented below the condyle to produce downward and backward rotation of the chin. As a result, lower anterior facial height is increased but chin prominence is reduced simultaneously. In essence, the appliance works in exactly the same way as functional appliances for mandibular prognathism. As a significant amount of force from the chincup is transferred to the base of the lower alveolar process, the lower incisors are also uprighted.

If the patient is not keen to try growth modification or the parents express concern about the need for prolonged retention of the corrected incisor relationship, the malocclu-

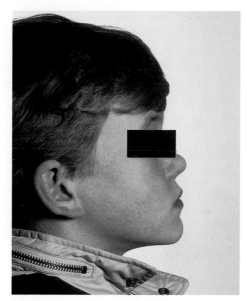

Fig. 11.5 (A) Post-treatment: profile view.

Fig. 11.5 (B) Post-treatment: occlusion.

sion should be accepted for the present. Arrangements should be made to review occlusal development and to monitor facial growth. In Alistair's case it would be wise to review his occlusion in 18 months (at age 10 years) to check particularly on the position of the unerupted permanent maxillary canines and to measure the reverse overjet.

Once the permanent dentition is established, provided the reverse overjet has not worsened markedly and the chin prominence has not increased greatly, consideration could be given to removal of $\overline{4|4}$ only, in conjunction with upper and lower fixed appliance therapy to correct the incisor relationship. If the upper arch is crowded, $5|5$ may be removed also, but it is wise to delay the decision regarding the need for any upper arch extractions until the reverse overjet has been corrected. It is important to assess the pattern of mandibular growth from an updated cephalometric radiograph prior to this treatment approach, and if there is any concern about it, treatment should be delayed until growth is almost complete.

If the reverse overjet increases considerably with further growth, a combined orthodontic and surgical approach may be required for correction, depending on the patient's concerns. This treatment would not be undertaken until mandibular growth is complete in the late teens.

Prognosis

■ *What factors will influence stability of the corrected incisor relationship?*

The amount of overbite is important in the short term but the pattern of facial growth, in particular the magnitude and direction of mandibular growth, will influence longer-term stability.

The profile and occlusion following crossbite correction are shown in **Figure 11.5**.

Recommended reading

Battagel JM 1993 The aetiological factors in Class III malocclusion. Eur J Orthod 15:347–370.

De Toffol L, Pavoni C, Baccetti T et al 2008 Orthopedic treatment outcomes in Class III malocclusion. A systematic review. Angle Orthod 78:561–573.

Levin AS, McNamara JA Jr, Franchi L et al 2008 Short-term and long-term treatment outcomes with the FR-3 appliance of Frankel. Am J Orthod Dentofacial Orthop 134:513–524.

Miethke RR, Lindenau S, Dietrich K 2003 The effect of Fränkel's function regulator type III on the apical base. Eur J Orthod 25:311–318.

For revision, see Mind Map 11, page 173.

12

Increased overbite

SUMMARY

Harry, aged 10 years and 6 months, presents with crowded upper teeth and a deep traumatic overbite (Fig. 12.1). What has caused these problems and how may they be treated?

History

Complaint

Harry does not like the appearance of his upper teeth and has recently complained about the gum behind his upper front teeth being sore. His mother is keen for treatment.

History of complaint

His primary teeth were mildly irregular. His permanent upper front teeth erupted in a 'crooked' position and have not changed since.

Medical history

Harry is fit and well.

Dental history

Harry is a regular attender at his general dental practitioner and has not required any dental treatment so far.

Family history

Harry's father has the same arrangement of the upper anterior teeth as his son. He had four teeth removed and treatment with fixed appliances as a teenager. However, the treatment result relapsed and the upper front teeth have largely returned to their original position. Harry's mother is keen that this does not happen to her son.

Examination

Extraoral

■ *Harry's profile view is shown in Figure 12.2. What do you notice about the anteroposterior skeletal pattern and the lips?*

Harry has a Class II skeletal pattern with slightly reduced FMPA.

The lips are competent.

Intraoral

■ *The appearance of the mouth is shown in Figures 12.1 and 12.3. What do you see?*

Soft tissues appear healthy apart from mild gingival erythema related to the upper incisors.

The oral hygiene is fair with no visible carious lesions.

There are no restorations visible.

Harry is in the mixed dentition with the following teeth visible: $\frac{6e4321|124e6}{6e43|3456}$ ($2\overline{1|1}2$ are erupted but covered by the upper incisors).

Mild upper labial segment crowding.

Class II division 2 malocclusion with deep complete overbite.

Buccal segment relationships are a half-unit Class II bilaterally.

Fig. 12.1 Anterior occlusion at presentation.

Fig. 12.2 Profile at presentation.

Fig. 12.3 (A) Right buccal occlusion.

Fig. 12.3 (B) Left buccal occlusion.

■ *What are the possible causes of the traumatic overbite?*

In a Class II division 2 malocclusion several factors contribute to an increased overbite. These are listed in **Table 12.1**.

Table 12.1 Causes of increased and traumatic overbite in Class II division 2 malocclusion

Cause	Aetiology
Skeletal: anteroposterior and vertical	A Class II skeletal pattern in combination with a reduced lower facial height
Growth pattern	An anterior mandibular growth rotation tends to increase overbite
Soft tissues	Effects are via the skeletal pattern – reduced lower facial height leads to a high lower lip line that will retrocline the upper incisors, leading to overbite increase
	A hyperactive high lower lip in association with a reduced lower facial height leads to bimaxillary retroclination
Dental factors	Absence of a well-defined cingulum stop on the upper incisors leads to continued eruption of the lower incisors, increasing overbite

■ *What further investigations would you undertake?*

1. *Assessment of the extent of soft tissue trauma palatal to the upper incisors and labial to the lower incisors from the increased overbite.* Periodontal pocket depth should be probed in these areas and gingival recession should be noted. Incisor mobility should also be assessed. Although there was evidence of tooth impingement on the gingivae palatal to 1|1 and labial to 1|, periodontal probing depths did not exceed 2 mm and there was no incisor mobility or gingival recession.

2. *Assessment of tooth surface wear on the upper and lower incisors* – this may be on the labial aspect of the lower

and/or the palatal aspect of the upper incisors as well as the incisal edges. Harry should be asked about any bruxing habit and his mother should be asked if she is aware of him having any nocturnal bruxing habit. If wear of the incisors is observed, site and extent should be noted for future monitoring; as this is better undertaken from dental casts, impressions should be recorded of the dental arches to allow these to be constructed. There was no noticeable incisor wear and no bruxing habit was reported.

3. *Assessment of the amount of upper and lower arch crowding.* Space may be obtained to relieve mild/moderate lower arch crowding and level an increased curve of Spee by some proclination of the lower labial segment and by a small amount of intercanine width expansion, which appear to be stable in this malocclusion. Therefore, in Class II division 2 malocclusion, lower arch extractions should generally only be undertaken if crowding is severe. In this case, lower arch extractions should be considered with great reservation as this will allow the lower labial segment to drop lingually and aggravate an already traumatic overbite. There was 2 mm of lower labial segment crowding and space analysis indicated sufficient space for the canines and premolars (21 mm present in each quadrant; 21 mm is required, on average, to accommodate 3̄, 4̄, 5̄).

> **Key point**
>
> In Class II division 2 malocclusion:
> - Beware of lower arch extractions only, as a deep overbite may become traumatic.
> - Some proclination of 2 1|1 2 and mild lower intercanine expansion are often possible and stable.

4. *Radiographic investigations.* The following views are required:
   - Dental panoramic tomogram, to account for the presence/absence, position, form of all unerupted teeth. This showed: normal alveolar bone height; normal developing dentition with a full complement of teeth. No tooth appeared to be in an ectopic position or to be of abnormal size or shape.
   - A lateral cephalometric radiograph to assess the anteroposterior and vertical skeletal relationships and the angulation of the incisor teeth to their underlying dental bases.

■ *What is your interpretation of the following cephalometric findings (see p. 204)?*

SNA = 81°; SNB = 74°; ANB = 7°; MMPA = 22°; 1 to maxillary plane = 99°; 1̄ to mandibular plane = 88°; interincisal angle = 162°; facial % = 51%.

This indicates SNA is average; SNB is reduced; ANB is increased, indicating a Class II skeletal pattern; MMPA is reduced, which in conjunction with the Class II skeletal pattern is contributing to the increased overbite; 1 to maxillary plane is retroclined; 1̄ to mandibular plane is retroclined, and not compensating completely for the reduced MMPA; interincisal angle is increased; facial % is reduced.

■ *What is your diagnosis?*

Class II division 2 malocclusion in the late mixed dentition on a Class II skeletal base with reduced FMPA. Mild marginal gingivitis related to the upper incisors. Traumatic overbite onto gingivae palatal to 1|1 and labial of 1̄. Mild upper and lower arch crowding. Buccal segment relationship half-unit Class II bilaterally.

■ *What is the IOTN DHC grade (see p. 203)?*

4f – due to the traumatic overbite.

Treatment

■ *What are your aims of treatment?*

Aims of treatment are to:

Relieve upper and lower arch crowding.

Reduce the overbite.

Correct the incisor relationship to Class I.

Correct the molar relationship to Class I.

Retain the corrected occlusion.

■ *How do you propose to achieve these aims?*

As Harry is growing and has Class II and deep bite skeletal problems, growth modification by a functional appliance would be the treatment of choice. A preliminary phase of upper removable appliance therapy will be required to align 1|1 by proclination and to expand the upper arch slightly, allowing the mandible to be postured forward with the arch widths coordinated for the construction bite for the functional appliance. Following that treatment phase, final detailing of the occlusion with fixed appliances is likely to be required prior to proceeding to retention.

■ *Describe the design of appliances you would use.*

The upper removable appliance to procline 1|1 would have the following design:

- *Activation*: Z springs to 1|1 (0.5 mm stainless steel wire). Midline expansion screw.
- *Retention*: Adams clasps 64|6 (0.7 mm stainless steel wire). |4 is insufficiently erupted at present to clasp.
- *Anchorage*: From baseplate.
- *Baseplate*: Full palatal acrylic coverage with flat anterior biteplane, initially to half the height of 1|1. A measurement of the overjet plus 3 mm should be forwarded to the laboratory at the time of appliance construction to ensure adequate posterior extension of the biteplane.

As treatment progresses, addition of cold-cure acrylic to the flat anterior biteplane may be made at the chairside, until sufficient overbite reduction has been achieved. The upper incisor teeth should be overproclined slightly to allow for some retroclination under the influence of the functional appliance.

The patient should be instructed to turn the midline expansion screw one quarter turn per week. Arch coordination should be monitored at each recall by getting the patient to posture the mandible forward until the molars are

in a Class I relationship and checking to ensure that the buccal segment teeth are not in crossbite. As the upper arch in Class II Division 2 malocclusion is usually square-shaped and the lower arch is 'u'-shaped, only a small amount of upper arch expansion is generally required to achieve coordination of the arch widths with the mandible postured forward.

An activator-type functional appliance is particularly useful in this type of malocclusion. A Herbst appliance is less recommended as it may tend to depress upper molars and inhibit correction of the deep bite problem. For this case, the construction bite for the activator appliance should be taken with the mandible postured forward edge-to-edge with the incisors 3–4 mm apart and the centrelines correct. If the centrelines had been discrepant by several millimetres initially, the bite should not compensate for this.

The design of a medium opening activator to be used here would be as follows:

- Adams clasps and occlusal rests to 6|6 (0.8 mm stainless steel wire).
- Labial bow 3| to |3 (0.8 mm stainless steel wire); palatal bow 2| to |2 (0.8 mm stainless steel wire).
- Acrylic palatal baseplate, deep acrylic capping of the lower incisors and canines with acrylic struts joining the upper to the lower part of the appliance. The acrylic should be heat-cured.

An alternative to using an upper removable appliance to procline the upper incisors, followed by an activator-type appliance, is to use a modified Twin-Block appliance to achieve the desired tooth movements. The design of this appliance incorporates Z springs to procline 1|1, and has no labial bow.

■ *What are the goals of the functional appliance treatment?*

To correct the skeletal Class II problem by differential growth of the jaws, in particular addressing the mandibular retrusion.

To increase the lower facial height and to correct the deep bite by preventing incisor eruption, controlling eruption of the upper posterior teeth while allowing eruption of the lower posterior teeth. This differential control of incisor/molar eruption aims to rotate the occlusal plane in a manner that allows Class II correction.

Key point

Class II division 2 malocclusion in the mixed dentition may be amenable to functional appliance correction, taking advantage of facial growth to aid overbite reduction.

■ *Why may a later phase of fixed appliance therapy be required?*

Rotational correction, especially of 2|2, and detailing of the buccal segment occlusion require the use of fixed appliance therapy.

■ *What aspects of the corrected occlusion are prone to relapse? How may you try to prevent/minimize relapse?*

Rotations of 2|2 – pericision (severing of the free gingival fibres) should be undertaken a few months prior to fixed

Fig. 12.4 (A) Post-treatment. Profile.

Fig. 12.4 (B) Post-treatment: left buccal occlusion.

Fig. 12.4 (C) Post-treatment: anterior occlusion.

Key point

The corrected aspects of Class II division 2 malocclusion most prone to relapse are:
- Rotational correction of 2|2.
- Overbite reduction.

The facial profile and the occlusion after functional appliance followed by fixed appliance therapy are shown in **Figure 12.4**.

Recommended reading

Dyer FM, McKeown HF, Sandler PJ 2001 The modified twin block appliance in the treatment of Class II division 2 malocclusions. J Orthod 28:271–280.

Kim TW, Little RM 1999 Postretention assessment of deep overbite correction in Class II division 2 malocclusion. Angle Orthod 69:175–186.

Lapatki BG, Mager AS, Schulte-Moenting J, Jones IE 2002 The importance of the level of the lip line and resting lip pressure in Class II division 2 malocclusion. J Dent Res 81:323–328.

Millett DT, Cunningham SJ, O'Brien KD et al 2006 Orthodontic treatment for deep bite and retroclined upper front teeth in children. Cochrane Database Syst Rev Issue 4 Number CD005972.

Selwyn-Barnett BJ 1996 Class II/Division 2 malocclusion: a method of planning and treatment. Br J Orthod 23:29–36.

For revision, see Mind Map 12, page 174.

appliance removal as it reduces relapse tendency. A bonded retainer, however, will be required to maintain upper labial segment alignment in the long term.

Overbite – the tendency for anterior mandibular growth rotation to continue into late teens and beyond will encourage overbite increase. To combat this, a flat anterior biteplane should be incorporated on an upper Hawley retainer (designed to fit around the upper bonded retainer) to be worn at night until growth has reduced to adult levels.

Anterior open bite

SUMMARY

Gerald is 11 years old. He presents with no contact of his incisor teeth (Fig. 13.1). Identify the cause(s) and discuss the treatment options.

History

Complaint

Gerald complains that his front teeth do not meet. This embarrasses him when eating as he cannot bite into food. His parents are also concerned by this and by lisping during speech, which they attribute to the position of his front teeth. They are anxious for treatment.

History of complaint

Gerald's parents report that his primary incisors did not meet either, but the space between the upper and lower permanent incisors appears to have increased in the past year. His lisp has also become more noticeable. He has no history of thumb or digit sucking.

Medical history

Gerald is fit and well.

Fig. 13.1 Anterior occlusion at presentation.

Dental history

Gerald is a regular attender at his general dental practitioner and has cooperated well with previous dental treatment.

Examination

Extraoral

■ *Gerald's facial profile is shown in* Figure 13.2*. What do you notice?*

Gerald has a mild Class II skeletal pattern with increased FMPA and increased lower anterior facial height. The lips are competent.

There was no facial asymmetry. Mouth opening was within normal dimensions and there was no temporomandibular joint tenderness or crepitus. No masticatory muscle tenderness was noted.

■ *What other features should you assess? Explain why.*

1. *The swallowing pattern.* Where there is a space between the upper and lower anterior teeth, swallowing is likely to be achieved by forward positioning of the tongue between the anterior teeth to achieve an oral seal. This is particularly so where the vertical facial proportions are increased as the likelihood of lip incompetence is greater. Although such behaviour of the tongue is in most cases adaptive, in rare instances an endogenous (primary) tongue thrust exists. It has been suggested that this is associated with lisping and some proclination of the upper and lower incisors. Any attempt in these cases to close the open bite is doomed to fail as the tongue will return the incisors to their original positions.

2. *Speech.* By asking Gerald to count from 60 to 70 aloud or to say 'Mississippi', the degree of sibilance (lisping) can be detected. The tongue position during speech should also be observed.

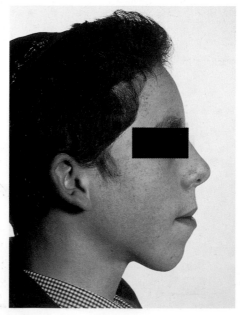

Fig. 13.2 Profile.

Gerald had a tongue to lower lip swallowing pattern and the lisp was deemed to be mild.

■ *What occlusal anomalies are associated with speech problems? Are the latter likely to resolve if any underlying malocclusion is treated?*

Although speech problems are associated with incisor spacing, Class II division 1 malocclusion, Class III malocclusion and anterior open bite, they do not occur in all individuals with these occlusal anomalies. Furthermore, correction of these occlusal problems is no guarantee that the associated speech problem will resolve satisfactorily. Where sibilance is judged to be marked, referral to a speech therapist would be prudent, although treatment may do little to mitigate the defect.

Intraoral

■ *What other features do you see (Figs 13.1 and 13.3)?*

Mild marginal gingival erythema related especially to the incisors and 4|.

No caries is visible.

Mild spacing of the upper and lower labial segments; mesiolabial rotations of 1|1.

Class I incisor relationship.

Anterior open bite (measured clinically = 6 mm from the mesioincisal aspects of $\left|\frac{1}{1}\right.$.

Class III molar relationship bilaterally.

Fig. 13.3 (A) Right buccal occlusion.

Fig. 13.3 (B) Left buccal occlusion.

■ *What are the possible causes of an anterior open bite?*

These are given in **Table 13.1**.

Table 13.1 Causes of anterior open bite

Cause	Aetiology
Skeletal	Increase in lower anterior facial height such that the compensatory ability of the incisors to erupt into contact is exceeded. This may be worsened by a downward and backward pattern of facial growth
Soft tissues	Rarely endogenous tongue thrust
Habits	Persistent digit-sucking habit, which often leads to an asymmetrical anterior open bite
Localized failure of alveolar development	Occurs in cleft lip and palate, although in other cases there may be no known cause

Key point

A persistent digit-sucking habit often produces an asymmetrical anterior open bite.

■ *What are the effects of a persistent digit-sucking habit on the occlusion other than creating an anterior open bite?*

It may result in retroclination of the lower incisors, proclination of the upper incisors, increased overjet and a unilateral buccal segment crossbite with associated mandibular displacement (see Chapter 14).

Investigations

■ *What special investigations would you require? Explain why.*

A *dental panoramic tomogram* is required to indicate what other teeth have yet to erupt and to check their developmental position and form.

A *lateral cephalometric radiograph* is required to assess more fully the extent of the anteroposterior and vertical skeletal discrepancies as well as the relationship of the incisors to the underlying dental bases.

The dental panoramic tomogram showed:

Normal alveolar base height.

A normal dentition. The developmental age matches Gerald's chronological age.

Third molars are present.

The cephalometric analysis revealed:

SNA = 82°; SNB = 76°; ANB = 6°; MMPA = 34°; 1 to maxillary plane = 111°; 1̄ to mandibular plane = 86°; interincisal angle = 126°; facial % = 60%.

■ *What is your interpretation of these findings?*

Relative to mean values for Caucasians, SNA is slightly increased and SNB is slightly reduced but both are within the normal range; the skeletal pattern is mildly Class II; 1 to maxillary plane shows that it is proclined relative to the mean but within the normal range; 1̄ to mandibular plane shows that it is retroclined relative to the mean but it is at the correct angulation to compensate for the increased MMPA (120° − 34° = 86°) ; relative to mean values, the interincisal angle is reduced but within the normal range and the facial proportion is increased.

Diagnosis

■ *What is your diagnosis?*

Class I malocclusion on a mild Class II skeletal base with increased FMPA. Marginal gingivitis related to the incisors and 4|. Mild mesiolabial rotations of 1|1 with spacing of the upper and lower labial segments. Anterior open bite. Buccal segment relationship Class III bilaterally.

■ *What is the IOTN DHC grade (see p. 203)?*

4e – due to the anterior open bite.

Treatment

■ *What treatment would you consider?*

As the anterior open bite is not due to digit sucking, treatment is likely to be complex. Gerald has anteroposterior and vertical skeletal problems, the latter being more marked, with a downward and backward pattern of facial growth that has produced the anterior open bite. An *attempt*, therefore, to achieve incisor contact may be by growth modification aiming for effective control of maxillary vertical skeletal and dental growth.

This would require specialist care. A functional appliance with posterior bite blocks, e.g. a Twin-Block appliance, would be optimal. As the incisor relationship is Class I and the molar relationships are Class III, no forward posturing of the mandible for the registration bite is advisable. The bite, however, must be opened beyond the normal resting vertical dimension so that molar eruption is prevented. As the appliance holds the mandible in this position, a vertical intrusive force is exerted on the posterior teeth mediated by the stretch of the muscles and other soft tissues. Gerald should be instructed to wear the appliance full-time including for meals. The anterior teeth are allowed to erupt while eruption of the posterior teeth is inhibited, thereby reducing the anterior open bite. This is supplemented by a tendency for mandibular growth to be projected anteriorly while vertical control of maxillary skeletal and dental growth is effected. In this case, high-pull headgear should not be added to the appliance. As the molar relationships are Class III, any molar distal movement is not indicated.

Currently, there is weak evidence that Function Regulator IV (FR IV) with lip-seal training and palatal crib associated with high-pull chincup are able to correct anterior open bite.

Key point

Unless anterior open bite is due to a habit, treatment is complex.

■ *If the anterior open bite had been due to thumb sucking, what treatment would you recommend?*

Gentle persuasion to discontinue the habit is usually best (**Fig. 13.4**). If unsuccessful, consideration could be given to

Fig. 13.4 (A) Another case with anterior open bite due to thumb sucking.

Fig. 13.4 (B) Following cessation of the habit and fixed appliance therapy. Note that acid pumice microabrasion was used to improve the appearance of 1|1 (see Chapter 34).

provision of a habit-breaker, such as an upper removable appliance or palatal arch modified to break the 'pleasure cycle' associated with the sucking habit. If the habit ceases, the anterior open bite will usually reduce spontaneously although this is likely to take several years.

■ *What is the likely prognosis of treatment?*

As the anterior open bite is quite marked and the vertical skeletal pattern is moderately increased, the prognosis is guarded. Gerald and his parents should be made aware of this before treatment commences. Provided there is excellent cooperation with appliance wear and vertical facial growth is favourable, functional appliance treatment has a reasonable chance of success at this stage. However, a second phase of treatment with fixed appliances is likely to be required to detail the occlusion. As these appliances do not control eruption so favourably, posterior bite blocks or similar components will be required during that phase of treatment as well, to maintain the correction achieved in the earlier phase. Thereafter, bite blocks will also need to be incorporated in any retainer. Long-term retention will be required to avert the possible unfavourable effects of subsequent vertical facial growth.

The lisp may improve with closure of the anterior open bite, but Gerald and his parents should not have high expectations regarding this.

■ *Are there any other treatment options?*

If Gerald does not cooperate with functional appliance wear, treatment for the anterior open bite may be considered by a specific type of fixed appliance mechanics (Kim mechanics), most likely in conjunction with the removal of second or third molars. This approach to appliance treatment requires specialist training. The objective is to correct the cant of individual occlusal planes, uprighting the teeth in relation to the bisecting occlusal plane. Impressive and stable correction of marked anterior open bite, in adolescents and adults, has been reported using this technique. Should the anterior open bite worsen considerably, a combined orthodontic surgical approach may be sought when growth is complete.

Key point

Management options for anterior open bite may be:
- Accept.
- Habit breaker.
- Growth modification.
- Orthodontic camouflage.
- Surgery.

Recommended reading

Johnson NC, Sandy JR 1999 Tooth position and speech – is there a relationship? Angle Orthod 69:306–310.

Kim YH 1987 Anterior openbite and its treatment with multiloop edgewise archwire. Angle Orthod 57:290–321.

Lentini-Oliveira D, Carvalho FR, Qingsong Y et al 2007 Orthodontic and orthopaedic treatment for anterior open bite in children. Cochrane Database Syst Rev Issue 2 CD005515.

Lopez-Gavito G, Wallen TR, Little RM, Joondeph DR 1985 Anterior open-bite malocclusion: a longitudinal 10-year postretention evaluation of orthodontically treated patients. Am J Orthod 87:175–186.

Mizrahi E 1978 A review of anterior open bite. Br J Orthod 5:21–27.

For revision, see Mind Map 13, page 175.

14

Posterior crossbite

SUMMARY

Kirsten is 7. She presents with a crossbite of the right buccal segments (Fig. 14.1). What will be your assessment and management options for this problem?

History

Complaint

Kirsten's mother is concerned about the way her daughter's teeth bite together. She has noticed that Kirsten's jaw moves to one side as she closes her mouth. This makes her face appear crooked, a further cause of anxiety for her mother.

History of complaint

Kirsten used to suck her thumb until 5 months ago when $\overline{1|1}$ started to erupt. Her mother has become more aware of her daughter's 'deviated bite' in the past year and wondered if the thumb-sucking habit could have contributed to the problem.

Medical history

Kirsten is fit and well.

Family history

There is no family history of facial asymmetry.

Fig. 14.1 Anterior occlusion at presentation.

Examination

Extraoral

Kirsten has a mild Class III skeletal pattern with slightly increased FMPA; the chin point is displaced slightly to the right. The lips are incompetent but habitually held together. There is a tongue to lower lip swallowing pattern. There is no masticatory muscle tenderness, temporomandibular joint tenderness or crepitus, and mouth opening is not restricted.

■ *What other feature would you check for, bearing in mind the history? Explain why.*

It is important to check if there is mandibular displacement on closure as this would indicate that the facial asymmetry is more an apparent than a true skeletal asymmetry. For the former, orthodontic correction of an associated crossbite should be straightforward but for the latter further investigations would be required to determine if the asymmetry is progressive and more complex treatment would be required to address the facial and occlusal problems.

Early correction of a crossbite with a mandibular displacement is indicated to allow the occlusion to develop in an undisplaced position. It is likely also to reduce the possibility of development of temporomandibular joint dysfunction syndrome, which may occur in susceptible individuals in whom this occlusal discrepancy exists.

An anterolateral mandibular displacement on closure was detected on $\frac{c}{c}$ with an associated 3 mm shift between retruded contact position (RCP) and intercuspal position (ICP).

Key point

Early correction of a posterior crossbite with associated mandibular displacement is advisable.

Intraoral

■ *What features are evident on the intraoral views (Figs 14.1 and 14.2)?*

Mild marginal gingival erythema related to the erupting permanent incisors but otherwise the soft tissues appear healthy. There is no caries visible.

Fig. 14.2 (A) Right buccal occlusion.

Fig. 14.2 (B) Left buccal occlusion.

6edcb1 are present in both upper quadrants and in the lower right quadrant; 12cde6 are present in the lower left quadrant.

Spacing of the upper and lower incisors with distopalatal rotation of 1| .

Class III incisor relationship.

Anterior open bite.

Lower centreline shift to the right.

Half-unit Class II right molar relationship with buccal crossbite of the right buccal segments (note palatal inclination of the teeth).

Class III left molar relationship.

■ *How would you assess the centrelines?*

The upper and lower centrelines should be coincident with each other and with the midline of the face. Both of these aspects should be assessed, the latter by first looking at the patient anteriorly and then down on the face from above. With study models alone, it is not possible to determine the relation of the dental midlines to the facial midline.

In this case, the lower centreline is displaced to the right by about half the width of a lower incisor.

■ *What are the possible causes of a lower centreline shift?*

These are listed in **Box 14.1**. In this case, it is due to the lateral aspect of the mandibular displacement on closure.

Box 14.1 Causes of a lower centreline shift

- Unbalanced loss of c, d and possibly e; the age at extraction, the degree of crowding and the tooth extracted (the more anterior, the greater the effect) influence the extent of centreline shift.
- Unilateral retained primary incisor, canine or molar.
- Hypodontia of an incisor or premolar.
- Supplemental incisor or premolar.
- Lateral mandibular displacement on closure producing unilateral buccal segment crossbite (often secondary to digit- or thumb-sucking habit).
- Early unilateral condylar fracture leading to deficient growth on the affected side.
- Hemifacial microsomia.
- Hemimandibular hypertrophy (known formerly as condylar hyperplasia). Cause is entirely unknown. Most likely in females between the ages of 15 and 20 but may occur in either sex as late as the early thirties.

■ *What factors may be implicated in the aetiology of the crossbite?*

These are summarized in **Table 14.1**.

Table 14.1 Causes of buccal segment crossbite

Cause	Aetiology
Skeletal	Mismatch in the widths of the dental arches and/or an anteroposterior skeletal discrepancy – buccal and anterior crossbites are most commonly found in Class III malocclusion. Rarely, mandibular growth restriction following condylar trauma or hemimandibular hypertrophy may be implicated, both producing asymmetry
Soft tissues/habit	With a digit-sucking habit, the tongue position is lowered with the teeth apart, and cheek contraction is unopposed during sucking, narrowing the upper arch slightly

■ *What is the most likely cause of the posterior crossbite in this case?*

The thumb-sucking habit.

Key point

A digit-sucking habit may lead to posterior crossbite with associated mandibular displacement.

Investigations

■ *What special investigations would you undertake and why?*

A dental panoramic tomogram (**Fig. 14.3A**) is required to survey the developing dentition for any abnormalities of tooth number, size and position.

Impressions of the dental arches and a wax registration in maximum intercuspation should be taken to allow study models to be constructed. These will allow a thorough occlusal assessment to be performed and will act as a baseline record of the malocclusion.

■ *What does the dental panoramic tomogram show?*

Normal alveolar bone height.

All permanent teeth developing apart from third molars.

No apparent caries or other pathology.

■ *What is the most likely reason for the blurred image of the right half of the dental panoramic tomogram?*

Movement of the patient during image capture, most probably due to swallowing, is the likely cause.

Fig. 14.3 (A) Dental panoramic tomogram.

Fig. 14.3 (B) Repeat of right half dental panoramic tomogram.

■ *Why was a right half, rather than a full, dental panoramic tomogram retaken? (Fig. 14.3B)?*

In line with current radiology guidelines, the radiation dosage to the patient should be as low as reasonably achievable for the diagnostic purposes required. Retaking the right-half image only satisfies diagnostic needs here.

Diagnosis

■ *What is your diagnosis?*

Class III malocclusion on a mild Class III skeletal base with slightly increased FMPA; anterolateral mandibular displacement on closure on $\frac{c}{c}$. Mild marginal gingivitis related to the erupting incisors. Spacing of the upper and lower incisors with 1| distopalatally rotated. Anterior open bite; lower centreline shift to the right. Buccal segment relationship half-unit Class II on the right and Class III on the left. Buccal crossbite of the right buccal segments associated with the mandibular displacement.

■ *What is the IOTN DHC grade (see p. 203)?*

4c – due to mandibular displacement >2 mm between the RCP and the ICP.

Treatment

■ *What treatment plan would you propose?*

Oral hygiene instruction to improve gingival health.
Correction of the right buccal segment and anterior crossbites.
Regular review of the developing occlusion.

■ *How may the crossbites be corrected? Describe the design of any appliance you would use.*

Possible approaches to treatment are as follows:

1. As the digit-sucking habit has been abandoned and the mandibular displacement arises from premature contact on $\frac{c}{c}$, judicious grinding of their cusp tips may remove the occlusal interference and correct the buccal segment crossbite. A systematic review on management of posterior crossbites concluded that removal of premature displacing contacts on primary teeth prevents perpetuation of the posterior crossbite into the permanent dentition. The permanent incisors are erupted insufficiently, at present, to consider their proclination and which means will be best.

2. As the upper buccal segment teeth are not tilted buccally, upper arch expansion by a midline screw in an upper removable appliance may be considered. The appliance may be clasped on 6d|d6 (Adams clasps: 6|6 0.7 mm stainless steel wire; d|d 0.6 mm stainless steel wire). Buccal capping will facilitate tooth movement by disengaging the posterior occlusion. Kirsten should be encouraged to turn the screw one quarter turn twice weekly (0.25 mm of activation with each turn) until the crossbite is corrected. A small amount of overexpansion is advisable as some relapse is to be expected. Then the capping should be reduced to half its height at one visit and removed completely at the following visit to allow the buccal segment teeth to erupt into occlusion. The appliance should then be worn for 3 months full-time followed by 3 months at night only as a retainer.

3. Alternatively, upper arch expansion may be undertaken using a quadhelix. This consists of bands cemented to the first permanent molars with soldered arms, in this case, extending forward to the palatal aspects of the c's. Alternatively, a preformed quadhelix may be employed that fits into sheaths soldered to the palatal aspects of the molar bands, allowing easy removal for adjustment. Activation is usually half a tooth width on each side. To facilitate crossbite correction, it may be necessary to disengage the buccal occlusion temporarily by placing glass ionomer cement on the occlusal surfaces of the molars. Once the crossbite has been corrected, the cement may be removed and the quadhelix should be rendered passive prior to cementation for 3–6 months as a retainer. Research has shown that the expansion achieved by an upper removable or a quadhelix appliance is similar but the latter is more cost-effective.

The final occlusion following crossbite correction by an upper removable appliance is shown in **Figure 14.4**. Correction of the incisor relationship and improvement in 1| alignment occurred spontaneously.

Key point

Management options for a unilateral posterior crossbite with associated mandibular displacement in the mixed dentition:
- Grind c's.
- URA with midline screw.
- Quadhelix.

■ *What will determine if the corrected buccal segment crossbite is likely to be stable?*

Good buccal segment interdigitation and absence of any displacing occlusal contacts.

Fig. 14.4 (A) Post-treatment. Right buccal occlusion.

Fig. 14.4 (B) Post-treatment. Anterior occlusion.

Recommended reading

Harrison JE, Ashby D 2001 Orthodontic treatment for posterior crossbites. Cochrane Database Syst Rev Issue 1: CD000979.

Hermanson H, Kurol J, Ronnerman A 1985 Treatment of unilateral posterior crossbites with quadhelix and removable plates. A retrospective study. Eur J Orthod 7:97–102.

Primozic J, Ovsenik M, Richmond S et al 2009 Early crossbite correction: a three-dimensional evaluation. Eur J Orthod 31:352–356.

For revision, see Mind Map 14, page 176.

Bilateral crossbite

Case 1

SUMMARY

Jean has just turned 12. She presents with bilateral buccal crossbites** (Fig. 15.1)**. What are the possible causes and how could it be managed?

History

Complaint

Jean does not like the 'narrow' appearance of her upper teeth, especially when she smiles.

History of complaint

Her mother says that Jean's 'baby' teeth had the same appearance and she also has a similar appearance of her upper teeth to her daughter. Jean's teeth erupted in the position they are in at present. There is no history of trauma to her upper jaw and birth was normal.

Medical history

Jean is asthmatic and uses a salbutamol (Ventolin) inhaler. She is prone to upper respiratory tract infections and is unable to breathe through her nose. Her mother reports that she snores and is prone to day-time drowsiness, which her teachers have noticed. Otherwise she is well. Her mother

Fig. 15.1 Case 1: Anterior occlusion at presentation.

wonders if the narrow appearance of Jean's upper teeth is related in any way to her mouth breathing and snoring. She is keen to know if Jean's mouth breathing and snoring could be improved by any brace treatment.

■ *What is the relevance of Jean's mode of breathing to snoring and to her complaint?*

Compulsive mouth breathing, due to inability to breathe through the nose, may contribute to an altered head posture and low tongue position; this may lead to unopposed action of buccinator musculature and bilateral narrowing of the upper arch creating bilateral buccal crossbites.

Inability to breathe through the nose is also linked with snoring, which is associated with sleep apnoea, a major cause of day-time drowsiness. Prolonged inflammation of the nasal mucosa associated with allergies (in Jean's case there is a history of asthma) or chronic infection (she is prone to upper respiratory tract infections) could produce some degree of nasal obstruction and lead to mouth breathing. The normally large pharyngeal tonsils or adenoids in children may also contribute.

Key point

Mouth breathing may contribute to altered head posture, low tongue position and bilateral buccal crossbite, but it is not the sole or even the major cause of such crossbites.

Dental history

Jean is an irregular attender at her general dental practitioner. She has fissure sealants to several molar teeth and one filling. There is no history of digit-sucking.

■ *How may a digit-sucking habit cause a buccal segment crossbite?*

This is given in **Table 14.1** (p. 63).

Social history

Jean has two younger sisters. Neither of them have had orthodontic treatment and neither of them have teeth like hers.

Examination

Extraoral

Jean has a Class 1 skeletal pattern with slightly increased FMPA and no facial asymmetry. Lips are incompetent. There are no signs or symptoms associated with the temporomandibular joints.

Intraoral

■ *The appearance of the teeth on presentation is shown in Figures 15.1 and 15.2. Describe what you see.*

Fair oral hygiene with generalized marginal gingival erythema.
$\frac{654321 \mid 123456}{7654321 \mid 1234567}$ visible (please note 7|7 are also erupted).

All teeth visible appear caries-free; amalgam restoration in 6̄.

Moderate lower arch crowding; 1̄1̄ appear slightly small (contact point displacements were 3 mm between 1̄ and 2̄; also between 2̄ and 3̄); mild upper arch crowding

Fig. 15.2 (A) Case 1: Right buccal occlusion.

Fig. 15.2 (B) Case 1: Left buccal occlusion.

Class I incisor relationship; average and complete overbite; upper and lower centreline shifts (upper appears to the left, lower to the right); 2|2 in crossbite.

Molar relationship Class I on right and Class III on left with bilateral buccal crossbite affecting $\frac{6543\,|\,456}{6543\,|\,56}$.

■ *What are the possible causes of bilateral buccal crossbite?*

Factors implicated in the aetiology of a bilateral buccal crossbite are given in **Table 15.1**.

Table 15.1 Possible causes of bilateral buccal crossbite

Bilateral buccal crossbite	Possible causes
Skeletal	Mismatch in relative widths of arches or anteroposterior discrepancy (commonly associated with Class III malocclusion)
Soft tissues	Possible role of adenoids/tonsils (see text)
	Low tongue position possibly due to altered head posture associated with mouth breathing
	Scar tissue of cleft repair restraining growth in upper arch width

Investigations

■ *What investigations would you undertake in relation to the bilateral buccal crossbite? Explain why.*

Clinical

It would be important to ascertain if there is an associated mandibular displacement, although this is rare with bilat-eral crossbites. It is more usual to have a mandibular displacement associated with a unilateral buccal crossbite.

No mandibular displacement was noted.

Radiographic

A dental panoramic tomogram would be useful to determine the presence, position and form of unerupted third molars. A lateral cephalometric radiograph will also be required (to ascertain the angulation of the upper and lower incisors to their respective dental bases).

The dental panoramic tomogram indicated four third molars of good form and position to be present.

The cephalometric findings were as follows:

SNA = 81°; SNB = 79°; MMPA = 28°; $\underline{1}$ to maxillary plane = 113°; $\overline{1}$ to mandibular plane = 93°; interincisal angle = 138°; facial % = 56%.

■ *What is your interpretation of these findings?*

Relative to mean values for Caucasians, SNA is normal; SNB is slightly increased; ANB (SNA – SNB) = 2°, indicating a Class I skeletal pattern; MMPA is slightly increased, $\underline{1}$ to maxillary plane is increased, so upper incisors are slightly proclined; $\overline{1}$ to mandibular plane is normal; interincisal angle is slightly increased; facial % is slightly increased.

All values are within the normal range for Caucasians.

Diagnosis

■ *What is your diagnosis?*

Class I malocclusion on a Class I skeletal pattern with slightly increased FMPA and no facial symmetry. Generalized marginal gingivitis. Moderate lower labial segment crowding: mild upper labial segment crowding with 2's in crossbite; upper and lower centreline shifts. Molar relationship Class I on right; Class III on left with bilateral buccal crossbite affecting $\frac{6543\,|\,456}{6543\,|\,56}$.

■ *What is the IOTN DHC grade (see page 203)?*

3d – due to contact point displacement between $\overline{1}$ and $\overline{2}$; also between $\overline{2}$ and $\overline{3}$.

Treatment

■ *What are the aims of treatment?*

To improve oral hygiene.

To correct the bilateral buccal crossbite.

To relieve upper and lower arch crowding.

To align upper and lower arches with centreline correction.

To correct the left buccal segment relationship to Class I.

■ *What treatment would you provide?*

Oral hygiene instruction by hygienist. Provided the marginal gingivitis is corrected then proceed to correction of the bilateral buccal crossbite (the need for extractions for relief of crowding and centreline correction should be reviewed following crossbite correction).

■ *What options are there for management of the bilateral buccal crossbite? Which would you choose?*

Table 15.2 Management options for bilateral buccal crossbite

Management option	Indications	Comments
Accept and monitor	Patient not keen for correction.	Not an option here as Jean is keen for correction
	Part of underlying skeletal III problem which is likely to worsen with mandibular growth, especially in males	
Removable appliance with midline screw or heavy midline spring	Primary/early mixed dentition	Rate of expansion must be quite slow and force employed low: otherwise retention of appliance compromised by higher expansion forces
		Compliance with wear and activation may be problematic
		Not cost-effective as often lengthy time required to produce desired expansion
Quadhelix	Preferred approach in early mixed dentition	Made of 1 mm stainless steel wire attached to bands cemented to molar tooth on each side
	3–5 mm maxillary expansion required (mainly dental but some skeletal expansion)	Delivers few hundred grams of force
	Teeth preferably tipped palatally but molar inclination may be adjusted with fixed appliances later	Produces efficient slow expansion
		May derotate molars
		May be adjusted to give more expansion posteriorly or anteriorly
		May be custom-made or preformed types available
		Activation half a tooth width each side
Rapid maxillary expansion (RME)	Child/adolescent	Produces ~ equal amounts of dental/skeletal expansion
	Minimal/no palatal tipping of the buccal segment teeth, i.e. skeletal crossbite	May be undertaken using a banded or bonded appliance (the latter limits the amount of downward-backward rotation of the mandible)
	>5 mm transverse maxillary expansion required	
	Mild anterior maxillary crowding	The older the age at expansion, the less likely the increase in vertical facial height will be recovered by subsequent growth
Surgically assisted rapid maxillary expansion (SARPE)	Skeletally mature patient with severe skeletal crossbite in whom segmental expansion in Le Fort I osteotomy might compromise blood supply to segments	Not an attractive option if further maxillary repositioning in the anteroposterior or vertical plane is required later
	>5 mm transverse maxillary expansion required	

The options are given in **Table 15.2**. In view of the severity of the crossbite and the desire to simultaneously, if possible, improve nasal breathing, rapid maxillary expansion (RME) would be the preferred choice of treatment.

■ *What factors should be checked before using this treatment? What are the chances of opening the mid-palatal suture in this patient?*

It is particularly advisable to check that there is adequate buccal supporting bone and gingival tissues. Before the age of 15, the chances of successful opening of the mid-palatal suture are almost 100% but reduce after that due to greater interdigitation of the sutures.

> **Key point**
>
> Mid-palatal suture opening by RME is almost 100% guaranteed before age 15.

■ *Describe the design of the appliance you would use. What instructions would you give Jean regarding this appliance?*

The mechanism of mid-palatal suture separation is expansion by a screw built into a fixed appliance that is attached rigidly to as many teeth as possible.

The appliance may only comprise metal or acrylic framework against the teeth, which does not contact the palatal mucosa or may be made with acrylic palate-covering

Fig. 15.3 Case 1: Rapid maxillary expansion appliance with Hyrax screw.

shelves. The latter type may, in theory, produce more bodily positioning of the alveolar processes but may impinge on the palatal tissues. For that reason, appliances that are tooth-borne are preferred.

The appliance used in Jean's case was as follows (**Fig. 15.3**):

- *Activation*: mid-palatal expansion screw (Hyrax).
- *Retention*: bands on 4's and 6's.

- *Anchorage*: <u>4</u>'s and <u>6</u>'s and the joining metal struts between the bands on these teeth.
- *Baseplate*: No palatal acrylic or buccal capping.

■ *What should Jean be advised of regarding the effects of expansion?*

As the suture expands more anteriorly than posteriorly, an upper median diastema will usually develop within days of appliance activation. Following correction of the bilateral crossbite and several months retention, during which time the appliance is left in place, the pull of the gingival fibres and some skeletal relapse will close the diastema.

With transverse maxillary expansion, some molar extrusion is likely and cuspal interferences are created that cause the mandible to rotate downward and backward. This will reduce the overbite.

■ *Describe how the appliance works?*

It separates the mid-palatal suture as if on a hinge at the nasal base. Rapid expansion is achieved using forces of 10–20 lb (approximately 4.5–9 kg) over 2–3 weeks with the patient turning the screw twice daily (~0.5 mm movement per day). This contrasts with slow expansion (force of 2–4 lb (0.9–1.8 kg) over about 2.5 months with the screw being turned once every other day, 1 mm per week). Minimal suture disruption takes place with slow expansion.

With a screw device for rapid expansion, force is transmitted first to the teeth and then to the suture, producing microfractures of the interdigitating bone spicules. Because closure begins posteriorly in the midpalatal suture, and the other maxillary structures also exert a buttressing effect in this region, the suture opens wider and faster anteriorly, often producing a median diastema. Some overcorrection is advisable (maxillary palatal cusps in line with mandibular buccal cusps) as there is a strong relapse tendency due to palatal soft tissue elasticity.

Key point

Rapid midpalatal suture expansion:

- Exerts a force of 10–20 lb (approximately 4.5–9 kg) over 2–3 weeks.
- Produces ~0.5 mm movement per day.
- Creates a median diastema.
- Has a strong relapse tendency, requiring overcorrection.

■ *How will you retain the crossbite correction?*

The expansion appliance should be rendered passive and remain in place for 3 months as a retainer. On its removal, a removable retainer with palatal acrylic coverage should be fitted unless further treatment is being carried out immediately in which case a heavy expanded maxillary archwire may be placed for retention. A modified transpalatal arch with arms extending to the mesial of the <u>4</u>'s or a 1 mm stainless steel archwire through the headgear tubes are alternatives while light wires align the remaining teeth. On completion of treatment, an upper Hawley retainer (see p. 87) or a fitted palatal arch may be placed.

The occlusion at removal of the RME appliance and immediately prior to proceeding to fixed appliance therapy is shown in **Figure 15.4**.

Fig. 15.4 Case 1: Anterior occlusion following RME and prior to proceeding to upper/lower fixed appliance therapy.

Recommended reading

Battagel JM 1996 Obstructive sleep apnoea: fact not fiction. Br J Orthod 23:315–324.

Herold JS 1989 Maxillary expansion: a retrospective study of three methods of expansion and their long-term sequelae. Br J Orthod 16:195–200.

Lagravere MO, Major PW, Flores-Mir C 2005 Long-term dental arch changes after rapid maxillary expansion treatment: a systematic review. Angle Orthod 75:155–161.

Vig KWL 1998 Nasal obstruction and facial growth: the strength of evidence for clinical assumptions. Am J Orthod Dentofacial Orthop 113:603–611.

Case 2

SUMMARY

Aidan is 19 years old. He presents concerned about the appearance of his top teeth and his bite (Fig. 15.5). How may it be treated?

■ *What are the main features of note in Figure 15.5?*

Narrow maxillary arch.

Bilateral posterior buccal crossbite, extending to include <u>3|</u>.

Upper labial segment crowding with incisor rotations; very mild lower labial segment crowding.

Fig. 15.5 Case 2: Anterior occlusion at presentation.

Class III incisor relationship with 2|2 in crossbite (distal aspects of 1|1 also in crossbite).

Upper and lower centreline discrepancy (appears that lower centreline is shifted to the right).

Minimal overbite.

Lateral open bites.

History of complaint

Aidan has been concerned for some time regarding his dental appearance. He now has a new job with a retail firm and feels embarrassed when he smiles. A previous orthodontist told him that he would need to wait until he was in his late teens before anything could be done regarding the bite of his front teeth.

■ *What makes a smile attractive?*

On smiling, the full height of the upper incisors should be seen (usually at rest, there is 1 mm incisor show in males and 3 mm incisor show in females). Although some gingival display is acceptable, the interproximal gingivae only should be visible for optimal aesthetics. The contour of the upper incisor edges should match that of the lower lip (smile arc), with no upper incisor/lower lip contact. In the transverse dimension, the smile should include at minimum the upper first premolars. The distance between the inside of the cheek and the maxillary posterior teeth (buccal corridor), particularly the premolars, should be narrow.

Key point

An attractive smile comprises:

- Full length of the upper incisors.
- Related interproximal gingivae.
- Upper incisor edges contour matches that of the lower lip.
- Extends laterally to include no less than upper first premolars.
- Narrow buccal corridors.

Medical and dental history

Aidan is in good health. He is unable to breathe through his nose.

Treatment

■ *Why is RME not feasible?*

In adults, the midpalatal and lateral maxillary sutures are well-interdigitated, which afford increased resistance to the orthopaedic-type palatal expansion (RME) that may be used in adolescents.

■ *How is SARPE undertaken?*

Originally, surgically assisted rapid palatal expansion (SARPE) was undertaken using bone cuts only in the lateral maxillary buttress to decrease resistance such that in adults the midpalatal suture could be microfractured by forced

Fig. 15.6 (A) Case 2: Expansion appliance in situ after surgery.

Fig. 15.6 (B) Case 2: Completion of alignment by fixed appliances.

opening. Although this is commonly successful in patients under 30, in older patients there is a risk of unwanted fractures in other areas. Currently, the procedure is often undertaken using cuts as for a Le Fort I osteotomy but without maxillary down-fracture. The maxilla is thus able to widen in a process akin to distraction osteogenesis (see p. 72) as resistance is provided by the soft tissues only. The RME appliance is cemented prior to surgery and activation of the screw usually commences within 2 days at the same rate as for non-surgically assisted RME. Fixed appliances are required to complete alignment (**Fig. 15.6**).

The improved occlusion on completion of treatment is shown in **Figure 15.7**.

■ *How stable is SARPE?*

SARPE appears to be more stable than surgical widening of the maxilla. The latter has a high relapse tendency due to elastic rebound of the stretched palatal mucosa. Even following SARPE, wear of a palate-covering retainer for at least the first post-surgical year is recommended to control relapse.

Key point

SARPE:

- Is indicated for bilateral posterior crossbite correction in adults.
- Allows widening of the maxilla against only soft tissue resistance.
- Appears to be more stable than surgical widening of the maxilla.

Fig. 15.7 (A) Case 2 post-treatment: Anterior occlusion.

Fig. 15.8 (A) Case 3: At presentation: Right buccal occlusion.

Fig. 15.7 (B) Case 2 post-treatment: Left buccal occlusion.

Fig. 15.8 (B) Case 3: At presentation: Anterior occlusion.

Recommended reading

Koudstaal MJ, Poort LJ, van der Wal KG et al 2005
Surgically assisted rapid maxillary expansion (SARME):
a review of the literature. Int J Oral Maxillofac Surg
34:709–714.

Magnusson A, Bjerklin K, Nilsson P, Marcusson A 2009
Surgically assisted rapid maxillary expansion: long-term
stability. Eur J Orthod 31:142–149.

Parekh SM, Fields HW, Beck M, Rosenstiel SF 2006
Attractiveness of variations in the smile arc and buccal
corridor space as judged by orthodontists and laymen.
Angle Orthod 76:557–563.

Fig. 15.8 (C) Case 3: At presentation: Left buccal occlusion.

Case 3

SUMMARY

*Simon is 13 years old. He presents complaining about
the prominence of his top teeth and the crooked
lower back teeth (Fig. 15.8). What are the causes and
what options are there for management?*

■ *What are the main features of note in Figure 15.8?*

Enamel fracture in incisal third of ⌊1 with composite
restoration (⌊1 had suffered trauma 2 years previously but was
symptom-free).
Caries 5⌋ distally.
Mild upper arch crowding; moderate lower arch crowding.

Fig. 15.8 (D) Case 3: At presentation: Lower occlusal view.

Class II division 1 malocclusion; increased overjet; slightly increased overbite.

Canine relationship half-unit Class II bilaterally.

Bilateral lingual crossbite (also referred to as scissors bite or Brodie bite) affecting 54|5.

■ *Given the position of 5|45, what would you enquire about?*

It would be useful to know if there had been early loss of lower e̅'s which would encourage mesial drift of 6̅'s and lingual displacement of 5̅'s.

Simon had e|de removed when he was aged 7.

Key point

Lingual crossbites are associated with Class II malocclusions.

Extraoral

Simon has a Class II skeletal pattern with slightly reduced FMPA; there is no facial asymmetry.

No mandibular displacement or temporomandibular joint signs or symptoms were detected.

■ *What are the causes of bilateral lingual crossbite?*

These are given in **Table 15.3**. In Simon's case, a combination of local and skeletal causes are implicated in the bilateral lingual crossbite.

Table 15.3 Causes of bilateral lingual crossbite

Local	Bilateral early loss of e̅'s may allow 5̅'s to be displaced completely lingually
Skeletal	Mismatch in relative width of arches or a Class II skeletal discrepancy
Combination of local and skeletal	
Rarer causes	Pierre Robin anomaly (mandibular retrognathia, cleft palate, glossoptosis)

■ *What treatment options are there for correction of bilateral lingual crossbite?*

It is important to ascertain the number of teeth affected and to check the inclination of the affected teeth. These will help to indicate the severity of any underlying skeletal component and whether reciprocal movement of the affected teeth with the opposing teeth only will suffice for correction. Management options are given in **Table 15.4**.

In view of the underlying Class II skeletal problem, Simon was treated first by growth modification with a Frankel II appliance followed by non-extraction upper and lower fixed appliance therapy (**Fig. 15.9**).

Key point

Correction of a bilateral lingual crossbite:
- Single tooth affected on each side: consider extraction of displaced teeth.
- Several teeth affected on each side: consider combination of buccal movement of affected lower teeth/palatal movement of affected upper teeth.

Table 15.4 Management options for bilateral lingual crossbite

Option	Possible indications
Extraction	Single tooth on either side affected and completely excluded lingually
Reciprocal movement of affected upper and lower teeth	Depends on inclination of teeth, number of teeth affected and presence/absence of underlying Class II skeletal discrepancy
	Fixed appliances required
Growth modification	An appliance that influences soft tissue force balance may be useful, e.g. Frankel II
Orthodontic camouflage	Extraction/non-extraction therapy depending on local/skeletal components
	An appliance that facilitates lower inter-premolar expansion may be helpful, e.g. Damon appliance
Midline distraction osteogenesis	Severe mandibular crowding with well-aligned upper arch, v-shaped mandible and narrow mandibular arch with bilateral scissors bite affecting several teeth
Orthognathic surgery	Adult skeletal Class II with mandibular deficiency

Fig. 15.9 (A) Case 3: Mid treatment with Frankel II.

Fig. 15.9 (B) Mid treatment with fixed appliances.

■ *Simon was treated with the fixed appliances shown in Figure 15.9*. **What type of appliance is this? What are its claimed advantages compared with conventional fixed appliance systems?**

This is a self-ligating fixed appliance (Damon). The archwire is not pressed firmly against the bracket base but is held in place by either a rigid (as with the Damon system) or spring clip (Speed) or retaining springs (Smart-Clip). These replace the stainless steel ligatures or elastomeric modules that are used (the latter mainly) to retain the archwire in the bracket slot with conventional non-self-ligating systems. Claimed advantages include faster ligation, lower friction, faster treatment, less pain and fewer appointments. Compared with conventional pre-adjusted edgewise brackets, current prospective evidence for self-ligating brackets indicates: no clinically significant difference in treatment duration between the two systems; similar effects on arch form for each system; modest time-saving for tying and untying self-ligating brackets but time saving varies with bracket design. More well-designed prospective clinical trials using identical wire sequences and mechanics are required to provide more robust data regarding self-ligating brackets.

■ How does distraction osteogenesis work and what are the complication risks of mandibular midline distraction?

Based on the manipulation of a healing bone, distraction osteogenesis stretches an osteotomized site before calcification has taken place to generate formation of additional bone and investing soft tissue. As there is insufficient soft tissue in the mandibular symphyseal area to cover a bone graft necessary for widening the mandibular symphysis by orthognathic surgery, distraction affords the opportunity for formation of new bone (osteogenesis) and soft tissue (histogenesis) to create new periosteum over the distracted area. Although in concept, mandibular midline distraction is basically the same as SARPE, in contrast to the maxilla no lateral surgical disjunction is performed as the mandible is not connected rigidly to the skull. Distraction of the mandible, therefore, will not be parallel but will always rotate around the condyles. Vertical cuts are made through the mandibular facial and lingual cortical plates, usually extending all the way through the symphysis. Following a 5–7-day latency period, distraction begins by turning the screw twice per day (0.5 mm) until the desired movement is achieved. The distractor may be tooth-borne or screwed to the bone; in the latter case, it is removed about 4 months post-operatively.

Complications of mandibular midline distraction arising within 2 weeks post-operatively, but are relatively rare and mainly of a mild or transient nature. Only 3% of patients experience more serious damage due to fractured incisor roots or gingival recession. Mandibular midline distraction, thus, appears a relatively safe method for expansion of the mandible.

Simon's final occlusion is shown in **Figure 15.10**. A well-interdigitating buccal occlusion will facilitate stability of bilateral lingual crossbite correction.

Fig. 15.10 (B) Case 3 post-treatment: Anterior occlusion.

Fig. 15.10 (C) Case 3 post-treatment: Left buccal occlusion.

Recommended reading

Fleming PS, Johal A 2010 Self-ligating brackets in orthodontics: A systematic review. Angle Orthod 80:575–584.

Freeman DC, McNamara JA Jr, Baccetti T et al 2009 Long-term treatment effects of the FR-2 appliance of Frankel. Am J Orthod Dentofacial Orthop 135:570.e1–e6.

von Bremen J, Schafer D, Kater W, Ruf S 2008 Complications of mandibular midline distraction. Angle Orthod 78:20–24.

For revision, see Mind Map 15, page 177.

Fig. 15.10 (A) Case 3 post-treatment: Right buccal occlusion.

16

Late lower incisor crowding

SUMMARY

Graham is almost 20 years old. He presents with crowding of his lower incisors (Fig. 16.1). What is the cause and how would you treat it?

History

Complaint

Graham is concerned about the crowding of his lower front teeth and wonders if it will get worse.

History of complaint

His lower front teeth were straight until 18 months ago when he noticed crowding developing. He now finds it more difficult to keep his lower front teeth clean. Calculus build-up also seems to occur more easily on the inside of the lower teeth, which he finds annoying. He is also aware of the two wisdom teeth erupting at the back of his lower jaw for the past 18 months. These do not cause him any problems but he wonders if they are making his lower front teeth crooked.

Fig. 16.1 Lower occlusal view at presentation.

Medical history

Graham is fit and well.

Dental history

Two years ago Graham had a course of fixed appliance therapy to close a large space between 1|1 followed by composite build-up of 2|2 .

Examination

Extraoral examination

Graham has a Class I skeletal pattern with average FMPA and no facial asymmetry. Lips are competent. There are no signs or symptoms associated with the temporomandibular joints.

Intraoral examination

The appearance of the teeth on presentation is shown in **Figures 16.1** and **16.2**.

■ *What do you notice?*

Soft tissues appear healthy with the possible exception of mild gingival erythema related to |34 associated with slight plaque deposits; otherwise oral hygiene appears good; slight gingival recession on |4 .

All lower permanent teeth present; 1|123456 visible in upper arch; (note |7 was erupted).

Lower labial segment crowding with 8|8 erupting; worst incisor contact point displacement was 2.5 mm.

Upper left quadrant appears aligned.

Class I incisor relationship, although it appears to be tending towards Class III.

Left buccal segment relationship Class III.

■ *Is development of lower incisor crowding common in the late teens?*

In modern populations, there is a strong tendency for crowding of the mandibular incisor teeth to develop in the late teens. This occurs even if the teeth were well aligned or spaced initially, leading usually to mild crowding, whereas initial mild crowding tends to become worse. Lower labial segment crowding also occurs in patients in whom extractions for relief of crowding and fixed appliance therapy have been undertaken (unless a bonded lingual retainer has been placed).

Fig. 16.2 Left buccal occlusion.

What are the possible causes of late lower incisor crowding?

The aetiology is multifactorial and the major theories proposed are as follows:

- *Late mandibular growth.* Forward mandibular growth, especially if a growth rotation is also present, and where maxillary growth has stopped, aided by lip pressure, tends to reposition the lower incisors lingually, reducing arch length and causing anterior crowding. Currently it is thought that as the lower incisors, and perhaps the whole lower dentition, move posteriorly relative to the mandibular body late in mandibular growth, lower incisor crowding almost always develops. The greater the magnitude of late mandibular growth when other growth has essentially stopped, the greater the likelihood of developing late lower incisor crowding. On average, in a male patient, as is the case here, mandibular growth is complete by 19 years but it may continue for longer.
- *Gingival and/or occlusal forces.* Pressure from the transseptal fibres and/or the anteriorly directed component of occlusal forces lead to mesial migration of the dentition.
- *Lack of approximal attrition in modern diet.* This was thought to explain absence of lower labial segment crowding in Australian aborigines but has not been borne out by research findings.
- *Reduction in intercanine width.* The mandibular intercanine width reduces gradually during the teenage years, and this decrease progresses at a reduced rate into adult life. The result is an increase in lower labial segment crowding, most marked during the late teens.
  The presence of third molars. Their role is controversial. Two theories abound:
  - They may exert mesial pressure on the lower dentition during eruption, tending to produce lower labial segment crowding.
  - They may prevent the lower teeth from moving distally in response to forces generated by mandibular growth or soft tissues.
- However, late lower incisor crowding develops even when third molars are absent so their presence is not the critical factor in the aetiology of the problem. The amount of late mandibular growth is paramount.

Key point

Possible factors in the aetiology of late lower incisor crowding include:

- Late mandibular growth.
- Gingival and/or occlusal forces.
- Reduction in intercanine width.
- Third molars?

Investigations

What investigations would you undertake? Explain why.

Radiographic

A dental panoramic tomogram would be useful to assess the position and inclination of the partially erupted lower

---

third molars. As a radiograph was taken prior to commencing orthodontic treatment, this should be consulted first and the need for a further radiograph should be assessed based on the clinical assessment and the radiographic findings.

Study models

Upper and lower impressions and a wax registration in centric occlusion should be taken for study models to record accurately the current malocclusion and to aid further treatment planning.

What do you notice on the dental panoramic tomogram taken pre-orthodontic treatment (*Fig. 16.3*)?

Normal alveolar bone height.
All teeth present and of good quality.
$\overline{8|}$ is slightly mesioangularly impacted.
$\overline{|8}$ is upright.
Bone overlies the distal half of the crown of both lower third molars.

Diagnosis

What is your diagnosis?

Class I malocclusion on a Class I skeletal base with average FMPA; lower incisor crowding; impacted third molars; left buccal segment relationship Class III.

What is the IOTN (DHC) grade (see p. 203)? Explain why.

3d – based on the 2.5 mm worst contact point displacement between the lower incisor teeth.

What are the management options for late lower incisor crowding?

Accept and monitor. As this is a normal maturational change in the lower arch, it would be sensible in a late teenager, and where the crowding is mild, to keep it under observation. Where more marked crowding is present, intervention may be considered.

Interproximal stripping. This is only acceptable in an adult with mild lower incisor crowding. By removing 0.25 mm at most from the mesial and distal aspects of each incisor, up to 2 mm of space can be obtained for relief of crowding. Incisor alignment may then be achieved with a sectional fixed appliance. A removable appliance, with an acrylated

Fig. 16.3 Dental panoramic tomogram.

labial bow or Invisalign® (a clear vacuum-formed thermoplastic aligner) made to fit a duplicate study model with the incisors aligned with their mesial and distal surfaces reduced, are alternative approaches. With Invisalign®, however, several appliances will be required to achieve incremental change (~0.25–0.3 mm per aligner worn for about 20 hours per day and changed about every 2 weeks) until the final alignment has been realized. A bonded retainer will be required to maintain the result long term.

Extraction of a lower incisor. Where the lower labial crowding is marked, removal of a lower incisor may be indicated to give sufficient space for alignment of the remaining units. It is advisable to carry out a diagnostic wax-up on a duplicate set of study models to ascertain what the final result is likely to be and to ensure the patient is happy with this before proceeding with the extraction. The patient should be warned of the possibility of the upper labial segment moving palatally, with resultant misalignment, in response to the lower labial segment being aligned slightly lingually. Unless the incisor to be extracted is completely excluded from the arch and the remaining incisors are well aligned, fixed appliance therapy is inevitably indicated to detail the position of the remaining labial segment teeth. Bonded lingual retention will then be required.

Extraction of lower premolars. Where the buccal segment occlusion is well interdigitated and crowding is confined to the lower labial segment, it is preferable to avoid lower mid-arch extractions because these will disrupt the buccal occlusion. Instead removal of a lower incisor will expedite lower labial segment alignment while preserving the integrity of the buccal segments.

■ *Would you advise removal of the lower third molars?*

Lower third molars should not be removed in an attempt to prevent further increase in lower labial segment crowding, as their relation to this aspect of malocclusion is unproven.

Current guidelines advise removal of lower third molars only if they are associated with recurrent episodes of pericoronitis or other pathology. In this case, as neither of these apply at present, the lower third molars should be retained and their position reviewed if symptoms develop.

Key point

Management options for late lower incisor crowding:
- Accept and monitor.
- Interproximal stripping with appliance therapy.
- Lower incisor extraction with appliance therapy.

■ *How would you manage the lower incisor crowding?*

As the lower labial segment crowding is mild, Graham should be advised to accept it for the present. It should be kept under review and if the crowding increases, consideration could be given to treatment.

The eruption of the lower third molars should be monitored.

Recommended reading

Dacre JT 1985 The long-term effects of one lower incisor extraction. Eur J Orthod 7:136–144.

Harradine NW, Pearson MH, Toth B 1998 The effect of extraction of third molars on late lower incisor crowding: a randomized controlled trial. Br J Orthod 25:117–122.

Little RM, Riedel RA, Artun J 1988 An evaluation of changes in mandibular anterior alignment from 10 to 20 years postretention. Am J Orthod Dentofacial Orthop 93:423–428.

NHS Centre for Reviews and Dissemination, York 1999 Prophylactic removal of impacted third molars: is it justified? Br J Orthod 26:149–151.

Richardson ME 2002 Late lower arch crowding: the aetiology reviewed. Dent Update 29:234–238.

For revision, see Mind Map 16, page 178.

Prominent chin and TMJDS

SUMMARY

Jocelyn, aged 23, is referred by her general dental practitioner because of her prominent chin (Fig. 17.1) and pain in her left temporomandibular joint (TMJ). What are the causes and how would you manage these problems?

History

Complaint

Jocelyn's main concern is that she does not like the prominent appearance of her chin and her upper teeth biting inside her lower teeth. She has pain in her left jaw joint and has some difficulty chewing. She is also aware that she has a lisp, which she dislikes.

History of complaint

Jocelyn has been more aware of her prominent chin and her bite since she was in her last year at school. After

Fig. 17.1 Profile at presentation.

consultation with an orthodontist at age 12, she had two upper teeth removed to provide space for the upper eye teeth (she had both lower first permanent molars extracted at age 8 because of decay.) She did not wear any braces on her teeth. She was advised to wait until she was in her late teens to have the bite of her front teeth reassessed. In the past 6 months she has become quite self-conscious about her facial appearance, although she feels that her chin does not appear to have become more prominent in the past 4 years.

■ *What questions would you ask about the temporomandibular joint pain?*

When and how the pain started.

Type and duration of pain.

Frequency.

Is it localized? Site of radiation.

Associated symptoms, e.g. muscle pain, click, jaw locking, trismus.

Aggravating factors, e.g. stress.

Any habits, e.g. nail-biting, bruxism, pen-chewing.

Relieving factors, e.g. heat, analgesics (type and amount).

The pain started suddenly when Jocelyn was preparing for examinations in her first year at university. She has had intermittent discomfort in her left jaw joint since then but it has been of a mild nature. The discomfort is an ache that is principally in the left jaw joint area but radiates to the jaw muscles on that side. It does not keep her awake at night but she feels it is worse in the morning. Typically it lasts for a few hours and then disappears. It tends to return when Jocelyn is stressed by work. She is aware of grinding her teeth when stressed. She does not engage in chewing pencils or pens or nail-biting. She feels that in the past year the pain has recurred more frequently and has become worse. Chewing hard food or opening her mouth too wide makes the pain worse; one or two paracetamol tablets usually relieves the ache. Jocelyn is also aware that she has a jaw click.

Medical history

Jocelyn is fit and well.

Dental history

Jocelyn is a regular attender at her general dental practitioner and brushes twice daily.

Family history

Jocelyn's sister also has a prominent chin, but not as marked as hers, and her sister's bite was corrected with fixed braces.

Examination

Extraoral examination

■ *What do you observe from Jocelyn's profile view (Fig. 17.1)?*

Class III skeletal pattern with average FMPA. Competent lips.

Fig. 17.2 (A) Right buccal occlusion.

Fig. 17.2 (C) Left buccal occlusion.

Fig. 17.2 (B) Anterior occlusion.

■ *Based on the history, what other aspects would you assess extraorally?*

Temporomandibular joints. Opening and lateral mandibular movements should be assessed by first observing the patient from in front and second by palpation of the condylar heads while listening for the presence of crepitus or a joint click. As symptoms are present, the masticatory muscles should also be palpated. A left TMJ click and left masseteric tenderness were detected.

Mandibular path of closure. The path of closure from rest position to maximum interdigitation should be assessed, noting any anterior or lateral mandibular displacement produced by a premature contact.

In this case, there is an anterior mandibular displacement on closure on contact of $\frac{7}{8|}$ (centric relation to occlusion shift of ~3 mm).

Intraoral examination

The intraoral views are shown in **Figure 17.2**.

■ *What do you see?*

Gingival tissues appear healthy; gingival recession related to $\frac{63 \mid 356}{7 \mid}$.

Oral hygiene appears overall good apart from slight plaque deposit on $|3$

$\frac{765321 \mid 12356}{8754321 \mid 123457}$ are visible.

No obvious caries.

Very mild lower incisor crowding with spacing between the $\overline{4}$'s and $\overline{5}$'s.

Very mild upper arch crowding with slight mesiolabial rotations of $2|2$.

Class III incisor relationship with reverse overjet (measured 4 mm clinically), reduced overbite and coincident dental centrelines.

Class I canine relationship bilaterally.

Buccal crossbite affecting $\frac{7}{8|}$.

■ *What is the most likely cause of the considerable spacing in the lower premolar areas with $\overline{5}$'s drifted into contact with $\overline{7}$'s ?*

Early removal of $\overline{6e|e6}$ in an uncrowded arch is the most likely explanation for the spacing. An uncrowded lower arch is common in Class III malocclusion.

■ *What occlusal features may predispose to temporomandibular joint dysfunction syndrome?*

Crossbites, Class III malocclusion and anterior open bite have been shown to have a significant association with temporomandibular joint dysfunction syndrome (TMJDS) in some studies while others have found no link between signs and symptoms of TMJDS and mandibular displacement. The aetiology of TMJDS is multifactorial with the implicated involvement of psychological, traumatic and occlusal elements. The most salient factor is probably stress, which may transmit its effect by a parafunctional habit, stemming perhaps from a displacing occlusal contact in susceptible individuals. In this case, a displacement exists on $\frac{7}{8|}$ on closure. There are also anterior and posterior crossbites present.

■ *Why was Jocelyn advised to wait until her late teens for reassessment?*

In a Class III malocclusion, the amount of reverse overjet tends to increase with forward mandibular growth during teenage years. Waiting until mandibular growth is essentially completed, which is generally about 17 years in girls and 19 years in boys, has three advantages. First, it allows treatment planning to be undertaken with reasonably stable facial and occlusal characteristics. Second, if treatment is undertaken, it safeguards against relapse due to further growth. Third, the magnitude of occlusal change due to mandibular growth influences whether treatment can be undertaken by orthodontic means alone or whether a combined surgical-orthodontic approach is necessary. Orthodontic treatment involves inducing dentoalveolar compensation for the underlying skeletal pattern, but if unsuccessful due to continued adverse mandibular growth the compensation would need to be undone as part of pre-surgical orthodontics. This may involve opening up lower premolar extraction spaces. Hence the decision to treat a Class III malocclusion in early teenage years by orthodontic camouflage that includes lower arch extractions must be made with great caution.

In this case the severity of the anteroposterior skeletal pattern, the likely pattern of mandibular growth, the amount of dentoalveolar compensation, the amount of overbite and the relative absence of crowding (following the removal of upper first premolars and lower first permanent molars) would all have been considerations in delaying any further orthodontic intervention. Whether the patient could achieve an edge-to-edge incisor relationship would also need to have been assessed.

Key point

Waiting until at least late teens before considering an orthodontic/orthognathic approach is desirable as:
- Facial and occlusal characteristics stabilize.
- It safeguards against relapse due to further growth.
- Camouflage or surgery is determined by the extent of mandibular growth.

Investigations

■ *What investigations are required and why?*

The patient's primary concern is about her facial appearance and she has a malocclusion which is likely to be untreatable by orthodontic means alone. A combined orthodontic-surgical approach is required. The investigations required, in such cases, together with reasons for their selection, are listed in **Table 17.1**. If possible, three-dimensional (3D) facial images, at rest and smiling, should also be recorded at this stage to act as a baseline from which to monitor robustly 3D facial changes produced by surgery and during subsequent follow-up. Similarly, if feasible, cone beam computed tomography (CBCT) may be undertaken.

- The TMJ assessment has already been undertaken for Jocelyn (p. 78).
- The dental panoramic tomogram showed no condylar pathology.

The cephalometric values are as follows:

SNA = 79°; SNB = 85°; ANB = −6°; $\underline{1}$ to maxillary plane = 113°; $\overline{1}$ to mandibular plane = 82°; interincisal angle = 139°; MMPA = 26.5°; SN to maxillary plane = 11°; facial % = 56%.

Table 17.1 Investigations required in combined surgical-orthodontic planning*

Investigation required	Reason
Thorough clinical assessment of facial form in full face and profile	To locate any cranial, maxillary, nasal, mandibular or chin deformities
	To assess the height and width proportions of the face, interalar distance, nasolabial angle, upper incisor exposure, relation of upper dental midline to other facial midlines, the form and tone of the soft tissues
Assessment of TMJ	To record signs and/or symptoms of TMJ dysfunction. Treat these conservatively if possible prior to treatment; if marked occlusal problems contributing to dysfunction, aim to correct these with treatment
Dental panoramic tomogram (DPT)	To assess the general dental status and prognosis of the dentition as well as the position of unerupted third molars (bitewing or periapical radiographs may be required depending on clinical and/or DPT findings)
Lateral cephalometric radiograph	To ascertain the aetiology of the malocclusion and to facilitate surgical planning
Facial and dental photographs	To record the facial and dental characteristics of the malocclusion
	To allow surgical planning by matching the digital profile facial image with the lateral cephalometric tracing
Study models and duplicates mounted on an articulator	To allow thorough orthodontic/occlusal assessment and model surgery

*Three-dimensional (3D) facial images, where possible, and when combined with cone beam computed tomography, allow 3D surgical planning, although further development is required to optimize this.

■ *What is your interpretation of these findings (see p. 204)?*

Moderately severe Class III skeletal pattern due to a combination of maxillary retrognathia and mandibular prognathism. As SNA is 2° less than the mean of 81°, application of the Eastman correction adds 1° to the ANB to give a revised ANB value of −5°.

Slightly proclined upper incisors (although inclination is within the normal range) and markedly retroclined lower incisors indicating dentoalveolar compensation for the Class III skeletal pattern. The lower incisor angulation must be considered with the MMPA – this has been explained on page 43.

Interincisal angle is increased but within the normal range for Caucasians.

MMPA, SN to maxillary plane and facial % are all slightly outwith the mean values but lie within the normal range for Caucasians.

Diagnosis

■ *What is your diagnosis?*

Class III malocclusion on a Class III skeletal base with average FMPA. TMJDS with left TMJ click. Gingival recession on $\underline{63|356}$ and $\overline{7}$. Previous loss of $\overline{6}$'s and $\underline{4}$'s. Very mild upper and lower labial segment crowding. All of the upper arch in crossbite with the exception of $\underline{65|56}$. Buccal crossbite on $\dfrac{7|}{8|}$ with associated mandibular displacement.

What is the IOTN DHC grade (see p. 203)? Explain why.

5m – due to reverse overjet greater than 3.5 mm with reported masticatory and speech difficulties.

Treatment

What are the aims of treatment?

- Relief of the TMJDS.
- Control of the gingival recession.
- Correction of the underlying skeletal Class III problem.
- To establish Class I incisor and molar relationships.
- To correct the buccal segment crossbites.
- To restore the lower buccal segment spaces.

What treatment is required? Explain why.

A combined orthodontic-surgical-restorative approach is needed due to:

The patient's concern relating to facial and dental appearance.

The severity of the underlying Class III skeletal pattern.

Despite the degree of dentoalveolar compensation, a reverse overjet of 4 mm exists.

An ANB angle of greater than −4° and lower incisor angulation to the mandibular plane of less than 83° have been found indicative of an orthodontic-surgical approach.

Pre-surgical lower arch decompensation (see below) will open up more space between the premolars and then require restorative management to optimize the final occlusion.

In addition, lower incisor decompensation may run the risk of creating gingival recession, particularly as Jocelyn already has several teeth affected by minor gingival recession. A specialist periodontal opinion should be sought before embarking on pre-surgical orthodontics.

It was decided that the spacing in the lower buccal segments would be managed by resin-retained bridgework following uprighting of the premolars. The periodontist advised Jocelyn to adjust her toothbrushing technique and she was given appropriate oral hygiene instruction aimed to prevent any deterioration in the areas affected by gingival recession. A pre-treatment gingival graft to the lower incisors was not deemed necessary; maintenance of good oral hygiene practices during orthodontic appliance therapy was emphasized. Periodontal review was arranged 6 months into orthodontic treatment.

How will this case be managed?

Short term

A hard full coverage upper acrylic splint should be made and Jocelyn should be instructed to wear this full-time until the TMJ symptoms subside. She should also be advised to take a soft diet and to avoid straining her jaw joints by, for example, yawning widely. Mild analgesics should also be taken as required.

Longer term

A combined orthodontic-surgical-restorative approach is required to correct the facial and occlusal problems. The

TMJDS symptoms may ease with orthodontic treatment. This is due to tooth movement rendering the teeth tender on biting, so parafunctional activity stops because tooth clenching/grinding does not produce the same subconscious pleasure as previously. The improvement in symptoms may be transient, even if displacing occlusal contacts (present here on $\frac{7}{8}$|) are eliminated.

The patient should be warned about the unpredictable impact of orthognathic surgery on TMJDS to avoid unreasonable expectations of treatment.

Key point

Orthodontic treatment and/or orthognathic surgery cannot be guaranteed to eliminate TMJDS.

Explain how you would proceed with surgical planning for this case.

1. A team approach is required involving the orthodontist and the oral and maxillofacial surgeon. The input of a restorative specialist is also required in relation to management of the lower premolar spacing. The involvement of a clinical psychologist with an interest in orthognathic surgical cases would also be helpful. Jocelyn must understand that to obtain the best facial and occlusal result possible, fixed appliance therapy is essential to the overall plan.

2. Surgical planning may be undertaken by various means. To provide information about the inter-relationships of the dentofacial complex components, namely the cranium and cranial base, nasomaxillary complex and maxillary dentition, mandible and related dentition, specialized cephalometric analyses exist. These allow comparison of individual cephalometric data with 'normal' data that should be matched for age, gender and racial background. Computer programs then allow surgical, skeletal and dental movements to be planned and displayed visually on screen before printing.

3. By linking the patient's digital profile image with the cephalometric tracing, specialized planning software can automatically morph the image in response to planned surgical and orthodontic movement undertaken virtually on the computer. The likelihood of different treatment options can thus be explored. In addition, the patient can view the final computerized prediction to appreciate more clearly the possible likely outcome in profile aesthetics although it should be understood that this is not guaranteed. Using reference lines to measure distances, planned surgical movements should then be transferred to a duplicate set of study models, mounted on a semi-adjustable articulator in this case as maxillary surgery is planned. The ability to plan orthognathic surgery in 3D (superimposing 3D facial images and CBCT scans) is being developed and offers exciting possibilities.

4. The final plan should be explained to Jocelyn, ensuring that she is aware that her profile will be worsened by pre-surgical orthodontics and that she realizes what her final facial appearance is likely to be. If she wishes, arrangements should be made for her to meet and discuss the process with another patient for whom a successful outcome was achieved.

Key point

Planning surgical-orthodontic treatment:
- Requires a team approach.
- May be assisted by: matching the digital facial profile image with the lateral cephalometric tracing and using computer prediction software.

■ Describe the phase of pre-surgical orthodontics.

This phase of fixed appliance treatment aims to allow the jaws to be moved to their desired location without interference from tooth positions. The upper and lower arches are aligned and coordinated as well as establishing the vertical and anteroposterior position of the incisors. This involves decompensating for any existing dentoalveolar compensation. For Jocelyn, this will involve primarily labial movement of the lower incisors, which will eliminate the mild crowding and slight uprighting of the upper incisors. The full extent of the skeletal discrepancy is thus revealed, maximizing the extent of possible surgical correction. Class II intermaxillary traction may be required to aid decompensation. No extractions are indicated in this case to achieve the desired tooth movements. The gingival status labial to the lower incisors should be monitored during decompensation to ensure that gingival recession does not ensue.

When the requisite tooth movements have been achieved, rigid rectangular stainless steel archwires should be used to passively stabilize tooth position. Final pre-surgical records – study models, photographs and a cephalometric film – will then be taken to assess the changes that have occurred and to decide if the original surgical plan will be followed or require some amendment. Hooks should be attached to the archwires just prior to surgery. These facilitate intermaxillary fixation and/or elastic traction post-operatively.

Key point

Pre-surgical orthodontics:
- May involve extractions.
- Usually involves decompensation for any dentoalveolar compensation.
- Aligns and coordinates arches or arch segments.
- Establishes the vertical and anteroposterior position of the incisors.
- Place rigid rectangular archwires with ball-hooks immediately pre-surgically.

■ What surgical procedures are likely to be required?

- Le Fort I advancement.
- Mandibular setback.

■ What form of splint and fixation is likely to be required?

An interocclusal acrylic wafer, fabricated to fit articulator mounted casts positioned to the desired occlusal result, is recommended routinely to ensure accuracy of the post-surgical result. Following Le Fort I advancement and mandibular setback osteotomies, mini-plates and lag screws are likely to be required respectively for fixation. Intermaxillary fixation may also be required. If not, and a jaw exercise programme is commenced immediately after surgery, mouth opening will be satisfactory 2–3 weeks later. This will allow the use of light elastic traction to guide jaw function while maintaining the acrylic splint in place to key the occlusion.

■ Describe the post-surgical orthodontic phase.

When a satisfactory range of mandibular movement and stability of the osteotomy sites have been achieved, the acrylic splint should be removed. Light round archwires should be placed immediately to allow occlusal settling, often aided by the use of posterior box elastics with an anterior force vector, which helps maintain the sagittal corrections. When good interdigitation has been achieved, elastic wear should be discontinued. Rarely will this phase of treatment take longer than 6 months to complete. A period of retention is then required, no different from that for other adults who have completed routine orthodontic treatment. Surgical follow-up should be for a minimum of 2 years.

■ What factors influence post-surgical stability?

Stability will be influenced by:
- Orthodontic and surgical plans being correct, realistic, well-integrated and undertaken competently.
- Modest surgical movement – no greater than 6 mm in any direction in the maxilla or 8 mm in the mandible. This does not place the soft tissues under tension, and the condyles are not distracted at surgery.
- Absence of tongue thrust, previous surgical scarring.
- Patient compliance with all aspects of treatment, particularly post-surgical wear of elastic traction. Adequate fixation.
- The post-surgical profile and occlusion are shown in **Figure 17.3**.

Key point

Stability is enhanced when surgical movement is modest and does not induce soft tissue tension.

Fig. 17.3 (A) Post-treatment. Profile.

Recommended reading

Hajeer MY, Millett DT, Ayoub AF, Siebert JP 2004 Applications of 3D imaging in orthodontics: Part II. J Orthod 31:154–162.

Hunt NP, Rudge SJ 1984 Facial profile and orthognathic surgery. Br J Orthod 11:126–136.

Fig. 17.3 (B) Post-treatment. Occlusion.

Luther F 2007 TMD and occlusion part I. Damned if we do? Occlusion: the interface of dentistry and orthodontics; TMD and occlusion part II. Damned if we don't? Functional occlusal problems: TMD epidemiology in a wider context. Br Dent J 202:E2, Br Dent J 202:E3.

Proffit WR, White R, Sarver D 2003 Contemporary treatment of dentofacial deformity. Mosby, St Louis.

For revision, see Mind Map 17, page 179.

18

Drifting incisors

SUMMARY

Iain, a 51-year-old man, presents with spacing and mobility of his upper incisors (Fig. 18.1). What is the cause and what can be done?

History

Complaint

Iain complains of the spacing of his upper front teeth and looseness of all his front teeth, particularly of 2⌋ and ⌊2. He is self-conscious of the spacing and is worried in case his front teeth fall out.

History of complaint

He has noticed increasing mobility of his upper front teeth over the past few months. The spacing between the teeth appeared at the same time and is becoming progressively worse. There is no pain associated with the mobility of the teeth but eating has become uncomfortable. He is also aware of mobility of his lower front teeth and of several upper and lower back teeth. Recently he has experienced an unpleasant taste in his mouth, which appears to originate from the upper front teeth.

Dental history

Iain has been a regular attender at another dental practice for many years, before moving to your area. He is highly motivated and does not wish any tooth to be lost. ⌊1 was traumatized in his early twenties and has become progressively darker but he is unconcerned by this.

Medical history

Iain has diabetes which is well controlled by insulin. He is otherwise fit and well.

Social history

Iain smokes 10 cigarettes a day and has done so for 30 years.

Examination

Extraoral

There are no palpable submandibular or cervical lymph nodes.

Intraoral

■ **What do you notice in** *Figures 18.1* **and** *18.2?*

Oral hygiene appears fair with generalized interproximal staining. Interdental gingivae related to the lower central and lateral incisors appears slightly oedematous.

Fig. 18.2 (A) Lower occlusal view.

Fig. 18.1 Occlusion at presentation.

Fig. 18.2 (B) Upper occlusal view.

Fig. 18.2 (C) Right buccal occlusion.

Fig. 18.2 (D) Left buccal occlusion.

Generalized gingival recession.

Heavily restored dentition with |1 discoloured.

7654321 present in all quadrants; 8 also in lower right quadrant.

Mild lower incisor crowding.

Uncrowded upper arch with incisor spacing.

Class III incisor relationship with minimal overbite and overjet except for 2|1; upper and lower centrelines are not coincident.

Class I molar relationship bilaterally.

■ *Based on what you know so far, what are the possible factors implicated in respect to mobility and drifting of 21|12 ?*

Chronic periodontal disease is a definite possibility when the overall periodontal condition is observed.

Periapical periodontitis is another possibility but this would also tend to lead to extrusion of these teeth, which is not markedly evident.

Root resorption. This would have to be extensive to produce such spacing and mobility.

Root fractures. This is not a possibility in view of the history.

Other pathology such as radicular cyst or bony lesions are rarer possibilities.

■ *What would you check for specifically in relation to the history?*

Degree of any tooth mobility.

Presence, extent and location of plaque and/or supragingival/subgingival calculus deposits.

Fig. 18.3 Full-mouth periapical radiographs.

Presence/site of bleeding on probing.

Presence/site of periodontal purulent exudate.

Presence/site of a sinus and/or associated exudate.

Presence/site of any deep carious lesion.

Occlusal factors that may contribute to tooth mobility, e.g. displacing occlusal contacts and/or a bruxing habit.

Other habits, e.g. pen-chewing, nail-biting.

Calculus is present subgingivally on all teeth with generalized 4–6 mm pocketing and delayed bleeding on probing. There is a purulent discharge from the periodontal pocket on the mesial aspect of 2| . No sinuses are present. There are no carious teeth.

Upper and lower molars, premolars and canines exhibit grade I mobility buccolingually but not vertically. Upper and lower incisors have grade I mobility buccolingually but *not* vertically except for |2 , which exhibits grade II mobility buccolingually and vertically.

Iain has right and left group function in lateral excursions. There are no occlusal interferences in protrusion.

Investigations

■ *What other investigations would you carry out? Why?*

Full-mouth periapical radiographs are required to assess accurately the periodontal status, particularly the alveolar bone height as well as the presence of any periapical pathology.

■ *Full-mouth periapical radiographs are shown in Figure 18.3. What do you see?*

Generalized horizontal bone loss of at least 50% with angular bone defects affecting $\frac{2 \mid 1}{63 \mid 26}$.

70–80% alveolar bone loss affecting the lower incisor teeth.

Heavily restored dentition but no caries visible.

Diagnosis

■ *What is your diagnosis?*

Chronic moderate periodontitis with localized areas of advanced disease. Class III malocclusion with mild lower incisor crowding and spacing/drifting of the upper incisors. Upper and lower centreline shifts. Buccal segment relationship Class I bilaterally.

■ *With loss of periodontal attachment, how may labial drifting of the incisors occur?*

Alveolar bone loss compromises the ability of the teeth to deal with soft tissue and occlusal forces, thereby leading to tooth movement.

A traumatic occlusion may result from extrusion as a consequence of periodontal inflammation. Drifting may occur where periodontal support is also reduced.

Labial shift of periodontally involved upper incisors may result also from a displacing occlusal contact on closure producing a forward mandibular slide.

Undue forces may be placed on the incisors, where posterior tooth support is lacking due to tooth loss, and these can lead to upper incisor proclination.

Key point

Migration of periodontally involved incisors may be exacerbated by:
- A forward mandibular displacement on closure.
- Deficient posterior occlusal support.

■ What is the significance of the medical history and social history to the diagnosis?

Diabetes affects the host response to periodontal pathogens by altering polymorph chemotaxis. Although the diabetes is well controlled in Iain's case, periodontal disease is chronic and generalized due to inadequate oral hygiene measures exacerbated by the host response.

Smoking contributes significantly to periodontal disease through a variety of means. Gingival blood flow is reduced; salivary flow is slowed also, leading to poorer removal of periodontopathic bacteria and encouraging calculus build-up.

Treatment

■ What treatment would you advise?

Cessation of smoking. The patient should be encouraged to stop smoking to prevent any further insult to his periodontal health imposed by this habit.

Referral for joint periodontal/orthodontic consultation. Iain's condition requires specialist care in view of the advanced nature of the periodontal disease.

■ What periodontal treatment do you envisage will be required?

Oral hygiene instruction, particularly in the use of interproximal cleaning aids.

Full-mouth scaling and root planing.

Reassessment.

Consider localized surgery to those areas where response to primary phase therapy is inadequate, i.e. bleeding/purulent exudate on probing persists.

■ How would you describe the prognosis of Iain's dentition?

Prognosis depends on the response to initial therapy and patient factors such as motivation towards maintenance of a very high standard of oral hygiene and cessation of the smoking habit.

Based on the amount of alveolar bone loss, the prognosis of the upper incisors is likely to be better than that of the lower incisors.

■ What are the treatment options for the upper labial segment spacing?

1. Orthodontic alignment of the upper labial segment teeth with space closure. Six months after completion of periodontal therapy, the periodontist should re-evaluate the periodontal status. Provided it has not deteriorated and Iain is not averse to the prospect of wearing an orthodontic appliance, orthodontic treatment could be considered.

2. Extraction of 2| or of 21|12 and replacement on a partial upper denture or adhesive bridgework. Extraction of 1̄|1̄2̄ may be required also with similar prosthetic replacement to the extracted upper units.

Iain opted for fixed appliance therapy to align the upper teeth (**Fig. 18.4**).

■ What options are there with regard to improving appliance aesthetics in an adult patient?

Options are: aesthetic brackets (polycarbonate or ceramic), clear aligner therapy (Invisalign®) and lingual orthodontics. Each, however, is not without its shortcomings (**Table 18.1**).

Table 18.1 Shortcomings of aesthetic orthodontic appliances

Treatment option	Shortcomings
Aesthetic brackets	
Polycarbonate brackets	Stain, deform, poor torque control (improved with metal insert)
Ceramic brackets	Cannot bond to composite unless use silane-coupling agent which increases bond strength and risk of enamel damage at debond (overcome by different base designs to allow mechanical bond)
	Enamel damage at debond (problem overcome with different base design but must follow manufacturer's instructions specific for different bracket designs)
	Bracket breakage
	Wear of opposing enamel
	Increased friction compared to metal (overcome by insertion of metal slot)
Clear aligner therapy	Control of root movement and possible intermaxillary correction limited unless add bonded attachments appropriately
	Extraction site space closure difficult
Lingual appliances	Tongue discomfort
	Speech adjustment
	Difficult to place (indirect bonding required) and adjust (operator/patient time and cost implications)

Fig. 18.4 Upper fixed appliance.

Fig. 18.5 Final occlusion (bonded palatal retainer in place).

■ *What special considerations are there with orthodontic treatment in a periodontally compromised dentition?*

Bands should be avoided due to the risk of further compromising periodontal support by placement of the band margin subgingivally, creating a nidus for plaque accumulation. Bonded attachments, therefore, should be placed on all teeth including molars. It is also preferable to use stainless steel ligatures rather than elastomeric modules to retain orthodontic archwires, as modules have higher levels of plaque micro-organisms.

If several posterior teeth have been lost, anchorage for the tooth movements required may not be sufficient and reinforcement with a bonded transpalatal arch or a temporary anchorage device may be necessary.

With reduced alveolar bone support, light forces should be applied to the teeth.

When gingival recession is evident pre-treatment, the patient should be warned as to the possibility of this being aggravated by orthodontic tooth movement.

Regular periodontal recall should be undertaken throughout orthodontic treatment.

Due to loss of periodontal attachment and alveolar bone, permanent bonded retention will be required.

The final occlusion is shown in **Figure 18.5**.

Key point

For orthodontic treatment in a periodontally involved dentition:

- Avoid bands.
- Use light forces.
- Ensure regular periodontal recall during treatment.
- Retain permanently.

Recommended reading

Gustke CJ 1999 Treatment of periodontitis in the diabetic patient. A critical review. J Clin Periodontol 26:133–137.

Joffe L 2003 Invisalign®: early experiences. J Orthod 30:348–352.

Johnson GK, Hill M 2004 Cigarette smoking and the periodontal patient. J Periodontol 75:196–209.

Nattrass C, Sandy JR 1995 Adult orthodontics – a review. Br J Orthod 22:331–337.

For revision, see Mind Map 18, page 180.

Appliance-related problems

Case 1

SUMMARY

Leanne, a 12-year-old girl, presents for a routine check of her upper retainer. You notice a reddened palate (Fig. 19.1A). What is your diagnosis and what management would you institute?

History

Complaint

Leanne's only complaint is that her upper retainer is loose. She is not aware of any problem with her palate.

History of complaint

Leanne has been wearing the upper removable retainer for the past 10 weeks. 5|5 were absent and she had e|e removed to provide space for relief of upper arch crowding. She was offered upper fixed appliance treatment to produce the best occlusal result but she was not keen for this. Instead, she opted for upper removable appliance therapy. She has worn one previous appliance. The current appliance has been getting progressively looser over the past month.

Medical history

Leanne is asthmatic and has used a salbutamol (Ventolin) inhaler for the past 4 years. Her asthma is well controlled.

Examination

Extraoral

Leanne has a Class I skeletal pattern with average FMPA and no facial asymmetry. Her lips are competent, with the lower lip just covering the incisal third of the upper anterior teeth. There are no temporomandibular joint signs or symptoms.

Intraoral

The soft tissues appear normal except for generalized mild marginal gingivitis and the palatal mucosa, which is shown in **Figure 19.1A**. Oral hygiene is fair.

■ *Describe the appearance of the palate.*

The lesion affecting the palate can be described as follows:
  Site – palatal mucosa and attached gingivae.
  Size – area affected relates to that covered by the baseplate of the upper removable retainer (**Fig. 19.1B**).
  Shape – the posterior limit of the lesion is semilunar and defined, as is the rest of the lesion, by the baseplate outline.
  Colour – uniformly reddened appearance of the palate and attached gingiva underlying the baseplate with some petechial areas along the right posterior palatal extension.
  Background – mucosa and gingivae not covered by the baseplate appear of normal colour.

■ *What are your observations regarding the retainer?*

  The appliance is a Hawley retainer with Adams clasps on 6|6 and a labial bow from 3| to |3.
  The baseplate is made of clear acrylic.
  Appliance hygiene does not appear optimal – food debris and plaque deposits are visible, through the baseplate, on the fitting surface of the appliance.

■ *What is the most likely diagnosis based on the information you have so far?*

Fig. 19.1 (A) Appearance of the palate at presentation.

Fig. 19.1 (B) Upper removable retainer.

Palatal (denture) stomatitis, as the patient is symptom-free.

■ *What other condition would produce a similar appearance?*

Acrylic allergy. This, however, is unlikely as a 'burning' sensation of the mucosa underlying the baseplate would have been reported early after insertion of the first upper removable appliance and there would be erythema of all of the soft tissues adjacent to the acrylic.

■ *What is the aetiology of 'denture' stomatitis?*

Candida is the principal cause. Although a normal oral commensal, proliferation of *Candida* is facilitated by local environmental or systemic factors, thereby allowing it to become pathogenic (**Table 19.1**).

Table 19.1 Causes of denture stomatitis

Factor	Aetiology	
Local	Infection with *Candida* (~90% due to *Candida albicans*)	
	Poor denture/appliance hygiene	
	Night-time wear of denture/appliance	
	Possible trauma	
	Poor salivary clearance of oral commensals	
	High sugar intake providing substrate for *Candida* proliferation	
Systemic	Iron and vitamin deficiencies	
	Steroids	
	Drugs that cause xerostomia	predispose to *Candida* infection
	Endocrine abnormalities, e.g. diabetes	
	Antibiotic therapy	

Key point

Candida is the principal cause of palatal stomatitis related to an upper removable appliance.

■ *What factors in this case may have predisposed to 'denture' stomatitis?*

The use of a steroid inhaler, poor appliance hygiene and full-time wear of the appliance are likely to be the main contributory factors. A direct relationship has been shown between the presence of an upper removable appliance, *Candida* and low salivary pH levels. In addition, upper removable appliance therapy has a positive, though transient, influence on the prevalence of *Candida* and density of oral candidal carriage, suggesting that the carrier state may be initiated by the appliance.

Investigations

■ *How would you confirm the diagnosis?*

The ideal investigation is a smear from the palatal mucosa underlying the baseplate for microbiological testing.

Saliva sampling for *Candida* counts.
Culturing for accurate identification and sensitivity testing may also be undertaken.

■ *What stains identify Candida?*

Gram stain: *Candida* is strongly Gram positive.
Periodic acid–Schiff (PAS): the magenta stain locates carbohydrate in fungal cell walls.

Treatment

■ *How would you treat this condition?*

Leanne should be advised to:

1. Leave the appliance out at night. Timing is fortuitous as she is in the retention phase of treatment, and in 2 weeks time she is due to progress to night-only wear of the retainer. Due to the infection, it would be wise to wear the appliance throughout the day but remove it at night until the palatal mucosa returns to health.
2. Improved appliance hygiene – brush the fitting surface and soak it in a 1% hypochlorite solution.
3. Improve oral hygiene – teeth, gingivae and palatal mucosa should be brushed thoroughly after every meal.
4. Reduce sugar intake – alter diet to low carbohydrate consumption.
5. Antifungal agents (nystatin or amphotericin suspension or miconazole oral gel) should be applied to the fitting surface of the appliance four times daily. A 0.2% chlorhexidine mouthwash may also be beneficial due to its antifungal effect.

As the asthma is well controlled, there is no need to refer Leanne to her general medical practitioner.

Key point

Management of palatal stomatitis:
- Leave appliance out at night.
- Improve appliance and oral hygiene.
- Reduce carbohydrate consumption.
- Antifungal agents.

■ *What is the prognosis for this condition?*

Provided all the above strategies are followed, the condition should resolve completely within a few weeks.

Recommended reading

Arendorf T, Addy M 1985 Candidal carriage and plaque distribution before, during and after removable orthodontic appliance therapy. J Clin Periodontol 12:360–368.

Wilson J 1998 The aetiology, diagnosis and management of denture stomatitis. Br Dent J 185:380–384.

Cases 2 and 3

SUMMARY

Two common fixed appliance problems are shown. What is the cause of each and what treatment would you provide?

■ ***What problem do you notice in*** *Figure 19.2A****?***

A bracket has become debonded from 5̅|.

■ ***Why has this occurred?***

Bond failure may occur for various reasons (**Table 19.2**).

Table 19.2 Causes of bracket bond failure

Factor	Aetiology
Operator	Insufficient etch time
	Poor etch pattern*
	Poor moisture control during bonding
	Non-adherence to manufacturer's instructions with the bonding adhesive chosen
	Movement of the bracket after initial placement, which interferes with bond formation within the adhesive
	Application of high force to the bracket to accomplish archwire engagement
Patient	Eating hard/sticky foods
	Possibly use of phenolic-containing mouthrinses that soften composite
	Occlusal trauma/bruxing habit
	Pen-chewing/nail-biting

*Etch pattern is poorer on premolars than on canine or incisor teeth. This contributes to the greater bond failure rate on premolars (note failure in Fig. 19.2A is on 5̅|).

Treatment

■ ***What treatment would you provide? Explain why.***

The patient should be advised first to contact their orthodontist for repair of the appliance (**Fig. 19.2B, C**).

Fig. 19.2 (A) Lower occlusal view.

If this is not possible and the loose bracket is at risk of being swallowed or inhaled, it should be removed. In this case, however, this risk is less likely as the bracket remains attached to a ligature wire and elastometric module.

Should the loose bracket be a source of discomfort to the patient, as a general dental practitioner, you could remove the loose bracket and the loose ligature. The patient should be appointed with their orthodontist at the earliest opportunity.

■ ***What problem do you notice in*** *Figure 19.3A****?***

Fig. 19.2 (B) Following removal of ligature wire and 5̅| bracket.

Fig. 19.2 (C) Following replacement of ligature wire and rebonding of a 5̅| bracket.

Fig. 19.3 (A) Upper occlusal view.

The cheek mucosa is ulcerated due to trauma from the over-extended round archwire.

■ *How has this problem arisen?*

The amount of projection of the archwire beyond the molar band may have been overlooked at the time of archwire placement, or the archwire may have moved to its current position following insertion, as the teeth aligned, or due to loss/bond failure of another appliance component.

■ *How would you manage this problem?*

As a general dental practitioner, you should, first, advise the patient to contact their orthodontist to deal with this problem. If this is not possible then you should provide emergency care.

■ *As a general dental practitioner, what emergency care would you provide?*

The distal end of the archwire should be cut flush with the terminal aspect of the molar tube or the archwire end turned underneath the molar tube or angled inward away from the cheek. As a round nickel titanium wire is in place, with the terminal end heat-treated (note blackened appearance), this is easily cut to the desired length or positioned to avoid cheek trauma (**Fig. 19.3B**).

The patient should be advised to maintain a high standard of oral hygiene and to rinse with lukewarm salty water after meals until the ulceration heals. Provision of a supply of soft wax to apply over the molar tube and the adjusted wire end may also be helpful in the intervening period. The patient should also schedule an appointment in the near future with their orthodontist.

Fig. 19.3 (B) Following shortening and adjustment of upper archwire.

Key point

Emergency treatment for:

- Loose bracket: remove if risk of ingestion/inhalation.
- Overextended archwire: cut wire and/or turn wire end inward away from the cheek.

Recommended reading

Hobson RS, Rugg-Gunn AJ, Booth TA 2002 Acid-etch patterns on the buccal surface of human permanent teeth. Arch Oral Biol 47:407–412.

Mandall NA, Millett DT, Mattick CR et al 2002 Orthodontic adhesives: a systematic review. J Orthod 29:205–210.

For revision, see Mind Map 19, page 181.

Tooth movement and related problems

Case 1

SUMMARY

Darren, a 13-year-old boy, has been undergoing upper removable appliance therapy for 6 months to retract and align 3|, following extraction of 4|. Tooth movement has been very slow with no movement recorded at the last two visits.

■ *What are the possible reasons for a slow rate of tooth movement?*

These can be divided broadly into patient, appliance and operator factors.

Patient factors

The patient is not complying with appliance wear as instructed.

Incorrect positioning of the spring on appliance insertion or distortion of the spring.

Contact of the tooth with the buccal cortical plate or with a retained root part of 4|.

The occlusion with the opposing arch may prevent tooth movement.

Appliance factors

Acrylic and/or wire may be interfering with tooth movement.

Operator factors

Design flaws, underactivation, overactivation or activation of the spring such that 3| is directly buccally into contact with the cortical plate rather than through the cancellous corridor of bone.

■ *What force range is optimal for retraction of 3| by tipping movement?*

The optimal force range is 30–50 g or 0.3–0.5 N.

■ *What cellular response is there following activation of the spring to retract 3| by tipping movement?*

The consequence of the spring activation is the setting up of pressure and tension zones within the periodontal ligament. Half of the periodontal ligament is stressed with maximum pressure created at the alveolar crest in the direction of movement and at the diagonally opposite apical area (**Fig. 20.1**).

> ### Key point
> Tipping movement, typically, requires forces of 30–50 g or 0.3–0.5 N.

Pressure zones

The cellular response depends on whether a light or heavy force is applied. With a light sustained force, tooth movement occurs within a few seconds as periodontal ligament fluid is squeezed out and the vascular supply is compressed, setting off a complex biochemical response. Within 2 days, osteoclast invasion occurs and frontal resorption follows.

When a heavy sustained force is applied, the periodontal ligament is compressed to such a degree that the blood supply is cut off completely, producing an area of sterile necrosis (hyalinization). Small areas of hyalinization are inevitable even with light forces, but the area of hyalinization is extended with forces of greater magnitude. Osteoclast differentiation is impossible within the necrotic periodontal ligament space, but after several days osteoclasts appear adjacent to and within the adjacent cancellous spaces. From there they invade the bone adjacent to the hyalinized area and tooth movement eventually occurs by undermining resorption.

Tension zones

Following initial application of a light force, the blood vessels vasodilate and the periodontal ligament fibres are stretched, while fibroblast and preosteoblast proliferation

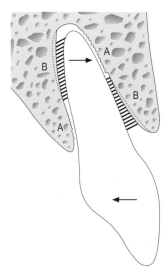

Fig. 20.1 Diagram illustrating zones of pressure (A) and tension (B) in the periodontal ligament induced by a tipping force.

occurs. The stretched fibres become embedded in osteoid, which later mineralizes. The normal periodontal ligament width is eventually regained by simultaneous collagen fibre remodelling.

With heavy forces, rupture of blood vessels and severing of the periodontal ligament fibres are likely but both are restored with the remodelling processes.

Key point

Application of a sustained force to a tooth creates areas of pressure and tension within the periodontal ligament, which ultimately lead to bone resorption and deposition, respectively.

■ *What is the mechanism for tooth movement?*

Although the histological response to an applied orthodontic force has been investigated extensively, the mechanism by which a mechanical stimulus is transferred to a cellular response is complex and is at present unresolved. It is likely that vascular changes in the periodontal ligament in areas of pressure and tension, electrical signals in response to alveolar bone flexing following force application, as well as prostaglandins and cytokine release interact in the process.

■ *How would you manage the problem in this case?*

Management is specific to each cause. The action taken may be one or more of the following:

    The need for full-time wear of the appliance must be emphasized to the patient/parent. They must be made aware that treatment will be ceased unless full cooperation is forthcoming.

    Show the patient how to insert the appliance with the spring positioned correctly and explain the action of the spring. Ensure that the appliance is not being removed by the spring. Check the activation of the spring and adjust it appropriately.

    Remove any acrylic or wire obstruction to tooth movement. This may involve remaking the appliance to an improved design.

    Add to a flat anterior biteplane or buccal capping to disengage the occlusion, if this is hampering tooth movement.

    Ask the patient and check their case records regarding any noted problem with the extraction of 4|. If indicated, take a periapical radiograph of 4| extraction site to check for a retained root fragment. If this is detected, seek an oral surgical opinion regarding its removal or whether it could be left in situ and its position monitored radiographically.

    Check 3| is not ankylosed. This is unlikely in this case as some movement of 3| has occurred since 4| was extracted.

    Darren admitted to intermittent wear of the appliance and, in particular, to leaving it out at meals. He was advised accordingly.

Key point

Full-time wear of an upper removable appliance is required for an optimal rate of tooth movement.

Fig. 20.2 Periapical radiograph.

■ *What do you notice on the periapical radiograph of another case (Fig. 20.2)?*

There is a small retained apical root fragment of 4|.

■ *What treatment would you advise?*

Complete retraction of 3| is unlikely due to the presence of this root fragment. However, its removal would require a surgical procedure, which would take away a considerable amount of alveolar bone and may damage the roots of the adjacent teeth. The root fragment may resorb in time and become confluent with the alveolar bone.

In view of the surgical risks, it would be wise to leave the root fragment in situ, monitor its status radiographically and accept the limitation this poses to complete retraction and alignment of 3|. The patient should be advised accordingly.

Recommended reading

Henneman S, Von den Hoff JW, Maltha JC 2008. Mechanobiology of tooth movement. Eur J Orthod 30:299–306.

Ren Y, Maltha JC, Kuijpers-Jagtman AM 2003 Optimum force magnitude for orthodontic tooth movement: a systematic literature review. Angle Orthod 73:86–92.

Roberts-Harry D, Sandy J 2004 Orthodontics. Part II: orthodontic tooth movement. Br Dent J 196:391–394.

Case 2

SUMMARY

Alan is reviewed 3 months after completion of a 2-year course of upper and lower fixed appliance therapy. He is wearing upper and lower removable retainers full-time. On removal of the retainers, you detect grade 2 mobility of the upper incisors and grade 1 mobility of all other teeth anterior to and including the first permanent molars in both arches. His oral hygiene is good and there is no bleeding on probing. You order a dental panoramic tomogram.

■ *Why is the radiograph ordered?*

It will allow a general screen of alveolar bone height and root length of all teeth.

■ *What do you notice on the film (Fig. 20.3A)?*

Generalized apical blunting (root resorption) of all teeth, anterior to and including the first permanent molars with

Fig. 20.3 (A) Dental panoramic tomogram.

Fig. 20.3 (B) Periapical radiographs of upper incisors taken 6 months into treatment. Note no apical root resorption apparent on |12 but slight apical resorption of 21| roots.

the possible exception of the second premolars. The upper incisors appear to have the most root resorption.

■ *Which teeth experience most orthodontically-induced root resorption?*

The upper incisors, followed by the lower incisors and first permanent molars, have consistently more root resorption than other teeth irrespective of suggested genetic or treatment-related risk factors.

■ *What risk factors have been suggested in relation to orthodontically-induced root resorption?*

Suggested patient-related risk factors include patient age and sex, root shape, history of previous trauma, teeth with short roots and previous root resorption, cortical bone proximity to the root, genetic factors and systemic factors.

Suggested treatment-related risk factors include length of treatment, force magnitude and method of application, direction of movement, appliance type, treatment mechanics and extent of apical movement.

■ *What does current evidence suggest with regard to orthodontically-induced root resorption?*

A recent systematic review identified that previous trauma and unusual tooth morphology are unlikely causes. An increased incidence and severity occurs with comprehensive orthodontic treatment with total root resorption reduced by a 2–3 month pause in treatment. Bracket prescription, self-ligation and archwire sequence do not affect it. Heavy forces produce most root resorption and evidence supports the use of light forces, especially for incisor intrusion.

Alan sustained coronal fractures to 1|1, involving enamel and dentine, 3 months before starting orthodontic treatment.

■ *Could root resorption have been prevented?*

Root resorption is regarded as an unavoidable sequela of orthodontic tooth movement. Although, on average 1 mm of root length will typically be lost over a 24-month course of orthodontic treatment, wide individual variation exists. Determining risk factors to identify those susceptible to orthodontically-induced root resorption and the means by which its severity and prevalence may be reduced, requires further well-designed clinical research studies.

During treatment excessive force application should be avoided. Where early root resorption is detected on progress radiographs, taken 6 to 12 months into treatment (**Fig. 20.3B**), further root resorption may be reduced by a 2–3 month pause (with a passive archwire). Where severe root resorption is detected (>4 mm or one third of the original root length), the treatment goals should be reconsidered with the patient and other options explored.

■ *What must the orthodontist ensure before treatment commences?*

The risk of apical root resorption as a consequence of orthodontic treatment must be explained to the patient/parents and discussed with them. In addition, an informed consent form signed by patient/parents and the orthodontist must describe, in particular, the risk of apical root resorption. Treatment should not be offered unless the anticipated benefits far outweigh the risk of minor apical resorption seen in most patients.

Appropriate radiographs should be available and the need for progress radiographs, as required, should be explained.

Key point

Root resorption;
- Increases in incidence and severity with comprehensive orthodontic treatment.
- Is promoted by the use of heavy forces.

Key point

- Root resorption is a common consequence of orthodontic treatment.
- Explain the risk to the patient before treatment starts and obtain consent.
- Monitor radiographically as required.

Fig. 20.3 (C) Periapical radiographs indicating marked root resorption of 21|12.

Fig. 20.4 Right buccal occlusion.

■ *What would you do in this case?*

Ask the patient if he is aware of marked mobility of any teeth and/or any other symptoms.

Clinically, the mobility of all teeth should be recorded. Alan was aware of upper incisor mobility.

Enquire about bruxism or other habits, such as nail-biting. None were reported.

Sensibility testing of the incisors and canines should be undertaken. All teeth were responsive to sensibility testing and no marked differences in recordings were detected between each tooth and its opposite number in each arch.

■ *What treatment would you provide?*

Alan should continue with full-time wear of his retainers for another 3 months and then proceed to night-only wear for at least a further 6 months.

Periapical radiographs should be taken of the upper incisors as these exhibit grade 2 mobility (**Fig. 20.3C**). Follow-up radiographic examinations and sensibility tests are recommended at 6 months to ascertain if the apical root resorption is progressive. This, however, should be unlikely as 'active' orthodontic treatment has been concluded. In the long term (10–25 years) after orthodontic treatment, teeth with root length of ≥10 mm and a healthy periodontium have been shown to remain stable.

Recommended reading

Brezniak N, Wasserstein A 2002 Orthodontically induced inflammatory root resorption. Part I. The basic science aspects. Angle Orthod 72:175–179.

Brezniak N, Wasserstein A 2002 Orthodontically induced inflammatory root resorption. Part II. The clinical aspects. Angle Orthod 72:180–184.

Hartsfield JK Jr, Everett ET, Al-Qawasmi RA 2004 Genetic factors in external apical root resorption and orthodontic treatment. Crit Rev Oral Biol Med 15:115–122.

Jonsson A, Malmgren O, Levander E 2007 Long-term follow-up of tooth mobility in maxillary incisors with orthodontically induced apical root resorption. Eur J Orthod 29:482–487.

Weltman B, Vig KWL, Fields HW et al. 2010 Root resorption associated with orthodontic tooth movement: A systematic review. Am J Orthod Dentofacial Orthop 137:462–476.

Case 3

SUMMARY

Lisa, an 18-year-old girl, had previous extraction of four first premolars and fixed appliance therapy to successfully correct her Class II division 1 malocclusion.

■ *What do you notice in* Figure 20.4*?*

Soft tissues appear healthy; slight decalcification on buccal aspect of 6| and 6|

Lower arch aligned (note lingual retainer to 5|5 bands in place).

Space in 4| area.

Increased overjet.

Molar relationship about quarter-unit Class II.

■ *What does this indicate?*

There has been relapse in the position of Lisa's teeth following treatment.

■ *Why has this occurred?*

The following factors are likely to destabilize the final orthodontic result.

Forces from the supporting tissues

Reorganization of principal periodontal ligament fibres and supporting alveolar bone occurs within 4–6 months after cessation of active tooth movement. At least 7–8 months, however, is required for the supracrestal fibres to reorganize because of the slow turnover of the free gingival fibres. Rotational correction and space closure are, therefore, liable to relapse.

Forces from the orofacial soft tissues

Following appliance therapy, the teeth should be in a position of soft tissue balance. The original mandibular arch form should remain unchanged as marked alteration in the inclination of the lower incisors will promote relapse. Limited proclination of the lower labial segment may be stable, however, in Class II Division 2 malocclusion, if the lower incisors were retroclined by a thumb-sucking habit or by a lower lip trap.

If a thumb- or digit-sucking habit is not ceased before treatment commences, its persistence will promote overjet relapse.

One-third to half of the labial surface of the upper incisors should be covered by the lower lip to give the best chance of stable overjet correction. Where the lips are grossly incompetent post-treatment, the upper incisor position will be inherently unstable and the mechanism by which an anterior oral seal is achieved will aggravate this further.

Occlusal factors

A poor buccal segment interdigitation with displacing occlusal contacts and an unfavourable interincisal angulation will encourage instability.

Post-treatment facial growth

Facial growth continues into adult life and, although of lesser magnitude than that observed during childhood, it varies among individuals. On average, females tend to demonstrate a backward mandibular rotation and this will not aid overjet stability. Late facial growth also impacts on the development of late lower incisor crowding.

Retention regimen

Firm rules do not exist for retention following active tooth movement but rather the retention regimen should be decided individually for each case. A case-specific duration of retention is unknown at present. It is common practice, however, following fixed appliance therapy, to retain with removable retainers for a minimum of 3–6 months full-time followed by 6 months of night-only wear. However, it is acknowledged that the only means of guaranteeing that tooth position is maintained unchanged long-term following completion of fixed appliance therapy is to advise long-term retention. Instead of a removable retainer, a bonded lingual retainer may be fitted to the lower incisors and canines; increasingly this is left in place permanently to prevent the development of late lower incisor crowding.

An inappropriate design of retainer, retention regimen and/or inadequate compliance by the patient will facilitate relapse.

Key point

Relapse may be due to:
- Forces from:
  - Supporting tissues.
  - Orofacial soft tissues.
  - Occlusion.
  - Facial growth.
- Inappropriate retainer design or retention regime, and/or patient compliance.

■ *What management options are there for this problem?*

The following options exist:

1. Accept and monitor. Study models should record the current tooth position and occlusion, to allow comparison with the pre- and post-treatment study casts, and to act as a baseline from which to assess future occlusal change. If there is further relapse, then consider options 2 or 3 below.

2. Re-treatment. Full case assessment is required with appropriate radiographs and study models. Further space, possibly by upper arch extractions, and fixed appliance therapy may be required for comprehensive recorrection of the malocclusion. Prolonged retention will be required thereafter.

3. A compromise plan would be to use an upper fixed appliance to retract the upper labial segment into the space that has opened in the first premolar extraction sites, accepting a slightly increased overjet. Then, prolonged retention would be required to maintain the result.

As Lisa is now a university student, she was not keen for further fixed appliance therapy and opted to accept and monitor the position of her teeth.

Recommended reading

Littlewood SJ, Millett DT, Doubleday B et al 2006 Orthodontic retention: a systematic review. J Orthod 33:205–212.

Melrose C, Millett DT 1998 Toward a perspective on orthodontic retention? Am J Orthod Dentofacial Orthop 113:507–514.

For revision, see Mind Map 20, page 182.

Cleft lip and palate

SUMMARY

Karen, a 9-year-old girl, is unhappy about the appearance of her teeth (Fig. 21.1). What is the cause and how will it be treated?

History

Complaint

Karen does not like the crookedness and spacing of her upper front teeth. Her mother is aware that the bite of Karen's side teeth is not correct also and feels that she moves her jaw to the side when she closes her teeth together.

History of complaint

Karen's baby front teeth were also crooked and spaced. Her mother has noticed the problem with her bite for several months.

Medical history

Karen was born with a cleft lip and palate, which has been repaired.

Family history

There is no family history of cleft lip and palate.

Fig. 21.1 Anterior occlusion at presentation.

■ *What is the prevalence of cleft lip and palate?*

It affects about 1 in 750 live births among Caucasians but the prevalence varies between racial groups as well as geographically, and is increasing. Cleft lip only is found in about 9% of all clefts whereas cleft of the lip and alveolus comprises about 3% of all clefts. Complete unilateral cleft lip and palate is the most common type of cleft and represents 50% of all clefts.

■ *Is there a sex and side variation for cleft lip and palate?*

Females are affected less frequently than males and the right side is involved less commonly than the left.

■ *How does this malformation occur?*

Failure of fusion of the median and lateral nasal processes and the maxillary process at about 4–6 weeks of intrauterine life leads to a cleft of the primary palate (the upper lip and the alveolus in the anterior region as far posteriorly as the incisive foramen). Cleft of the secondary palate (hard palate from incisive foramen back and soft palate) is due to failure of the palatal shelves to elevate and fuse at about 8 weeks.

Genetic and environmental factors, e.g. steroid therapy, folic acid deficiency or anticonvulsant drugs, interact in the aetiology.

Key point

Cleft lip and palate:

- Prevalence 1 in 750 live Caucasian births.
- Aetiology due to genetic and environmental factors.

Karen has been attending a cleft clinic at the regional dental teaching hospital since birth.

■ *Why is this? What treatment will have been provided to date and what role have you to play as her general dental practitioner?*

Due to the multidisciplinary care required, treatment is facilitated for the patient and family by coordinating management in a specialized centre by a team comprising an orthodontist, speech therapist, health visitor and clinical psychologist as well as plastic, ENT and maxillofacial surgeons.

Treatment until now is likely to have been as follows.

Neonatal period to 18 months

Parental counselling by a member of the Cleft Lip and Palate Association and /or clinical psychologist as well as reassurance of the future treatment by an orthodontist and member of the surgical team.

Advice and support to the parents by a specialized health visitor, particularly in relation to feeding. In this case, feeding problems are likely to have been modest as the cleft only involves the primary palate.

Planning of lip repair: this usually occurs at 3 months. In this case, closure of the alveolar defect may be undertaken at the same time. Where a palatal cleft exists, on average, this is repaired at around 9 months.

Primary dentition

First formal speech and hearing assessment at around 18 months and then speech therapy as required.

Regular speech and hearing assessments should be undertaken; consider closure of any palatal fistulae to assist speech development. Consider pharyngoplasty to reduce velopharyngeal incompetence at 4–5 years, thereby attempting to improve any nasal intonation to speech.

Consider lip revision at 4–5 years only if clearly indicated.

As a general dental practitioner your role is to:

Liaise with the cleft palate team.

Provide dietary advice and oral hygiene instruction to the parents, at regular intervals, from eruption of the primary incisors.

Consider the use of fluoride tablets if the level of fluoride in the local domestic water supply is below 1 ppm.

Attend to any dental treatment required.

Your particular aim in dental care is to promote and maintain excellent dental health for Karen, thereby avoiding the need for restorative treatment or enforced loss of primary teeth through dental caries.

Key point

Management of cleft lip and palate requires a team approach.

■ **What skeletal/dental/occlusal problems are commonly found with cleft lip and palate?**

Skeletally, there is a tendency for the maxilla and mandible to be retrognathic, the upper facial height to be reduced and the lower facial height to be increased. A Class III skeletal pattern is common.

On the cleft side, 2 is either absent, of abnormal size and/or shape, hypoplastic or as two conical teeth on either side of the cleft.

A supernumerary or supplemental tooth may exist on either side of the cleft.

1 is often rotated and tilted toward the cleft and may be hypoplastic.

Eruption is delayed.

Tooth size elsewhere in the mouth is small.

Class III incisor relationship is common with crossbite of one or both buccal segments and a lateral open bite on the cleft side.

Key point

Incisor and buccal segment crossbites are common in repaired cleft lip and palate.

Examination

Extraoral

■ **What do you notice from** Figure 21.2?

Karen has a Class I skeletal pattern with average FMPA and no obvious facial asymmetry. The lips are competent with a scar on the right side of the upper lip.

Fig. 21.2 (A) Profile.

Fig. 21.2 (B) Full face.

No clicks, locks or crepitus of the temporomandibular joints were detected.

■ **How is lip closure achieved?**

A Millard repair with or without its modifications is the most popular, aiming, after dissection, to place the lip muscles and alar base in their correct anatomical location. Whether subperiosteal or supraperiosteal dissection and skin-lengthening cuts are used to obtain tissue movement, remains controversial. The extent of alar cartilage dissection or the use of a vomer flap also remains unresolved.

Intraoral

■ **The appearance of the teeth is shown in** Figures 21.1 **and** 21.3. **What are your observations?**

Oral hygiene is fair. Plaque deposits are visible on several teeth. There is marginal gingival erythema related to most teeth.

$\frac{\text{edcb1} \mid \text{12cde}}{\text{6edc21} \mid \text{12cde6}}$ visible (6|6 were erupted but not shown)

e| restored; possible caries in e|de; 1| slightly hypoplastic.

Fig. 21.3 (A) Lower occlusal view.

Fig. 21.3 (B) Right buccal occlusion.

Fig. 21.3 (C) Left buccal occlusion.

Mild lower labial segment crowding.

Spaced upper labial segment with 1| distolabially rotated.

The cleft repair involves the right upper lip and alveolus – a bony depression is evident in the 2| area.

Class III incisor relationship with average overbite; b| in crossbite; lower centreline shift to the right.

Right molar relationship half-unit Class II with buccal segment crossbite involving cde|; (6| was also involved but not shown); left molar relationship Class I.

■ *In view of the unilateral crossbite of the right buccal segment, what should you check for? How would you do this?*

It would be important to check if there is a mandibular displacement on the path of closure associated with the crossbite. As Karen's mother has already noticed a shift of the lower jaw on closure, a displacement is likely. To detect this, Karen should be instructed to maintain the tip of her

Fig. 21.4 (A) Dental panoramic tomogram.

Fig. 21.4 (B) Upper anterior occlusal radiograph.

tongue in contact with the back of her palate as she closes her teeth together. Careful observation should be made of first tooth contact on the path of closure and the extent and direction of any mandibular displacement into maximum intercuspation should be recorded.

There is a mandibular displacement to the right on closure resulting from premature contact of $\frac{c|}{c|}$.

Investigations

■ *What investigations are required? Explain why.*

A dental panoramic tomogram should be taken to account for the presence and position of any unerupted teeth and to ascertain whether there are any permanent teeth absent.

An upper anterior occlusal radiograph is required to determine the extent of the alveolar cleft and the position of the permanent maxillary canine on the cleft side.

■ *Karen's dental panoramic tomogram and upper anterior occlusal radiograph are shown in* Figure 21.4. *What do you notice?*

The dental panoramic tomogram shows:

· Normal alveolar bone height except for the alveolar cleft in the 2| area, which extends to involve 3|.

· All permanent teeth are present except for 2| and third molars, ed|de are slightly infraoccluded.

· 1| is hypoplastic; e|e appear to have secondary caries underneath the restorations with possible furcation radiolucencies.

· There is carious involvement of d|d distally.

• The upper anterior occlusal radiograph confirms the extent of the alveolar cleft, and when assessed in combination with the dental panoramic tomogram, it shows 3| to be lying in the line of the arch.

Diagnosis

■ What is your diagnosis?

Repaired right unilateral cleft lip and alveolus.

Class III malocclusion on a Class I skeletal base with average FMPA.

Mandibular displacement to the right on closure on $\frac{c}{c}$.

Generalized mild marginal gingivitis.

Caries ed|de.

Mild lower labial segment crowding.

Spaced upper labial segment with 1| distolabially rotated; absent 2|.

Lower centreline to the right.

Right molar relationship half-unit Class II with buccal crossbite of the right buccal segments; left molar relationship Class I.

■ What is the IOTN DHC grade (see p. 203)? Explain why.

5p – due to cleft lip and palate.

Treatment

■ What are the aims of treatment at this stage?

Caries control.

Elimination of the mandibular displacement with correction of the right buccal segment crossbite.

Elimination of the alveolar cleft defect.

■ What would you do at this stage?

Reinforce oral hygiene practice in preparation for forthcoming orthodontic treatment.

Restore the lower primary molars.

Fissure seal the first permanent molars.

Liaise with the orthodontist on the cleft team regarding the planned orthodontic treatment.

■ What form do you envisage the orthodontic treatment to take?

Upper arch expansion, by a quadhelix appliance, to correct the right buccal segment crossbite is likely to be undertaken prior to alveolar bone grafting.

■ When is secondary alveolar bone grafting usually undertaken and what advantages does it confer?

Optimally, it is usually undertaken at around 9–10 years. It provides bone through which 3 can erupt, restores arch integrity, improves alar base support, aids closure of an oronasal fistula and allows orthodontic space closure.

■ The occlusion prior to bone grafting is shown in Figure 21.5. What may you consider at this stage?

Due to the advanced state of root resorption of c| (see also Figure 21.4) it would be useful to remove this at least 3 weeks before grafting to allow time for socket healing, thereby improving the likelihood of graft success as an access route for oral infection is removed.

Fig. 21.5 Right buccal occlusion following crossbite correction with quadhelix.

■ What treatment will be required following alveolar bone grafting?

Once 3| erupts, move the right upper buccal segment forward so 3| replaces 2|.

Consider relief of crowding in the non-cleft quadrant and in the lower arch. Delay any lower arch extractions if orthognathic surgery is planned at a later date.

Fixed appliance therapy will be required for the active tooth movement described above.

Bonded retention will then be required to maintain upper labial segment alignment, and restorative treatment will be required to make 3| simulate an upper lateral incisor. In late teenage years consideration may be given to further lip revision or orthognathic surgery with rhinoplasty later, if a marked anteroposterior and/or vertical skeletal discrepancy exists.

In Karen's case, provided facial growth is reasonably favourable, orthognathic surgery may not be required.

Key point

Secondary alveolar bone grafting:

• Provides bone for 3 eruption.

• Restores arch integrity.

• Improves alar base support.

• Aids oronasal fistula closure.

• Allows orthodontic space closure.

For revision, see Mind Map 21, page 183.

Recommended reading

Bergland O, Semb G, Abyholm FE 1986 Elimination of the residual alveolar cleft by secondary bone grafting and subsequent orthodontic treatment. Cleft Palate J 23:175–205.

Rivkin CJ, Keith O, Crawford PJM, Hathorn IS 2000 Dental care for the patient with a cleft lip and palate. Part 1: From birth to the mixed dentition stage; Part 2: The mixed dentition stage through to adolescence and young adulthood. Br Dent J 118:78–83, 131–134.

Thom AR 1990 Modern management of the cleft lip and palate patient. Dent Update 17:402–408.

Nursing and early childhood caries

SUMMARY

Kelly-Ann is only 3. She has been brought to the dentist by her mother because her upper front teeth are 'wearing away' (Fig. 22.1). What has caused this and how may it be treated?

History

The teeth apparently never came through properly and were never white like the rest of her teeth. There has been no pain from the teeth and Kelly-Ann is eating and drinking normally.

Medical history

Kelly-Ann is a healthy infant. She has had all her vaccinations and has had no illnesses. She has never been on any medication.

Examination

Extraorally there is no swelling and no facial asymmetry. Intraorally she is in the full primary dentition with the second primary molars having just erupted. There is caries affecting the upper incisors and cavitation in all first primary molars.

■ *What is the cause of this pattern of decay?*

'Nursing caries', or 'nursing bottle mouth' or 'bottle mouth caries'.

■ *What can cause this?*

Consumption of a sweetened drink or fruit-flavoured drink from a bottle or dinky feeder, especially if the feeder is constantly in the mouth or the child falls asleep with it in the mouth.

Persistent on-demand breastfeeding at night after 12 months of age (child is allowed to sleep on the breast) may cause caries in exceptional circumstances. There are many biological and social variables that confound this complex relationship.

As can be seen, the term 'nursing caries' is probably the most accurate as it encompasses both breastfeeding and bottle feeding.

■ *Why are the teeth affected in this pattern?*

Teeth become carious in the order in which they erupt (**Fig. 22.2**) with the exception of the lower primary incisors, which are protected by two major mechanisms: the position of the submandibular ducts that open adjacent to these teeth; the position of the tongue in suckling, which covers the lower incisors.

■ *What additional factors make the upper primary incisors more predisposed to caries?*

High bow-shaped upper lip in infants which does not cover the upper incisors and results in an increased evaporation of any saliva on these teeth.

Gravity, which keeps submandibular saliva pooled around the lower incisors and less likely to reach the upper incisors.

Any liquid with sugar that is allowed to bathe the teeth on a frequent basis will cause caries. This is especially so at night when the protective function of saliva reduces as less saliva is produced. Even breast milk, formula milk or cows' milk with their lowered natural sugars can still be cariogenic on this basis.

Key point

Nursing caries:
- Affects teeth in order of eruption.
- Lower incisors are protected by saliva.
- Can be caused by any sugar-containing liquid.

Fig. 22.1 Early cavitation in nursing caries.

Fig. 22.2 Classical distribution of affected teeth in nursing caries in upper arch.

■ What should be your advice about night-time feeding?

Only water should be given during the night after 12 months of age.

The term early childhood caries (ECC) is an additional term used to describe any caries presenting in the primary dentition of young children. Some children present with extensive caries that does not follow the 'nursing caries' pattern and have multiple carious teeth, and may be slightly older at 3, 4 or 5 years of age at initial presentation.

■ How could you identify pre-school children in need of dental care?

Encourage parents to bring their children for a dental check-up as soon as the child has teeth.

Make contact with local health visitors, baby clinics, and mother and baby groups via the local general medical practice.

Treatment

■ Kelly-Ann is in a high risk for caries group. List all the main factors you can think of for placing someone in the high risk group for dental caries.

See **Table 22.1**.

Table 22.1 'High-risk' factors for caries

Risk factor	Aetiology
Clinical evidence	New lesions
	Premature extractions
	Anterior caries or restorations
	Multiple restorations
	No fissure sealants
	Fixed appliance orthodontics
	Partial dentures
Dietary habits	Frequent sugar intake
Social history	Social deprivation
	High caries in siblings
	Low knowledge of dental disease
	Irregular attendance
	Ready availability of snacks
	Low dental aspirations
Use of fluoride	Drinking water not fluoridated
	No fluoride supplements
	No fluoride toothpaste
Plaque control	Infrequent, ineffective cleaning
	Poor manual control
Saliva	Low flow rate
	Low buffering capacity
	High *Streptococcus mutans* and *Lactobacillus* counts
Medical history	Medically compromised
	Physical disability
	Intellectual disability
	Xerostomia
	Long-term cariogenic medicine

■ What fluoride regimen would you suggest to Kelly-Ann's mother?

Fluoride paste. As a high risk subject, she should be given a 1000 or 1450 ppm fluoride paste rather than 450–600 ppm children's paste.

Fluoride supplements. These should be considered in high risk of caries subjects and in children in whom dental disease would pose a serious risk to general health (e.g. risk of infectious endocarditis). Such supplementation is only effective if given long term and regularly.

■ What information is essential before prescribing fluoride supplements?

The amount of fluoride in the local water. Telephone the local water supplier for this information.

■ What is the currently recommended fluoride supplementation regimen in the UK?

See **Table 22.2**.

Table 22.2 Recommended dosage schedule for fluoride supplements in areas where the water supply contains less than 0.3 ppm fluoride

Age	Fluoride per day (mg)
6 months to 3 years	0.25
3–6 years	0.50
6 years	1.00

Professionally applied fluorides

Site-specific application of fluoride varnish can be very valuable in the management of early, smooth surface and approximal carious lesions. Recent evidence suggests that passage of floss through a contact point between primary molars by parents can greatly enhance prevention and early treatment of approximal lesions. The most commonly used varnish – 5% sodium fluoride – has 22 600 ppm and should be applied very sparingly to specific areas three times a year.

■ Why can Kelly-Ann not have fluoride mouthwash?

These are contraindicated in children less than 6 years of age because more than half the mouthwash will be swallowed.

■ What other forms of preventive care does she need?

Toothbrushing instruction

Pre-school children need help from their parents if effective oral hygiene is to be maintained. Brushing needs to start as soon as the first tooth erupts. Standing or kneeling behind the child in front of a sink or mirror is often the best way to brush a young child's teeth. Supervision of brushing is important so that an appropriate amount of paste is placed on the brush to prevent/reduce ingestion of paste. Teeth should be cleaned at least once a day.

Diet analysis

The only way to effectively do this is by a 3- or 4-day written analysis. It is important to try to obtain 1 day's history from a weekend as they are invariably different from weekdays. In modern society it is common for most parents to work and the child to be looked after by a carer or nursery. It is critical to establish who is the carer on weekdays and weekends. Advice needs to be clear at all times, but if it has to be relayed from a parent in the surgery to a carer then it needs to be clear, succinct and written. Frequent consumption of sugar-containing drinks and feeds is the key aetiological feature in many pre-school children with caries. Reducing the frequency of sugar-containing snacks is the key message. If the child is a 'poor eater' there is need to build up the amount of food at mealtimes and, therefore, reduce the need for frequent snacking. Children do not need lots of fizzy drinks or fruit-based drinks. They often take them to make up for calories missed at mealtimes. Only milk and water should be taken between meals. A small amount of fruit-based drink can more safely be taken with a meal. As mentioned above, it is critical to stop the night-time bottle.

In your dietary advice you must be *practical*, *personal* and *positive*. Avoid making the parent feel excessively guilty but concentrate on practical strategies. It is probably unreasonable to give out more than four pieces of written advice. These should concentrate on day-time drinks, night-time drinks, between-meal snacks, and making sure the child has no food or drink for 1 hour before going to bed and then cleans the teeth just before bed.

Kelly-Ann has the early cavitation on her upper incisors that you see in **Figure 22.1**. She also has early cavitated occlusal caries in her first primary molars.

■ *How would you restore the upper incisors?*

These can be restored with a compomer or a composite. Both have a good bond strength to enamel and dentine. Compomers have good mechanical properties and in this situation will be as durable as composite.

■ *How would you restore the early cavitation in the first primary molars?*

Compomer or resin-modified glass ionomer cement similarly will be the restorative materials of choice.

All this work, because it is not extensive, could probably be achieved with a slow handpiece and excavator. However, if Kelly-Ann is apprehensive of the 'drill' then an alternative way of caries removal will have to be found.

■ *What method of caries removal, without a handpiece, may be applicable here?*

Carisolv, which accomplishes caries removal by chemo-mechanical means. Carisolv consists of a pink gel that contains mainly the amino acids leucine, lysine and glutamic acid, and hypochlorite. In addition there is cellulose and a colouring agent, erythrocin. The amino acids and hypochlorite work to separate carious dentine from sound dentine and the carious dentine is removed with the aid of special hand instruments that have different cutting edges and hand actions to excavators. They are used in a whisking, rotating, or up and down movement. Because the sound dentine is not stimulated by the temperature or vibration of a handpiece, or the temperature changes of a 3 in 1 spray, it is a painless procedure. The cavity should be dried by saline-dampened cotton wool, then dry cotton wool, prior to restoring with an adhesive material. Bond strengths to adhesive materials are the same as conventionally prepared cavities.

■ *How is pain relief best achieved in the child with nursing caries in* Figure 22.2*?*

This is a case where general anaesthesia for tooth removal is justified. This is covered in Chapter 26.

Recommended reading

Ripa LW 1988 Nursing caries: a comprehensive review. Paediatr Dent 10:268–282.

For revision, see Mind Map 22, page 184.

High caries risk adolescents

SUMMARY

Peter is 13 years old. He is concerned about the appearance of his teeth, especially the spaces between his front teeth and would like this improved (Fig. 23.1). He is not very keen on the prospect of complex restorative or orthodontic treatment. On presentation he is diagnosed as high caries risk. How would you plan treatment for this patient focusing initially on preventive care?

History

Complaint

Peter attends your surgery for the first time in a number of years. He advises you he would like the spaces between his front teeth corrected (**Fig. 23.1**).

History of complaint

Peter is a sporadic attendee with no pain in any teeth. He is now keen on having the appearance of his front teeth improved and is eager to learn how this can be achieved.

Medical history

Peter is fit and well, with no history of medication.

Dental history

Primary teeth removal under general anaesthesia at the age of 5 years.

Previous restorative care under local anaesthesia a number of years ago. You have not seen Peter for at least 3 years (**Fig. 23.1**).

■ *What aspects of the presentation and history help to determine the caries risk category so far?*

- Social history – irregular attendance and low dental aspirations to date (high caries risk).
- Medical history – fit and well (low caries risk).
- Dental history – primary tooth extraction under general anaesthesia (high caries risk).

Examination

Extraoral

Nothing relevant is revealed.

Intraoral

Peter's oral hygiene is not ideal. Normal saliva levels are noted. He is in the permanent dentition with missing lower central incisors and a retained lower left primary central incisor. His upper right first permanent molar has been extracted and the upper and lower first permanent molars and lower right first and second molars restored. No fissure sealants are present. There is evidence of mild buccal crowding in the lower arch with lower left second permanent premolar lingually placed. The lower left primary central incisor is retained and both lower permanent central incisors missing (see **Figs 23.2** and **23.3**).

■ *What further aspects of the clinical presentation help determine caries risk?*

Clinical evidence: Caries in lower left second permanent molar. Restorations present and removal of first permanent molar (high caries risk). This caries risk category will have the largest weighting in scoring overall caries risk.

Plaque control: Oral hygiene poor, especially upper anterior region (high caries risk).

Saliva – normal saliva levels noted (low caries risk).

Fig. 23.1 Anterior view of teeth at presentation.

Fig. 23.2 Upper occlusal view at presentation.

For a full list of caries risk factors, see Chapter 22, **Table 22.1**. This will help build up a picture of caries risk and formulate a prevention plan that is tailored to the patient's requirements.

■ *At present what caries risk category would you place Peter in?*

High caries risk.

■ *What further questions would you ask Peter to complete his caries risk assessment?*

Fluoride history

What level of fluoride toothpaste does he use? If Peter is not aware of the fluoride strength of the toothpaste he uses, he should be shown how to determine this on a toothpaste tube. He should be using 1450 ppm F (children 6 and older). He is presently using a brand which is adult strength.

How many times a day does he brush his teeth? He presently brushes twice daily but not effectively. Twice daily for 3 minutes should be recommended and the technique demonstrated.

Does he presently rinse with water after brushing? He rinses his teeth with water after brushing. The 'spit but don't rinse' with water policy should be recommended.

Is he presently using any fluoride supplements or mouthwash? If so, when does he do this? At present only toothpaste is used. Fluoride supplements or mouthwash should be used at a separate time to brushing his teeth. After coming in from school or after dinner is well remembered by many patients (high caries risk).

Dietary history

Frequency and timing of all food and drinks including milk and water? Carbonated drinks are consumed at least four times a week with diluted juice consumed on a daily basis.

Frequency and timing of food. Peter is a grazer and likes to eat well into the evening. Advice is given based on the completion of a 4-day food diary (high caries risk).

Peter's history, clinical assessment and further questioning combine to give a final caries risk assessment, which indicate high caries risk (**Table 23.1**).

Key points

Caries risk assessment
- The largest weighted caries risk assessment category is clinical evidence.
- The completion of a caries risk assessment helps formulate a prevention plan specific to the patient.

Preventive care and treatment

Peter is presently high caries risk. Prior to restorative work being undertaken, the preventive treatment plan should ensure that caries risk reduces, thus ensuring the patient's risk status is lowered and he remains caries free.

■ *After the initial bitewing radiographs are taken (see Fig. 23.4), when should Peter have radiographs taken again?*

In 6 months time if he remains high caries risk.

■ *What other forms of preventive care would he benefit from?*

Toothbrushing instruction.

Children of Peter's age should be shown how to brush their teeth using disclosing tablets or solutions. Disclosing tablets taken away should be used before going to bed when time can be devoted to improving brushing techniques.

Strength of fluoride toothpaste

In addition to the advice on adult toothpaste strength at initial presentation, were Peter to remain high caries risk for example, new lesions detected or commencing orthodontic treatment, he may then benefit from a higher strength 2800 ppm F toothpaste.

Fluoride varnish application

The evidence to date suggests an additional benefit from application 3–4 yearly in high caries risk children if using

Fig. 23.3 Lower occlusal view at presentation.

Fig. 23.4 Bitewing radiographs.

Table 23.1 Peter's caries risk assessment

Clinical Evidence	Dietary habits	Social history	Fluoride use	Plaque control	Saliva	Medical history	Caries risk
L **H**	L **H**	L **H**	L **H**	L **H**	**L** H	**L** H	L M **H**

daily fluoride toothpaste for both high and low caries risk children. Even if Peter's caries risk status were to subsequently reduce to low caries risk, twice-yearly application of a fluoride varnish (5% sodium fluoride 22 600 ppm F) would still be recommended.

Fluoride supplements

Fluoride mouthwash at 225 ppm F is recommended for daily use at a separate time to toothbrushing. Demonstrate to the patient on a mouthwash bottle where the fluoride concentration information is written. This then allows the patient to make an informed choice regarding the many brands of mouthwash available for use on a daily basis.

Diet analysis

As stated in Chapter 22, a 4-day food diary can highlight frequency and timing of foods that enable practical and patient-centred advice to be given.

Children of secondary school age can be given information that enables them to make informed choices regarding their eating and drinking practices, with, in many instances, simple changes made that reduce caries risk significantly.

Fissure sealants

Peter required fissure sealants on a number of his premolars (see **Figs 23.5** and **23.6**).

Table 23.2 helps highlight the complete package of preventive care that Peter should receive prior to any restorative work being undertaken.

Only on completion of this initial phase of prevention and simple restorative treatment should composite build-ups or other adhesive bridgework be considered (see **Figs 23.7** and **23.8**). In Peter's case the retained lower left primary central incisor was assessed and due to limited root length,

he was advised of its poor long-term prognosis. The primary incisor was extracted and a one-unit Maryland bridge provided. At a later stage, should Peter decide he would like more complex treatment such as fixed orthodontics or implants, this can still be provided.

Fig. 23.6 Fissure sealants in lower premolars.

Fig. 23.7 Final restorative treatment of the upper incisors.

Fig. 23.5 Fissure sealants in upper premolars.

Fig. 23.8 Final restorative care of the anteriors.

Table 23.2 Peter's prevention plan

Radiographs (Frequency)	Toothbrushing Instruction	Strength F⁻ toothpaste (F⁻ ppm)	F⁻ varnish (frequency)	F⁻ supplements (dose)	Diet analysis	Fissure sealants		Sugar-free medicines
6 months	With disclosing tablets and demonstration	1450 ppm F	3–4 monthly application	Daily use Fluoride Mouth wash 225 ppm F	4 day food diary	Yes / Yes	Yes / Yes	N/A

Key points

Preventive care:

- The evidence to date suggests an additional benefit from application of fluoride varnish 3–4 yearly in high caries risk children. Apply twice yearly in low caries risk children.
- Fluoride mouthwash at 225 ppm F is recommended for daily use at a separate time to toothbrushing.
- For some high caries risk adolescents higher strength fluoride regimens may be appropriate.

■ *What else might you suggest now that Peter is older that could help reduce his caries risk status further for the future?*

Higher strength fluoride toothpaste (2800 or 5000 ppm F) The effect of fluoride toothpaste is concentration dependent. The maximal over-the-counter product is 1500 ppm F. Two new prescription-only toothpastes containing 2800 and 5000 ppm F now allow the dental profession to target high caries risk adolescents. The results of a number of randomized clinical trials suggest that in the range 1000–2500 ppm F, every additional 500 ppm F, over and above 1000 ppm F, would provide a cumulative 6% reduction in caries increment. This dose response is highest in high caries risk children and those aged over 11 years. However, this would only be prescribed after assessing suitability and compliance with instructions for the use of higher strength fluoride toothpaste. It should be emphasized that such high-strength fluoride toothpastes should be kept out of reach of younger children, and individuals for whom this toothpaste is prescribed should be encouraged to expectorate after brushing. The 5000 ppm F toothpaste is used for children over 16 years of age and adults.

Tooth mousse or tooth mousse plus (CPP-ACP or CPP-ACFP) Tooth mousse is a water-based cream containing Recaldent (casein phosphopeptide-amorphous calcium phosphate or CPP-ACP). Tooth mousse plus, a stronger tooth mousse, is recommended at night only for patients who either have marked salivary dysfunction or increase risk of mineral loss from dental caries or erosion of teeth. Children should be at least 6 years of age before using tooth mousse plus. The proposed anticariogenic mechanism of CPP-ACP involves the enhancement of remineralization through the localization of bioavailable calcium and phosphate ions at the tooth surface. Casein phosphopeptides (CPP) stabilize high concentrations of calcium and phosphate ions as embryonic ACP nanoclusters together with fluoride ions at the tooth surface by binding to pellicle and plaque and act as a delivery vehicle to the tooth surface. The ions are freely bioavailable to diffuse down concentration gradients into enamel subsurface lesions, thereby effectively promoting remineralization.

Sugar-free chewing gum (xylitol/CPP-ACP nanocomplexes) Many chewing gums are now available as sugar-free with 50% sweetened with sugar substitutes. Oral bacteria do not use these sugar substitutes to produce the acids that demineralize enamel and dentine. Furthermore, the act of chewing stimulates saliva flow, which increases buffering capacity and enhances clearance of food debris and microorganisms from the oral cavity. Chewing gum containing xylitol, a polyol 5 carbon sweetener which reduces plaque salivary *Streptococcus mutans* levels and tooth decay, as well as enhancing remineralization. CPP-ACP sugar-free gum was shown to significantly slow progression and enhance regression of approximal caries relative to a control group in a 24-month clinical trial. This trial looked at the use of CPP-ACP gum in 2720 subjects randomly assigned to either the CPP-ACP gum or a control gum. Subjects chewing the CCP-ACP gum were 18% less likely to experience caries progression than those using the control gum.

Recommended reading

Cochrane NJ, Saranathan S, Cai F et al 2008 Enamel subsurface lesion remineralisation with casein phosphopeptide stabilised solutions of calcium, phosphate and fluoride. Caries Res 42:88–97.

Davies RM, Davies GM 2008 High fluoride toothpastes: their role in a caries prevention programme. Dent Update 5:320–323.

Kiet AL, Milgrom P, Rothen M 2008 The potential of dental-protective chewing gum in oral health interventions. JADA 139:553–563.

Morgan MV, Adams GG, Bailey DL et al 2008 The anticariogenic effect of sugar free gum containing CPP-ACP nanocomplexes on approximal caries determined using digital bitewing radiography. Caries Res 42:171–184.

Reynolds EC 2008 Calcium phosphate-based remineralisation systems: scientific evidence? Aust Dent J 53:268–273.

For revision, see Mind Map 23, page 185.

24

The uncooperative child

SUMMARY

Liam is 5. He is shaking and tearful as he is brought into the surgery. His mother says he has been in pain from his teeth for a long time. How would you manage Liam and his dental treatment?

■ **What do you understand by the term behaviour management?**

Based on scientific principles, the proper implementation of behaviour management requires an understanding of these principles. It requires skills in empathy, communication, coaching and listening.

The goals are to establish communication, alleviate fear and anxiety, deliver quality dental care, build a trusting relationship between dentist and child, and promote the child's positive attitude towards oral/dental health.

All decisions must be based on a benefit versus risk evaluation. Parents/legal guardians share in the decision-making process regarding treatment of their children.

■ **What history is important in Liam's case?**

Liam's dental history. It is crucial to identify any previous episodes either at the dentist, doctor or hospital, usually involving needles that may have frightened him. If there are no previous precipitating factors he may have been frightened by stories or comments from his peers or family.

Family dental history. Parental fear, and a negative attitude toward dental and oral health, can significantly affect the cooperation of a child.

Liam's development. Delayed development and poor cognition can affect the ability of a child to understand what you are trying to do to help. Children with a negative image of themselves who have never succeeded well at anything will be more difficult to treat. They often give up because they 'never succeed' and are often called 'failures' by their parents or peers.

Communicative management is the most fundamental form of behaviour management. It is the basis for establishing a relationship with a child that will allow you to successfully complete dental procedures and help the child develop a positive attitude toward dental health.

■ **What main forms of communicative management are there?**

Voice control.

Non-verbal communication.

Tell-show-do.

Positive reinforcement.

Distraction.

Parental presence/absence.

Voice control

Description: Voice control is a controlled alteration of voice volume, tone or pace to influence and direct the patient's behaviour.

Objectives:

To gain the patient's attention and compliance.

To avert negative or avoidance behaviour.

To establish appropriate adult–child roles.

Indications: May be used with any patient.

Contraindications: None.

Non-verbal communication

Description: Non-verbal communication is the reinforcement and guidance of behaviour through appropriate contact, posture and facial expression.

Objectives:

To enhance the effectiveness of other communicative management techniques.

To gain or maintain the patient's attention and compliance.

Indications: May be used with any patient.

Contraindications: None.

Tell–show–do

Description: Tell–show–do is a technique of behaviour shaping used by many paediatric professionals. The technique involves verbal explanations of procedures in phrases appropriate to the developmental level of the patient (Tell); demonstrations for the patient of the visual, auditory, olfactory and tactile aspects of the procedure in a carefully defined, non-threatening setting (Show); and then, without deviating from the explanation and demonstration, completion of the procedure (Do). The tell-show-do technique is used with communication skills (verbal and non-verbal) and positive reinforcement.

Objectives:

To teach the patient important aspects of the dental visit and familiarize the patient with the dental setting.

To shape the patient's response to procedures through desensitization and well described expectations.

Indications: May be used with any patient.

Contraindications: None.

Positive reinforcement

Description: In the process of establishing desirable patient behaviour, it is essential to give appropriate feedback. Positive reinforcement is an effective technique to reward desired behaviours and thus strengthen the recurrence of those behaviours. Social reinforcers include positive voice

THE UNCOOPERATIVE CHILD

modulation, facial expression, verbal praise and appropriate physical demonstrations of affection by all members of the dental team. Non-social reinforcers include tokens and toys.

Objective:

To reinforce desired behaviour.

Indications: May be useful for any patient.

Contraindications: None.

Distraction

Description: Distraction is the technique of diverting the patient's attention from what may be perceived as an unpleasant procedure.

Objectives:

To decrease the perception of unpleasantness.

To avert negative or avoidance behaviour.

Indications: May be used with any patient.

Contraindications: None.

Parental presence/absence

Description: This technique involves using the presence or absence of the parent to gain cooperation for treatment. A wide diversity exists in practitioner philosophy and parental attitude regarding parents' presence or absence during paediatric dental treatment. Practitioners are united in the fact that communication between dentist and child is paramount and that this communication demands focus on the part of both parties. Children's responses to their parents' presence or absence can range from very beneficial to very detrimental. It is the responsibility of practitioners to determine the communication methods that best optimize the treatment setting; recognizing their own skills, the abilities of the particular child and the desires of the specific parent involved.

Objectives:

To gain the patient's attention and compliance.

To avert negative or avoidance behaviours.

To establish appropriate adult-child roles.

To enhance the communication environment.

Indications: May be used with any patient.

Contraindications: None.

All these communication techniques integrate to enhance the evolution of a compliant and relaxed patient. It is an ongoing subjective process rather than a singular technique and is often the extension of the personality of the dentist.

Key point

The objectives of distraction are:
- To decrease the perception of unpleasantness.
- To avert negative or avoidance behaviour.

Examination

After spending some time talking to Liam and showing him that you are genuine in wanting to help, he allows you to look at his teeth. Both lower first primary molars are carious. All the other teeth are sound. Liam has been frightened by stories from his friends. His family are very supportive and are regular attenders.

Liam responds well to communicative management but, although he wants to have his treatment done he just cannot override his fear of the unknown.

■ *What additional help might you consider giving Liam?*

Sedation – there are two options for sedation, either oral or inhalational sedation.

Oral sedation is now an increasingly viable option using midazolam. A number of recent studies have shown that its use in a dose of 0.3–0.5 mg/kg, depending on age, has been therapeutically effective in producing effective sedation that has allowed subsequent dental treatment. The objectives, indications and contraindications for it are as follows

Objectives:

To reduce or eliminate anxiety.

To reduce untoward movement and reaction to dental treatment.

To enhance communication and patient cooperation.

To increase tolerance for longer appointments.

To aid in treatment of the mentally, physically or medically compromised patient.

To raise the patient's pain threshold.

Indications:

Fearful, anxious patients in whom basic behaviour management has not been successful.

Patients who cannot cooperate due to a lack of psychological or emotional maturity and/or mental, physical or medical disability.

Patients for whom the use of sedation may protect the developing psyche and/or reduce medical risk.

Contraindications:

The cooperative patient with minimal dental needs.

Predisposing medical conditions that would make sedation inadvisable.

Inhalational sedation has been known to be an effective and safe method of reducing anxiety and enhancing effective communication for the past 30 years. Its onset of action is rapid, the depth of sedation is easily titrated and reversible, and recovery is rapid and complete. Additionally, nitrous oxide mediates a variable degree of analgesia, amnesia and gag reflex reduction.

The need to diagnose and treat, as well as the safety of the patient and practitioner, should be considered before the use of nitrous oxide. The decision to use nitrous oxide must take into consideration:

Alternative behaviour management modalities.

Dental needs of the patient.

The effect on the quality of dental care.

The patient's emotional development.

The patient's physical considerations.

Written informed consent must be obtained from a legal guardian and documented in the patient's record prior to use of nitrous oxide.

The patient's record should include:

Informed consent.

Indication for use.

Nitrous oxide dosage:

- Per cent nitrous oxide/oxygen and/or flow rate.
- Duration of the procedure.
- Post-treatment oxygenation procedure.

Objectives:

To reduce or eliminate anxiety.

To reduce untoward movement and reaction to dental treatment.

To enhance communication and patient cooperation.

To raise the pain reaction threshold.

To increase tolerance for longer appointments.

To aid in treatment of the mentally/physically disabled, or medically compromised patient.

To reduce gagging.

Indications:

A fearful, anxious or obstreperous patient.

Certain mentally, physically or medically compromised patients.

A patient whose gag reflex interferes with dental care.

A patient in whom profound local anaesthesia cannot be obtained.

Contraindications:

May be contraindicated in some chronic obstructive pulmonary diseases.

May be contraindicated in certain patients with severe emotional disturbances or drug-related dependencies.

Patients in the first trimester of pregnancy.

May be contraindicated in patients with sickle cell disease.

Patients treated with bleomycin sulphate.

Liam had inhalational sedation, which enabled completion of his treatment and helped him overcome his fear of local anaesthesia. Unfortunately, there are some children for whom inhalational sedation will not work and general anaesthesia is the only option that will allow relief of pain and completion of dental treatment.

Key point

The patient's record in inhalational sedation should include:
- Informed consent.
- Indications for use.
- Nitrous oxide dosage.

■ *What are the indications for general anaesthesia?*

Patients who are unable to cooperate due to a lack of psychological or emotional maturity, and/or mental, physical or medical disability.

Patients for whom local anaesthesia is ineffective because of acute infection, anatomical variations or allergy.

The extremely uncooperative, fearful, anxious or uncommunicative child or adolescent.

Patients requiring significant surgical procedures.

Patients for whom the use of general anaesthesia (GA) may protect the developing psyche and/or reduce medical risks.

Patients requiring immediate, comprehensive oral/dental care.

■ *What are the contraindications for general anaesthesia?*

A healthy, cooperative patient with minimal dental need.

Predisposing medical conditions that would make GA inadvisable.

General anaesthesia is a controlled state of unconsciousness accompanied by a loss of protective reflexes, including the ability to maintain an airway independently and respond purposefully to physical stimulation or verbal command. It should only be provided in premises with resuscitation capability and intensive care back-up. All equipment must follow current guidelines.

Parental or legal guardian informed consent must be obtained and documented prior to the use of general anaesthesia. The patient's record should include:

- Informed consent.
- Indications for the use of GA.

Informed consent

Regardless of the behaviour management techniques utilized by the individual practitioner, all management decisions must be based on a subjective evaluation weighing benefit and risk to the child. Considerations regarding need of treatment, consequences of deferred treatment and potential physical/emotional trauma must be entered into the decision-making equation.

Delivery of dental treatment is often a complex decision. Decisions regarding the use of behaviour management techniques other than communicative management cannot be made solely by the dentist. Decisions must involve a legal guardian and, if appropriate, the child. The dentist serves as the expert about dental care, i.e. the need for treatment and the techniques by which treatment can be delivered. The legal guardian shares with the practitioner the decision whether to treat or not to treat and must be consulted regarding treatment strategies and potential risks. Therefore, the successful completion of diagnostic and therapeutic services is viewed as a partnership of dentist, legal guardian and child.

Although the behaviour management techniques included in this chapter are used frequently, parents may not be entirely familiar with them. It is important that the dentist inform the legal guardian about the nature of the technique to be used, its risks, benefits and any alternative techniques. All questions must be answered. This is the essence of informed consent.

Recommended reading

Guidelines for Behavior Management 1999 American Academy of Pediatric Dentistry Reference Manual 1999–2000. Paediatr Dent 21:42–46.

Hosey MT 2002 Managing anxious children: the use of conscious sedation in paediatric dentistry. UK National Clinical Guideline. Int J Paediatr Dent 12:359–372.

Pinkham JR 1995 Personality development. Managing behaviour of the cooperative pre-school child. Dent Clin North Am 39:771–787.

For revision, see Mind Map 24, page 186.

25

Disorders of eruption and exfoliation

Case 1

SUMMARY

Beth was only 20 days old when it was noticed she had two teeth at the front of the lower jaw (Fig. 25.1).

■ *What is the correct terminology for these early erupting teeth?*

If the teeth are present at birth, 'natal' is the correct term. If they are not present at birth but erupt within the first month of life, 'neonatal' is correct.

The prevalence rates for both natal and neonatal teeth are reported as 1 in 2000–3000 live births. The most commonly presenting tooth is the lower central incisor. More rarely, maxillary incisors or first molars have been reported. The early eruption is thought to be caused by the ectopic position of the tooth germ during fetal life. Natal and neonatal teeth may follow a sporadic pattern or they may be familial. However, they can be associated with specific syndromes:

Pachyonychia congenita.

Ellis–van Creveld.

Hallermann–Streiff.

Fig. 25.1 Natal teeth.

■ *What are the main problems associated with natal and neonatal teeth?*

Mobility.

Ulceration of ventral surface of tongue.

Nipple soreness (breastfeeding mothers).

The teeth are mobile because the development of the tooth is consistent with age. Only about five-sixths of the crown is formed and usually no root. Additionally, the crown is occasionally dilacerated and the enamel hypoplastic or hypomineralized.

Excessive mobility is a danger to the airway from aspiration and the tooth should be removed. Care should be taken to ensure that the entire tooth including the pulpal tissue is removed, otherwise dentine and a root will form, which will require eventual removal. If teeth can be left then continued root development will occur.

Nipple soreness may occasionally necessitate tooth removal.

Ulceration on the ventral surface of the tongue may respond to carmellose sodium oral paste. Smoothing of the incisal edges with sandpaper discs may also help.

■ *What factors can cause generalized premature eruption but still be considered as 'normal'?*

Familial – a family history is a common finding.

Children with high birth weights.

Race – generally Negroids tend to erupt their permanent teeth earlier than Mongoloids, who are in turn in advance of Caucasians. Racial group does not seem to affect eruption times of primary teeth but eruption patterns can vary in the primary dentition.

Sex – females tend to erupt permanent teeth several months ahead of males.

The opposite of premature eruption is delayed eruption.

■ *When is generalized delay in eruption of primary teeth expected?*

Preterm infants.

Very low birth weight infants.

■ *What conditions may lead to a generalized retarded eruption of teeth in both primary and permanent dentitions?*

Chromosomal abnormalities – Down's and Turner's syndromes.

Gross nutritional deficiency.

Hypothyroidism/hypopituitarism.

Hereditary gingival fibromatosis (HGF).

Acquired gingival overgrowth (drug-induced).

■ *What specific condition is associated with grossly delayed or failed eruption of teeth in the permanent dentition?*

Cleidocranial dysplasia – this is an autosomal dominantly inherited condition where, in addition to multiple supernumerary teeth causing delayed exfoliation of primary teeth and delayed eruption of permanent teeth, there is aplasia of commonly the distal end or total absence of the clavicles.

What local factors can account for delayed eruption of permanent teeth?

Supernumerary teeth or odontomes.

Ectopic crypt positions of permanent teeth.

Cystic change in the follicle of permanent teeth.

Crowding.

Thickened mucosa due to early primary tooth removal.

Key point
Natal and neonatal teeth may need to be removed if: • Mobility causes concern about inhalation. • Ulceration under the ventral surface of the tongue persists. • Nipple soreness is significant.

Exfoliation of teeth (like eruption) can be either premature or delayed.

Case 2

SUMMARY

George was 3 years of age when his mother first noticed that his lower primary incisors were loose.

History

George was born after a normal pregnancy and delivery but had problems after birth with recurrent coughs and colds, upper and lower respiratory tract infections, and oral ulceration. He was extensively investigated and was confirmed as having a cyclic neutropenia.

Dental history

George and his mother had regular toothbrush instruction and his oral hygiene was excellent. He also used 0.2% chlorhexidine gel at night instead of fluoridated toothpaste. Despite these efforts his lower primary incisors exfoliated between age 4 and 5 years and by his sixth birthday he had erupted his lower permanent central incisors and first permanent molars (**Fig. 25.2A, B**).

Premature loss of primary teeth is an important diagnostic event, as most conditions causing it are potentially serious and warrant immediate investigation (**Box 25.1**).

Box 25.1 Differential diagnosis of causes of premature exfoliation of primary and permanent teeth

- Neutropenias and qualitative neutrophil defects:
  - Cyclic neutropenia.
  - Congenital neutropenia (Kostmann disease).
  - Pre-pubertal periodontitis.
  - Juvenile periodontitis.
  - Leucocyte adhesion defect.
  - Papillon–Lefèvre syndrome.
  - Chediak–Higashi disease.
- Langerhans cell histiocytosis – leading to bony destruction.
- Hypophosphatasia with aplasia or hypoplasia of cementum.
- Self-injury in either a psychotic disorder or the congenital insensitivity to pain syndrome.
- Ehlers–Danlos syndrome (type VIII) – disorder of collagen formation causing progressive periodontal destruction.
- Scurvy – loss of tooth due to failure of proline hydroxylation and collagen synthesis.

Generally teeth may be lost early because of:

Metabolic disturbances.

Severe periodontal disease.

Loss of alveolar bone support.

Self-injury or non-accidental injury.

George will continue to have regular dental care and supervision of brushing. Even in the presence of immaculate plaque control we can expect that his neutrophil defect will predispose him to periodontal disease and premature loss of some if not all his permanent teeth.

The opposite of premature exfoliation is delayed exfoliation.

What causes delayed exfoliation of primary teeth?

Double primary teeth.

Hypodontia affecting permanent successors.

Ectopically placed permanent successors.

Trauma or periradicular infection of primary teeth causing interruption of physiological resorption.

Infraocclusion or ankylosis.

Double primary teeth are associated in 40% of cases with an abnormality of number of the permanent dentition. Parents should be advised of this and a dental panoramic tomogram should be taken around the age of 6.

Fig. 25.2 (A) Cyclic neutropenia.

Fig. 25.2 (B) Cyclic neutropenia.

Infraocclusion is the preferred term for either 'submerged teeth' or 'ankylosis' when describing teeth that have failed to achieve or maintain their occlusal relationship to adjacent or opposing teeth. Most commonly, primary teeth have reached a normal occlusal level before becoming infraoccluded. Rarely there may be primary failure of eruption of primary and permanent teeth in the same quadrant in the same person.

The tooth most commonly affected is the mandibular first primary molar. Males and females are affected equally. Infraoccluded primary teeth are associated with a higher incidence of absent permanent successors.

Key point

Infraocclusion:

- Mandibular first primary molar most commonly affected.
- More common in primary teeth than in permanent teeth.
- Equal sex ratio.
- Higher incidence of absent permanent successors.

▮ *How is infraocclusion graded?*

- Grade I – Occlusal level above contact point of adjacent tooth.

- Grade II – Occlusal level at contact point of adjacent tooth.

- Grade III – Occlusal level below contact point of adjacent tooth.

Grade III infraocclusions, if progressive, may be completely reincluded by the surrounding hard and soft tissues.

Radiographs of infraoccluded teeth show blurring or absence of the periodontal space.

Treatment options in infraocclusion

These are considered in Chapter 6.

Recommended reading

Crawford PJM, Aldred MJ 2005 Anomalies of tooth formation and eruption. In: Welbury RR, Duggal MS, Hosey MT (eds) Paediatric Dentistry, 3rd edn. Oxford University Press, Oxford, pp 297–318.

For revision, see Mind Map 25, page 187.

Pain control and carious primary teeth

SUMMARY

Paul is 5 years old. He is in pain from one of his upper back teeth. He has never had any treatment before. How would you manage Paul's problem?

■ *What questions do you need to ask regarding the pain?*

Site – ask Paul to point to the tooth.

Severity – does the pain stop him from playing or sleeping?

Onset – what causes it? Is it in response to hot, cold or sweet stimuli, or does it occur spontaneously? Does it wake him up from sleep?

Character – is it a sharp pain or is it dull and throbbing?

Duration – how long does it last?

The characteristics of the pain of reversible and irreversible pulpitis are shown in **Table 26.1**.

Table 26.1 Pain characteristics

Reversible	Irreversible
Transient or short duration (minutes)	Long duration
Response to hot, cold, sweet	Response to pressure (chewing)
Sharp	Spontaneous
Doesn't stop play or sleep	Throbbing
	Stops play or sleep

The initial management of a child attending in pain is often constrained by possible lack of sleep on behalf of the child or time available to the dentist to treat this extra 'emergency patient'.

■ *What dressings can help manage pulpitis initially?*

After gentle excavation of the softest layer of coronal caries:

Zinc oxide eugenol cement (e.g. Kalzinol or Intermediate Restorative Material (IRM)).

Poly-antibiotic and steroid pastes (e.g. Ledermix) placed underneath zinc oxide eugenol cement or glass ionomer cement (GIC).

If a tooth is abscessed, there is often significant coronal destruction. The pulp chamber of such teeth can often be accessed by gentle excavation, and a dressing of Ledermix on some cotton wool placed within the chamber and sealed with cement will often lead to resolution of the swelling.

An acute and/or spreading infection or swelling may require the prescription of antibiotics. This is discussed in Chapter 27. Antibiotics should only be prescribed for pain in the absence of swelling for immunosuppressed patients. Analgesics may be necessary for pain (**Table 26.2**).

Table 26.2 Dosages for common paediatric analgesics

Drug	Dosage
Paracetamol	20 mg/kg initially then 15 mg/kg every 4 hours
	Maximum 24-hour dosage 90 mg/kg
	Ensure adequate hydration
Ibuprofen (Non-steroidal anti-inflammatory drug (NSAID))	5–10 mg/kg every 8 hours
	Can be used in conjunction with paracetamol
	Best given with food and drink

Dressing open cavities has a number of advantages:

Simple introduction to dental procedures.

Oral mutans streptococci count is reduced when excavation of gross caries is accomplished. If the cavity is then completely sealed by a GIC there is evidence that the viability of the remaining organisms decreases and caries progression is greatly reduced. This buys the dentist time to institute preventive and behaviour management programmes before reassessing teeth with temporary restorations.

GIC cements act as a fluoride reservoir.

Makes toothbrushing and eating more comfortable.

History

Questioning suggested a reversible pulpitis in the upper left quadrant but with recent features of an irreversible nature.

Examination

Paul has no extraoral swelling or asymmetry. Intraorally he has all his primary teeth with the exception of a̅| and |a̅, which have just exfoliated. 1̅| and |1̅ are just erupting. There is mesial occlusal caries with loss of the marginal ridge on d|. The |e is grossly carious (**Fig. 26.1**). There is no associated soft tissue swelling.

■ *What investigation is essential to allow you to formulate a treatment plan?*

Bitewing radiographs are necessary to diagnose approximal caries in primary molars with their wide contact areas. Radiographs will increase the diagnosed yield of caries by

Fig. 26.1 Caries affecting d| and |e .

50%. Frequency of subsequent bitewing radiographs will depend on the classification of caries risk: high risk patients should have radiographs 6–12 monthly; medium risk 12–18 monthly; low risk 18–24 monthly. In Paul's case a small amount of occlusal caries was confirmed in e|.

Key point

Advantages of dressing open cavities are:

- Introduction to dental procedures.
- Reduction of Streptococcus mutans count.
- GIC acts as a fluoride reservoir.
- Eating and toothbrushing are more comfortable.

Treatment

Initial temporization of d| and |e was with Ledermix paste under IRM cement. A preventive and behaviour management programme was started. e| was restored with an adhesive restoration.

■ *What is your definitive treatment plan for d| and |e?*

Both these teeth require primary molar pulp treatment. Although d| is less affected by caries it has lost its mesial marginal ridge and will have histological evidence of inflammation in the coronal pulp.

■ *What types of primary molar pulp treatment are there?*

Vital pulpotomy. Coronal pulp is removed under local anaesthesia (LA) and the pulp stumps dressed for 15 seconds with 15.5% ferric sulphate. The chamber is then filled with zinc oxide eugenol cement.

Desensitizing pulp therapy. This is a two-stage procedure that is used when anaesthesia cannot be gained. A pledget of cotton wool with Ledermix paste is sealed into the cavity/chamber with temporary cement for 7–14 days. At the second visit the pulp can be removed and restored as in a vital pulpotomy or pulpectomy depending on the clinical finding.

Pulpectomy. This is used when there is non-vital tissue in the root canals. The canals are instrumented with files and the canals filled with either zinc oxide cement or a calcium hydroxide-iodoform paste.

The decision regarding which type of pulp treatment is applicable can often only be made once treatment starts and the clinical findings are taken into account. Pulp treatment should, ideally, always be completed under LA (with exception of desensitizing pulp therapy where LA has either not worked or cannot be given for behavioural reasons).

■ *The status of formocresol as a pulpotomy medicament.*

Formocresol has traditionally been used and widely recognized within the profession as a medium that has delivered the best long-term results. A one-fifth dilution of the original Buckley's formulation has been shown to be as effective as the full strength concentrate. However, Buckley's is not easy to obtain in the UK, and, in addition, there have been some international concerns over its toxicity both locally and systemically. These concerns have grown in the past 5 years with formaldehyde, one of the important components

of formocresol being linked to nasopharyngeal cancer. Attempts have been ongoing for the past few years to find a suitable replacement, and one material that has been shown in randomized controlled trials to be of equal efficacy for pulpotomies in primary molars is 15.5% ferric sulphate. Ferric sulphate has previously been used by the dental profession as an astringent (available commercially as Astringedent) to control gingival bleeding prior to impression taking, and also in endodontics. It is an excellent haemostatic agent, forming a ferric ion–protein complex on contact with blood, which then stops further bleeding by sealing the vessels. However, it must be remembered that ferric sulphate has no 'fixative' effect. For this reason, an accurate diagnosis of the state of the pulp tissue left behind and on which ferric sulphate is being applied will need to be made.

■ *What is the appropriate restorative material after pulp treatment?*

The techniques employed for definitive restorations in young children should take into account the active nature of the disease in the young child. The use of adhesive restorations should be limited to occlusal and small approximal cavities. Extensive cavities, teeth with two or more carious surfaces, and teeth after pulpotomy or pulpectomy should be restored with stainless steel crowns. Amalgam is still widely used as a restorative material but adhesive materials, especially polyacid-modified resins (compomers), and composite resins may be preferred as they have been shown to be as durable if they are placed under appropriate conditions with adequate isolation. Cermet cements are not appropriate restorations for primary teeth.

Extraction of teeth will be required if they are unrestorable or if there is acute pain and infection (Chapter 27). In pre-school children the extraction of one or two teeth may be able to be accomplished under LA with oral or inhalation sedation. However, if extractions are required in two or more quadrants then general anaesthesia (GA) in an appropriate setting will be the best way to accomplish the extractions. When GA is used in young children, treatment planning should be radical and aim to prevent a repeat GA in the future.

When planning extractions it is important to consider the need for balancing extractions. Factors such as the likelihood of continued future attendance and cooperation of the child should also be borne in mind. In pre-school children with extensive caries, extraction of first primary molars with maintenance and restoration of second primary molars where possible is often a good plan. This limits the risk of further decay by eliminating interproximal contact areas in the posterior teeth.

Key point

The main types of primary molar pulp treatment are:

- Vital pulpotomy.
- Desensitizing pulp therapy.
- Pulpectomy.

Recommended reading

Cameron A, Widmer R (eds) 2008 Pain control for children. In: Handbook of Pediatric Dentistry, 3rd edn. Mosby, Edinburgh, pp 19–23.

Duggal MS, Day PF 2005 Operative treatment of dental caries in the primary dentition. In: Welbury RR, Duggal MS, Hosey MT (eds) Paediatric Dentistry, 3rd edn. Oxford University Press, Oxford, pp 149–174.

Fayle SA 2005 Treatment of dental caries in the pre-school child. In: Welbury RR, Duggal MS, Hosey MT (eds) Paediatric Dentistry, 3rd edn. Oxford University Press, Oxford, pp 134–139.

For revision, see Mind Map 26, page 188.

Facial swelling and dental abscess

SUMMARY

Peter is 12 years old. He attended with a large facial swelling after an episode of trauma 3 weeks previously. He feels unwell and his right eye is closing (Fig. 27.1).

The presentation of *acute* infection, as demonstrated by Peter, is very different from *chronic* infection.

■ *List four symptoms and signs specific to each type of infection.*

Acute:

- Sick, upset child.
- Raised temperature.
- Red, swollen face.
- Regional lymphadenopathy.

Chronic:

- Buccal sinus may be present.
- Mobile tooth.
- Halitosis.
- Discoloured tooth.

Acute infections tend to present with facial cellulitis rather than a facial abscess with pus. Peter was febrile although he was not in any significant pain because the infection had perforated the cortical plate. The mainstay of

Fig. 27.1 Severe infection of canine fossa.

treatment is removal of the cause – either pulpal extirpation or removal of the tooth.

History

Peter traumatized his upper right lateral incisor 3 weeks ago, sustaining a deep enamel dentine fracture. The dentine was dressed with calcium hydroxide and a compomer dressing was placed over the exposed dentine and enamel. He had a review appointment with his dentist the following week.

On Saturday morning his mother noticed that his cheek was becoming swollen and the tissues around his right eye 'puffy and red'. He attended the accident and emergency department of the local hospital where he was prescribed amoxicillin 250 mg tablets to be taken three times daily for 5 days. Unfortunately, by Sunday evening Peter had become listless and his swelling had increased. He felt hot.

Examination

Extraorally there was facial asymmetry with a swelling of the right maxillary canine fossa. The overlying skin was red and hot. The right eye fissure was partially closed. Peter's temperature was 39°C. Maxillary canine fossa infections can spread via emissary veins, which have no valves, to the intracranial venous system causing either a cavernous sinus thrombosis or a brain abscess. The pathways of the IIIrd and VIth cranial nerves lie in the walls of the cavernous sinus. Thrombosis in the cavernous sinus can present with a squint due to involvement of the IIIrd and VIth cranial nerves, which are involved in control of the extraocular muscles.

■ *What is the major problem with mandibular infections?*

Spread alongside the fascial planes that surround the airway with subsequent narrowing of the airway and stridor.

Spread via the fascial planes to the mediastinum to cause a mediastinitis.

■ *What is the basic management of any infection?*

Removal of the cause – extraction or root canal therapy.

Local drainage and debridement – via root canal or incision and drainage.

Oral antibiotics if systemic involvement – amoxicillin or penicillin V are usually the drugs of first choice. Amoxicillin has the advantage that it is given with food and only needs to be taken three times per day. Metronidazole, which is active against anaerobes, can be added to either amoxicillin or penicillin if the infection is severe. Often the extraction of the abscessed tooth alone will bring about resolution without antibiotic therapy. It is important that antibiotics alone should not be considered as a first line of treatment unless there is systemic involvement. In a child a temperature of 39°C or higher can be considered significant (normal ≅ 37°C). Immunosuppressed patients and those with cardiac disease should receive antibiotics immediately if any infection is suspected.

■ *What are the criteria for hospital admission with orofacial infection?*

Dehydration. Ask whether the child has had a decreased frequency of micturition in previous 12 hours.

Significant infection or temperature greater than 39°C.

Floor of mouth swelling.

■ *What will the hospital management of a severe infection involve?*

Extraction of involved teeth. It is impossible to drain a significant infection solely through the root canals of a tooth.

Drainage of any pus. In addition to extractions there may be a need to incise and drain pus, often leaving a drain in situ for a few days to enhance drainage. With severe mandibular swellings or where the floor of the mouth is raised, it may be necessary to have an extraoral drain through a skin incision or a 'through and through' drain, which passes completely through the area of infection. Extraoral incisions are to be avoided if at all possible due to post-operative scarring.

Swabs of pus for laboratory culture to establish accurate sensitivities of the organisms concerned to common antibiotics.

Intravenous antibiotics. Benzyl penicillin is the drug of first choice or amoxicillin. Cephalosporins are effective if there is a penicillin allergy but there is some cross-allergenicity in those patients allergic to penicillin and so cephalosporins should be used with care, especially when there was a severe reaction to penicillin. In severe infections, metronidazole should be added as anaerobic organisms play a significant role.

Maintenance fluids will be given until the child is drinking normally again.

Warm saline mouthwashes.

Adequate pain control commonly with paracetamol or ibuprofen (**Table 27.1**).

Table 27.1 Common antibiotics and analgesics used in paediatric dentistry

Drug	Route	Dose	Frequency	Notes
Antibiotics				
Amoxicillin	PO	25–50 mg/kg/day	tds	Syrup or chewable tablets for young children
	IV	100–400 mg/kg/day	tds	
	PO, IV	50 mg/kg up to adult dose 3 g	1 hour before	Endocarditis prophylaxis. For highly susceptible patients, half dose 6 hours late
Amoxicillin plus clavulanic acid	PO	20–40 mg/kg/day	tds	For beta-lactam-resistant organisms only
Ampicillin	IV	50–100 mg/kg/day	qds	
	IV	50 mg/kg	stat	Endocarditis prophylaxis
Benzyl penicillin	IV	15–350 mg/kg/day		
		20 000–500 000 U/kg/day	qds	First IV drug of choice for odontogenic infections
Penicillin V	PO	< 5 years 500 mg/day		
		> 5 years 1–2 g/day	qds	Give 1 hour before meals
Cephalexin	PO	25–50 mg/kg/day	qds	
Cephazolin	IV	25–50 mg/kg/day		
Erythromycin	PO	25–40 mg/kg/day	qds	Ethylsuccinate is readily absorbed
Metronidazole	IV	22.5 mg/kg/day	tds	Not in pregnancy
	PO	10–15 mg/kg/day	tds	
Gentamicin	IV	2.5 mg/kg (children) up to 80 mg maximum	stat	Endocarditis prophylaxis in highly susceptible patients in conjunction with ampicillin. Follow-up dose of ampicillin or amoxicillin required 6 hours later
Clindamycin	PO, IV	15–40 mg/kg/day	qds	Risk of pseudomembranous colitis
	PO, IV	10 mg/kg up to adult dose 600 mg	oral 1 hour before, IV stat	Endocarditis prophylaxis. Susceptible patients. Follow-up dose half initial dose, 6 hours later (5 mg/kg up to 300 mg)
Vancomycin	IV	20 mg/kg up to adult dose 1 g	infused over 1 hour	Endocarditis prophylaxis, susceptible patients allergic to penicillin
Analgesics and sedatives				
Aspirin				Should not be used in children under 6 years of age because of the risk of Reye syndrome
Paracetamol	PO, PR	15 mg/kg	4-hourly	Hepatotoxic if overdose
Codeine phosphate	PO	1–1.5 mg/kg single dose 1–3 mg/kg/day	4–6 hourly divided doses	Similar side effects to narcotics, including nausea and constipation
Pethidine	IV, IM	1 mg/kg	3–4 hourly	Maximum 100 mg
Ibuprofen	PO	6–12 months 50 mg (5–10 mg/kg)	tds	
		1–3 yr 100 mg	tds	
		4–6 yr 150 mg	tds	
		7–9 yr 200 mg	tds	

Note: Current endocarditis prophylaxis guidelines should always be followed.

PO, per oral; IV, intravenous; IM, intramuscular; PR, per rectum; tds; three times daily; qds, four times daily; stat, at once.

If the eye is shut due to a swelling in the canine fossa it may be necessary to give chloramphenicol eye drops 0.5%, or chloramphenicol ointment 1.0% to prevent conjunctivitis.

Key point

Hospital admission in orofacial infection is necessary with:

- Dehydration.
- Temperature >39 °C.
- Floor of mouth swelling.

Treatment

Peter was treated by the following regimen:

1. Extirpation of 2|. The apex was not quite fully mature and good drainage of pus was achieved down the root canal.
2. Open drainage of the tooth for 2 days.
3. Amoxicillin 250 mg three times daily, metronidazole 200 mg twice daily for 5 days each.
4. Hot saline mouthwashes.

After 2 days Peter was reviewed. The swelling was virtually absent from his right cheek and his right eye was normal. The 2| was cleaned and filed and non-setting calcium hydroxide placed into the canal via a flexible tip. The access cavity was sealed with cotton wool and glass ionomer cement (GIC). The non-setting calcium hydroxide was replaced every 3 months until apical closure was achieved after 9 months. The tooth was obturated with gutta percha.

Recommended reading

Cameron A, Widmer R (eds) 2008 Paediatric oral medicine and pathology. In: Handbook of Pediatric Dentistry, 3rd edn. Mosby, Edinburgh, pp 169–214, 448–449.

For revision, see Mind Map 27, page 189.

The displaced primary incisor

SUMMARY

James, who is 3 years old, tripped over while playing outside. He hit his front teeth on the ground. How do you manage the immediate problem and what do you advise his parents about potential damage to the permanent teeth?

History

Complaint

James has been brought to your surgery straight from home by his mother. She says his upper front tooth has been pushed back (**Fig. 28.1**).

History of complaint

James tripped and fell forward hitting his teeth on the ground. One tooth is 'pushed backwards'.

Medical history

James is a healthy boy who has had no significant childhood illnesses and who is up-to-date with all his vaccinations.

Dental history

James has been a regular attender at his dentist since the age of 2 years. He has had his teeth polished and has no caries.

Fig. 28.1 Palatal luxation of |a .

■ *What specific questions would you ask and why?*

Was there any loss of consciousness? If there was, then this signifies intracranial trauma and the child should be referred to an accident and emergency department.

When did the accident occur? Delay in seeking help might arouse suspicions of a non-accidental injury.

Where did the accident occur? An accident outside raises the additional problem of potential wound contamination. Any child brought up in the UK should be immunized against tetanus. If a child has not been immunized seek the advice of a local GP or accident and emergency department.

What was the surface on which the accident occurred? Newly constructed playgrounds have to conform to British Standards and should be either of an energy-absorbing polymer or bark chippings. Older playgrounds and normal pathways will have non-yielding surfaces and are likely to produce greater damage and potentially greater risk of more underlying injuries.

How did the accident occur? This gives an indication of the force that produced the injury. The clinician needs to be highly suspicious of the high impact injury that looks simple. Always suspect a deeper underlying injury until proven otherwise.

Examination

Extraoral

James is distressed but there is no obvious extraoral swelling or facial asymmetry.

Intraoral

■ *The appearance of the upper anterior teeth is shown in Figure 28.1. What can you see?*

Palatal displacement of |a and associated gingival trauma.

■ *What specific signs will you look for in your examination?*

The mobility of the teeth. Are they a danger to the airway?

The occlusion. Do the injured teeth prevent normal occlusion?

Mobility of a segment of teeth. This indicates a dentoalveolar fracture.

■ *What question should dentists keep at the back of their minds when examining children?*

Are the injuries consistent with the history, and if you feel they are, is this normal behaviour?

Child physical abuse presents with orofacial signs of bruising, abrasions and lacerations, burns, bites and fractures in approximately 65% of cases.

Dentists should have a copy of their local area Child Protection Committee guidelines. This will tell them who they should contact for advice.

■ *What features in the history and examination would lead to suspicions of child physical abuse?*

There are 10 items to consider. Five are questions to ask yourself and five are observations about the behaviour of the child and the parent(s):

Could the injury have been caused accidentally and if so how?

Does the explanation for the injury fit the age and the clinical findings?

If the explanation of the cause is consistent with the injury, is this itself within the normally acceptable limits of behaviour?

If there has been delay in seeking advice are there good reasons for this?

Does the story of the accident vary?

The nature of the relationship between parent and child.

The child's reactions to other people.

The child's reactions to any medical or dental examinations.

The general demeanour of the child.

Any comments made by the child and/or parent that give concern about the child's upbringing or lifestyle.

Investigations

■ *What investigations would you perform for James? Explain why for each.*

Radiographs are required to visualize the traumatized area and assess whether there are any root fractures to either the traumatized or adjacent teeth. In addition, is a dentoalveolar fracture evident? Are permanent successor teeth present? In an intrusive injury a child may have been referred as an 'avulsed' incisor. It is imperative always to check in these circumstances that the tooth is not intruded. Re-eruption of an intruded tooth may occur and close review is necessary. If re-eruption has not occurred within 4–6 months an intruded primary incisor should be removed to minimize eruptive problems in the permanent dentition. An adult periapical film used as an anterior occlusal is the easiest way to obtain a periapical view of the upper anterior region in a young child. James's radiograph did not reveal any root fractures or dentoalveolar fractures.

Vitality testing of primary teeth is not indicated.

Diagnosis

■ *What is your diagnosis?*

James has a palatal luxation injury to his upper left primary central incisor.

Treatment

■ *What are the three key components of the history and examination in primary tooth trauma that will dictate if active treatment is required?*

Pain. Either spontaneous or on eating suggests pathosis.

Mobility. Is the tooth a danger to the airway?

Occlusal interference. A luxation injury that has prevented normal intercuspal occlusion will prevent normal eating.

■ *What treatments are usually required for displaced primary incisors?*

Concussion and subluxation: observation.

Lateral luxation: if no occlusal interference, the tooth is allowed to reposition spontaneously; if occlusal interference – extract.

Intrusion: if the apex is displaced toward the labial bone plate, then leave for spontaneous repositioning. If no movement within 4–6 months, extract. If the apex is displaced into the developing tooth germ, extract.

Extrusion: extract or reposition if only a minor extrusion.

Avulsion: replantation is not indicated.

Key point

Traumatized primary teeth may need to be extracted if:
- Pain interrupts eating or sleeping.
- Excessive mobility causes a danger to the airway.
- There is occlusal interference.

■ *What radiographs would you take for these displacement injuries?*

Concussion and subluxation: periapical.

Lateral luxation: occlusal view shows increased periodontal space apically.

Intrusion: periapical and extraoral lateral.

Extrusion: periapical.

Avulsion: periapical to ensure that missing tooth is not intruded.

■ *What are you going to tell James's mother about the risk to the permanent teeth?*

The reported incidence of damage to the developing permanent teeth as a result of trauma to primary incisors ranges from 17% to 64%. An easily remembered figure to tell all parents at the time of the initial presentation would be 50%. It is better to be pessimistic and then be pleasantly surprised on eruption of the permanent teeth rather than the opposite.

■ *What are the possible effects on the permanent successor teeth?*

- White or yellow-brown discoloration of enamel (hypomineralization).
- Enamel hypoplasia.
- Crown dilaceration.
- Crown-root dilaceration.
- Root dilaceration.
- Odontome formation.
- Partial/complete arrest of root formation.
- Sequestration of permanent tooth germ.
- Disturbance in eruption.

■ *Can you tell all of these sequelae on a periapical radiograph?*

No. Only structural abnormalities and abnormal root growth will be visible. White and brown areas of hypomineralization will only be evident on eruption of the permanent teeth.

■ *If you retain a luxated primary tooth how often would you review it?*

One week after the injury, 1 month, then 3-monthly.

How would you review it?

Historically: symptoms.

Clinically: colour, sinus, tenderness.

Radiographically: 6-monthly for one year and then when clinically indicated.

Key point

After primary tooth trauma:

- Damage to permanent teeth may occur in 50% of cases.
- Intrusive trauma causes most permanent tooth damage.

Does a discoloured primary incisor always need treatment?

When there is progressive worsening of discoloration then the tooth will be non-vital. When there is a grey discoloration that does not get worse then vitality may be maintained. In the absence of periapical pathosis a discoloured primary incisor can be reviewed. In the presence of pathosis extraction or root canal therapy with zinc oxide paste is indicated (**Fig. 28.2**).

Recommended reading

Curzon MEJ (ed) 1999 Handbook of dental trauma. Wright, Oxford.

Roberts G, Longhurst P 1996 Oral and dental trauma in children and adolescents. Oxford University Press, Oxford.

Fig. 28.2 Endodontically treated primary incisor.

Welbury RR, Whitworth JM 2005 Traumatic injuries to the teeth. In: Welbury RR, Duggal MS, Hosey MT (eds) Paediatric Dentistry, 3rd edn. Oxford University Press, Oxford.

For revision, see Mind Map 28, page 190.

The fractured immature permanent incisor crown

SUMMARY

Shay is 8 years old. While saving a penalty for his school team he collided with the goalpost and sustained enamel-dentine-pulp and enamel-dentine fractures to his upper central incisors. How would you manage the injuries? Outline a follow-up treatment plan.

History

Complaint

The upper right and left permanent central incisors are fractured (**Fig. 29.1**).

History of complaint

The injury was sustained during a game of soccer. There were no other injuries.

Medical history

Shay is a healthy boy with no history of illness. He has had all his vaccinations including a pre-school booster for tetanus.

Dental history

Shay is a regular attender at his dentist and has had local anaesthetic for a restoration.

Fig. 29.1 Trauma to the central incisors.

■ *What specific questions would you ask and why?*

Was there any loss of consciousness?

Was the fractured piece of tooth located?

A history of loss of consciousness together with a missing tooth fragment is an indication for a chest radiograph to check that there has not been inhalation of the tooth fragment.

When did the injury occur?

The time from the injury to presentation may affect the treatment options.

Did Shay cope well with his previous experience of local anaesthetic? The answer to this will dictate what treatment strategies will be possible.

Examination

Extraoral

■ *Why is the presence of lip swelling together with a mucosal laceration important?*

This could indicate that the missing tooth fragment is retained in the lip.

■ *How would you demonstrate there was a fragment of tooth in the lip?*

By soft tissue radiography using two views at right angles to each other. A simple anteroposterior view using a periapical film placed behind the lip and in front of the teeth, followed by a lateral soft tissue view using a lateral occlusal film (**Fig. 29.2**). Clinically, a fragment of tooth is often best located by 'feel' with a probe.

Key point

Missing tooth fragments could:
- Be within the soft tissues if there is a laceration.
- Have been inhaled if there was loss of consciousness.

Fig. 29.2 Fragments of tooth in lower lip (different case).

Intraoral

■ *What injuries are visible in* Figure 29.1*?*

There is an enamel-dentine fracture of |1 and an enamel-dentine-pulp fracture of 1| of greater than 1 mm in diameter.

■ *Are the roots of 1| and |1 likely to have open or closed apices?*

Open. Apices are not usually closed on upper permanent central incisors before the age of 11 years.

■ *How would you confirm apical status?*

Periapical radiograph.

■ *What other injuries must you exclude on the periapical radiograph?*

Root fractures.

■ *What other features of the anterior teeth are important at examination?*

Mobility. In a buccopalatal direction. Excessive mobility suggests either a periodontal ligament injury or a root fracture.

Colour. This will indicate whether any direct pulpal damage causing haemorrhage into the dentinal tubules has occurred.

Percussion. Tenderness suggests periapical damage and oedema. A dull note may suggest a clinically undiagnosed vertical crown fracture or root fracture.

Vitality. Following trauma there may be a period of apparent loss of vitality on testing with hot and cold stimuli or the electric pulp tester even in teeth without obvious crown fractures. Nevertheless, the readings serve as a baseline against which subsequent tests can be compared.

■ *What teeth should be examined after trauma affecting only the upper centrals?*

All upper and lower incisors should be included in an examination after any trauma to the anterior region.

Investigations

* *Radiographs* (previously mentioned) for:
  — Foreign body in soft tissues if applicable.
  — Apical status of teeth.
  — Presence or absence of root fractures.
* *Vitality testing* of all upper and lower incisors.

Treatment

■ *What is the prime consideration for both the upper central incisors?*

To maintain vital pulp within the root, which will allow physiological dentine deposition. This will result in full root growth with normal dentinal wall thickness, which will not be prone to fracture.

■ *What is the appropriate immediate treatment for |1 (that has an enamel-dentine fracture)?*

Reattachment of the fragment.

or

A bonded restoration/'bandage', which will produce a hermetic seal. Glass ionomer cement is not an adequate material for a 'bandage' and will fracture or be lost resulting in thermal damage to the pulp from hot and cold stimuli. A layer of setting calcium hydroxide cement should be placed over dentine where a pulpal shadow is visible prior to placement of an adhesive bandage.

■ *What are the treatment options for 1| (that has a pulpal exposure)?*

* Direct pulp capping.
* Complete pulpotomy.
* Partial pulpotomy.

Direct pulp capping, the placement of wound dressings on an exposed pulp, is considered very unpredictable by many authors. Partial pulpotomy (subtotal or Cvek) is the removal of only the outer layer of damaged and hyperaemic tissue in the exposed pulps and will also allow continued full root growth. Partial pulpotomy is a highly successful technique. Complete pulpotomy (cervical pulpotomy) is the removal of coronal pulp tissue and the placement of a wound dressing on the canal orifice. Complete pulpotomy will arrest dentine formation in the pulp chamber but allow full root growth. Complete endodontic treatment will then only be necessary in the future if the root canal is required for retention of a coronal restoration.

■ *What are the indications for permanent tooth pulpotomy?*

No history of spontaneous pain.

Acute minor pain that subsides with analgesics.

No discomfort to percussion, no sulcus swelling, no mobility.

Radiographic examination shows normal periodontal ligament.

Pulp is exposed during caries removal or subsequent to recent trauma.

Tissue appears vital.

Bleeding from the pulp excision site stops with isotonic saline irrigation within 2 minutes.

■ *How would you carry out a pulpotomy?*

Local analgesia and rubber dam. Flush exposed pulp tissue initially with isotonic saline. Then excise a 2 mm superficial layer of exposed pulp and surrounding dentine with a high speed diamond bur using a light touch under water spray cooling (partial pulpotomy). Irrigate the surface of remaining pulp with isotonic saline. If bleeding ceases then dry carefully with a dry sterile cotton pellet prior to applying a pulpal medicament with biologically available calcium hydroxide and seal coronal cavity with a bonded restoration. However, if there is either no bleeding at all or the bleeding does not cease then the remaining pulp tissue within the pulp chamber should be removed with a sharp excavator (coronal pulpotomy). Irrigate, dry and reassess. If healthy bleeding occurs which ceases then cover with a medicament as above. However, if after a coronal pulpotomy there is still either no bleeding at all or the bleeding does not cease, the remaining pulp tissue should be removed (pulpectomy).

Fig. 29.3 Fragments found at scene of incident.

Fig. 29.4 Fragments reattached.

The time from injury to presentation for treatment has been reported to be important with regard to the success of partial pulpotomy, with treatment within 24 hours giving the best results. However, proper treatment of pulp tissue and careful case selection are likely to be the key issues for a good outcome. Pulp tissue compromised by infection and inflammation must be removed to facilitate physiological haemostasis during saline irrigation. The larger and the deeper an access cavity needs to be to reach healthy tissue, the more likelihood there is of widespread infection and thus suggests a likely clinical contraindication to vital pulp therapy.

■ *How should the crown of 1| be restored?*

If the crown fragment has been retrieved then this can be stored in normal saline while the partial (subtotal) pulpotomy is completed. The fragment can then be reattached.

If the crown fragment is not available or the fracture extends significantly subgingivally, a bonded composite restoration should be provided.

Figures 29.3 and **29.4** show the crown fragments before and after reattachment in Shay's case. 1| had a partial pulpotomy as described.

■ *How should the upper centrals be reviewed and how often?*

Definitive crown morphology should be restored as soon as possible after emergency treatment to re-establish normal sagittal relations with the lower incisors.

One-, 3-, and then 6-monthly clinical and radiographic examinations should be done to check for continued vitality and normal root growth. If there is evidence of non-vitality then the immature tooth must be extirpated and non-setting calcium hydroxide used to stimulate root end closure prior to obturation with gutta percha.

Key point

Partial or complete pulpotomy:

- Has a high success rate.
- Is more successful if completed within 24 hours of an injury.
- Allows full root growth with a vital radicular pulp.

Recommended reading

Curzon MEJ (ed) 1999 Handbook of dental trauma. Wright, Oxford.

Roberts G, Longhurst P 1996 Oral and dental trauma in children and adolescents. Oxford University Press, Oxford.

Welbury RR, Whitworth JM 2005 Traumatic injuries to the teeth. In: Welbury RR, Duggal MS, Hosey MT (eds) Paediatric Dentistry, 3rd edn. Oxford University Press, Oxford.

For revision, see Mind Map 29, page 191.

The fractured permanent incisor root

SUMMARY

Andrea is 12 years old. She was trampolining at school when she fell and sustained middle third root fractures of 1⌋ and ⌊1. How do you manage this type of injury, and what do you advise her about the long-term prognosis for those teeth?

History

Complaint

Andrea is brought to your surgery by a schoolteacher. She is complaining that her upper permanent central incisors are loose and feel 'funny' when she bites together.

History of complaint

Andrea fell forward while on the trampoline at school and hit her teeth on the edge of the trampoline. Her mother arrives at the surgery soon after Andrea and her teacher. It appears Andrea was not being supervised on the trampoline and the foam protection was not in the correct position on the metal frame of the trampoline. Her mother is not very happy with the explanation by the teacher.

■ *What does this alert you to?*

The possibility of legal action against the school. It is especially important to make drawings of any external injuries on the face and keep accurate records of intraoral injuries and subsequent treatment. A photographic record will be an advantage.

Medical history

Andrea is under regular care with her dentist and has had local anaesthetic without problem.

■ *What specific questions would you ask and why?*

Was there any loss of consciousness? If there was, then Andrea should be referred to an accident and emergency department.

Is there any pain or discomfort while opening and closing the jaw? Absence of symptoms should rule out any condylar injury/fracture. When the force that produces an injury

is significant then it should raise suspicion of a deeper underlying bony injury. Bony injury would be more likely in Andrea's case compared to the scenario of root fractures on teeth that had been produced by less force.

Examination

Extraoral

There is some swelling of the upper lip and some bruising and swelling under the right eye.

■ *What questions and examination would you complete regarding the swelling and bruising under the right eye?*

Is there any double vision? Palpate the infraorbital margin for 'stepping' and then check for altered sensation over the distribution of the infraorbital nerve. Check that there is a full range of eye movements – especially upward gaze. Fracture of the infraorbital margin and infraorbital floor could lead to entrapment of the inferior oblique extraocular muscle preventing upward and outward movement of the globe of the eye.

Is there any altered sensation on the cheek? Oedema surrounding the infraorbital nerve or entrapment of the nerve in a fracture can result in paraesthesia.

If there is any doubt about a fracture then posteroanterior and occipitomental views will detect displacement of the infraorbital margin, and tomograms will detect orbital floor 'blow-out' fractures.

Intraoral

There is downward and palatal displacement of the crowns of 1⌋ and ⌊1, which are mobile. Centric occlusion is not possible because of the slightly palatal position of 1⌋ and ⌊1.

■ *What tests would you do prior to repositioning of the teeth?*

Radiographs. Intraoral periapicals (**Fig. 31.1**) or an anterior occlusal view are needed to diagnose root fractures compared to luxation injuries. The upper lateral incisors should also be checked for injury. Consideration should also be given to taking radiographs of the lower incisors, which may also have received either direct or indirect trauma. Where there is no significant displacement of the coronal portion of a tooth with a root fracture, then an anterior occlusal radiograph will often detect root fractures that may not be so evident on periapical views. These radiographs will serve as baseline views prior to repositioning.

Vitality tests of all upper and lower incisors.

Treatment

■ *What design of splint would you use for 1⌋, ⌊1? You have confirmed on radiography that they have middle third root fractures (Fig. 30.1).*

The splint should be flexible/functional and designed to have one sound abutment tooth on either side of the root-fractured teeth.

■ *How long should the splint be in place in root fractures?*

For 4 weeks in apical and middle third fractures until the majority of periodontal ligament fibres have healed. This

Fig. 30.1 Middle third root fractures.

time can be extended to 4 months in coronal third fractures. The old regimen of rigid splinting for root fractures has been shown to have no benefit. Rigid splinting was meant to give the fracture its best chance of a hard tissue union. Research has shown that hard tissue union is most likely to occur if there was little displacement at the time of the original injury rather than being a function of the type of splint employed. In other words, the larger the displacement at the fracture line at the time of the injury, the smaller the chance of a hard tissue union between the fracture ends after reduction and splinting.

■ *Do any forms of dentoalveolar injury need to be rigidly splinted?*

Only dentoalveolar fractures for a duration of 3–4 weeks. A rigid splint would involve two sound abutment teeth on either side of the injury. All other displacement injuries, root fractures and avulsions require flexible/functional splints.

> ### Key point
>
> Splinting in dentoalveolar trauma:
> * Flexible 2 weeks for avulsions.
> * Flexible 4 weeks for luxations and apical and middle third root fractures.
> * Flexible 4 months for coronal third root fractures.
> * Rigid 3–4 weeks for dentoalveolar fractures.

■ *Describe step by step your procedure for reduction and splinting Andrea's 1| and |1.*

Give topical and local anaesthesia labially and palatally.

While the local anaesthetic is taking effect, bend a section of 0.6 mm stainless steel wire to the shape of the upper labial segment to include the four incisor teeth.

Gently reposition 1|, |1 and hold these in approximate position with some red wax palatally, which extends over the incisal edges of 1|, |1.

Etch the labial surfaces of 2|, |2; wash, dry, place bonding resin and a spot of composite in the centre of the labial surface.

Place 0.6 mm wire into position on 2|, |2. Use a bonding brush to mould the composite already on the teeth over the wire. Add extra composite if required. Cure the composite.

Remove the wax and with a non-working hand, and bring 1|, |1 into an accurate position against the wire splint. Hold them in this position while etching, washing, bonding and adding composite with working hand. Cure the composite.

Smooth any rough areas with sandpaper discs.

■ *On removal of the splint how often would you review Andrea?*

After 1 month, then 3 months and then 6 monthly.

■ *What tests would you complete at each of these reviews?*

For all traumatized teeth, a regimen should be followed. If this is done in every case then omissions are less likely to be made.
* Clinical:
  — Colour (palatal surface best)
  — Buccal sulcus sensitivity to digital pressure
  — Sinus presence
  — Tenderness to percussion
  — Mobility
  — Sensibility testing.
* Radiography: long cone periapicals.

■ *Is sensibility testing accurate?*

No form of sensibility testing on its own is accurate. Electric pulp testing (EPT) is probably the most accurate but its real value lies in successive numerical readings with the same type of EPT. Numerical values can then be compared. In the future, the widespread use of Doppler in detecting blood flow in a traumatized tooth will inform all decisions regarding pulpal necrosis and the necessity for extirpation.

> ### Key point
>
> What types of healing occur in root fractures?
> * Hard tissue.
> * Connective tissue.
> * Osseous.

■ *What is the likely radiographic appearance at the fracture line if the coronal tooth portion becomes non-vital?*

There will be increasing widening and translucency between the fractured ends of root.

■ *If the coronal portion of an apical or middle third root fractured tooth became non-vital, how would you root treat the tooth?*

Extirpation to the fracture line.

Establish working length to fracture line.

Place non-setting calcium hydroxide 1 mm short of fracture line with aim of inducing barrier formation.

Change non-setting calcium hydroxide 3-monthly until barrier forms.

Fig. 30.3 Clinical appearance after 3 years.

Remove coronal fragment. Root treat apical fragment and cover with a mucoperiosteal flap. The width and height of the alveolus are thus retained for future implant placement. Prosthetic replacement required.

Remove all portions of tooth. Prosthetic replacement required. Future implant placement.

■ *Can root fractured teeth maintain vitality?*

Yes. The majority do so. **Figures 30.2** and **30.3** show Andrea's teeth 3 years after the original injury. The teeth maintained vitality and underwent progressive intracanal sclerosis. In addition the distal fragments are resorbing. Importantly, there has been no infection.

■ *Can root fractured teeth be moved orthodontically?*

Yes, but with caution. If there is not a hard tissue union between the fracture ends then the apical portion will remain static and only the coronal portion will move. Regular radiographic review will be necessary during any orthodontic treatment.

Recommended reading

Curzon MEJ (ed) 1999 Handbook of dental trauma. Wright, Oxford.

Roberts G, Longhurst P 1996 Oral and dental trauma in children and adolescents. Oxford University Press, Oxford.

Welbury RR, Whitworth JM 2005 Traumatic injuries to the teeth. In: Welbury RR, Duggal MS, Hosey MT (eds) Paediatric Dentistry, 3rd edn. Oxford University Press, Oxford.

For revision, see Mind Map 30, page 192.

Fig. 30.2 Radiographic appearance after 3 years.

Obturate with gutta percha to barrier.
Annual radiographic review.

■ *What happens to the apical fragment?*

In nearly all cases this will undergo intracanal sclerosis and will not need treatment. If there is infection of the apical fragment, it may require surgical removal. Root canal therapy across a root fracture is fraught with difficulty because of problems keeping the distal canal dry.

Is the prognosis good in coronal or gingival third root fractures?

No. Decisions need to be made early regarding options. Long-term stability and long-term retention of the whole tooth in these injuries is rare.

■ *What are the treatment options in coronal or gingival third root fractures?*

Retain crown temporarily with an endodontic post across the fracture line.

Remove coronal fragment. Root treat apical fragment and orthodontically extrude prior to post, core and crown placement.

31

The avulsed incisor

SUMMARY

Kathryn is 9 years old. She was playing with her friends at a brownie camp with a skipping rope, when the rope caught behind one of her upper central incisors and avulsed it. Her teacher has got the tooth. How would you manage this problem?

■ *Kathryn's teacher phones your surgery for advice. She has the tooth in a handkerchief. The accident occurred 10 minutes ago. What is your advice?*

- Check Kathryn has no other injuries, i.e. head injuries that require referral to an accident and emergency department.
- Check for any known medical history.
- Hold tooth by crown, wash gently under cold water to remove any debris for 10 seconds.
- Replant in socket ideally.
- Hold tooth in socket by biting on a handkerchief. Come to surgery.
- If replantation not possible, place tooth in either milk or normal saline (first aid box) and bring to surgery with Kathryn.

■ *The tooth is brought to the surgery in milk. How would you proceed?*

1. Check medical history. Heart defects, immunosuppression and a history of rheumatic fever are not reasons to deny replantation.
2. Place tooth in normal saline. Remove any foreign bodies. Check state of root development.
3. Give labial and palatal local anaesthesia.
4. Irrigate socket with normal saline.
5. Recontour labial plate with flat plastic instrument or Couplands elevator, if required.
6. Gently but firmly reposition avulsed tooth.
7. Bend a 0.6 mm stainless steel wire to include one tooth either side of avulsed tooth.
8. Follow guidelines in Chapter 30 for placement of the splint.
9. Prescribe chlorhexidine mouthwash and antibiotics. Amoxicillin 125 mg three times daily for 5 days is an appropriate antibiotic. If patient is allergic to amoxicillin, use erythromycin 125 mg four times daily for 5 days. Chlorhexidine 0.2% should be used twice daily to help normal oral hygiene.
10. Arrange a review appointment for 14 days.

■ *What factors are important when deciding whether root canal treatment is necessary in Kathryn's case?*

- Apical development.
- The time that the tooth was out of the mouth (extra-alveolar time).
- A tooth that has a mature apex will rarely undergo revascularization. The only tooth that has a chance of revascularization is the immature tooth with an open apex that is replanted within 30–45 minutes. All other teeth should be extirpated prior to splint removal at 7–10 days.

■ *What intracanal medicament should be placed in the extirpated tooth?*

There has been some in vitro work that has shown that if non-setting calcium hydroxide is inadvertently spun through the apex of a tooth with a damaged periodontal ligament (PDL), then instead of normal repair of PDL fibres there may be replacement resorption. With this in mind some authorities advocate that Ledermix/polyantibiotic paste should be the first dressing placed in root canals of teeth with PDL injuries if extirpation occurs within 14 days of the injury. However, other authorities claim that the above findings have never been shown to be a real risk in vivo and, therefore, place non-setting calcium hydroxide as the initial dressing to a calculated working length.

■ *What factors are important in predicting resorption?*

- Extra-alveolar dry time (EADT).
- Total extra-alveolar time (EAT).
- Recent research has shown that teeth with a dry time of greater than 5 minutes have a significantly increased risk of resorption. The two preferred storage media, milk and normal saline, are iso-osmolar and that is why they are recommended storage media. However, the PDL cannot retain vitality for long periods even in these media.

■ *What types of resorption are there?*

Surface: normally seen as blunting of tooth apices after application of excessive orthodontic forces or on the roots of upper lateral incisors as a result of canine tooth impaction. The teeth are usually vital in surface resorption.

External inflammatory: initiated in the PDL after traumatic injury. The surfaces of the roots have punched-out craters where multipotent PDL cells have become osteoclastic and started resorbing cementum and dentine. The walls of the root canal are intact. Exacerbated by a non-vital pulp.

Internal inflammatory: originating in the root canal. Usually due to inadequate mechanical and chemical debridement of a non-vital tooth.

Replacement: external replacement resorption is characterized by absence of the PDL and bone is fused to cementum and dentine. The tooth becomes part of bone and is constantly remodelled, resulting in progressive resorption of the root. In traumatology, external replacement resorption will inevitably follow external inflammatory resorption where there has been permanent damage to the PDL. Internal replacement resorption or progressive pulp canal obliteration or sclerosis is the response of a vital pulp to trauma.

Key point

Critical historical information in avulsion:
- EADT.
- EAT.
- Storage medium.

■ What is the treatment if inflammatory resorption occurs after trauma?

The only medicament we have that has the potential to stop the inflammatory resorption is non-setting calcium hydroxide. It is alkaline (pH 11–12), antibacterial and anti-inflammatory. It should be replaced within the root canal every 3–6 months, either until resorption has halted and a gutta percha root filling can be placed, or the tooth is lost as a result of progressive resorption.

Kathryn's |1 had an EADT of 10 minutes. Her tooth was then placed in milk and brought to the surgery prior to reimplantation. The total EAT was 1 hour 50 minutes. The tooth was extirpated prior to splint removal at 14 days and non-setting calcium hydroxide placed in the root canal (**Fig. 31.1**). A normal PDL re-formed and there was continued apexification and apical development as a result of 3-monthly changes in non-setting calcium hydroxide (**Fig. 31.2**). The tooth was subsequently obturated with gutta percha, and it should be retained as a functioning unit for life.

■ If resorption in |1 was progressive how would you plan for its ultimate loss?

Try to maintain |1 for as long as possible as its presence helps to maintain both the height and the width of the alveolus. This will be important in future prosthetic considerations.

Replace |1 with an immediate replacement denture when it is eventually lost. Maintain the denture until upper canines have erupted.

Resin-retained bridge to replace |1 until 18 years of age. Consideration for single osseo-integrated implant at age 18–20.

Key point

Types of resorption:
- Surface.
- Inflammatory – external and internal.
- Replacement – external and internal.

■ How does the EADT influence your treatment of the avulsed incisor?

Recent guidelines would suggest that 60 minutes is a critical time. If a tooth has been dry for less than 60 minutes then the PDL has potential to survive and conventional treatments should be followed including splinting for 14 days and elective extirpation prior to splint removal for all teeth except the tooth with an immature apex that has been out of the mouth for less than 30–45 minutes.

If a tooth has been kept dry for greater than 60 minutes then the following treatment should be instituted. If the apex is very immature then the tooth should not be reimplanted. In this circumstance the risks of ankylosis and resorption are high and the tooth will be lost quickly from the mouth. This is due to the high turnover rate of bone at this age. If the apex is mature then the PDL should be scraped off the root with a sharp excavator and the tooth immersed in 2.4% sodium fluoride solution, acidulated to pH 5.5 for 5 minutes prior to replantation if possible. The sodium fluoride solution will increase the resistance of the

Fig. 31.1 Pulp extirpation in replanted incisor.

Fig. 31.2 Root end closure achieved and normal periodontal ligament.

root to future resorption. In these cases where the PDL is removed prior to replantation, it is optional whether extirpation and obturation is done extraorally or once the tooth has been repositioned. Splinting after PDL removal should be for 4 weeks.

Recommended reading

Curzon MEJ (ed) 1999 Handbook of dental trauma. Wright, Oxford.

International Association for Dental Traumatology 2007 Guidelines for the management of traumatic dental injuries II. Avulsion of permanent teeth. Dent Traumatol 23:130–136.

Roberts G, Longhurst P 1996 Oral and dental trauma in children and adolescents. Oxford University Press, Oxford.

For revision, see Mind Map 31, page 193.

Poor quality first permanent molars

SUMMARY

Lisa is 9 years old. Her mother has brought her to your surgery because her new permanent teeth at the back of her mouth are brown and there are white and brown patches on her new incisors. What has caused these discolorations? How may they be treated?

History

Lisa has complained that for the past few months the teeth have been painful on eating hot and cold foods. The pain is of 1–2 minutes' duration. Toothbrushing also has caused sensitivity at the back of the mouth. There has been no pain on biting and eating foods. Very recently Lisa felt that one of the back teeth especially has started to crumble. Her mother has also noticed this when she has helped with brushing.

Lisa has not required any analgesics for the discomfort caused by her teeth.

Medical history

Lisa is a healthy child who has never been in hospital.

Dental history

Lisa and her family are regular dental attenders. The family all have a low caries risk. Lisa has no restorations in her primary dentition. She used a children's toothpaste (500 ppm) until recently and is now using the same adult toothpaste as her parents (1450 ppm).

Examination

Intraoral examination revealed that all four first permanent molars (FPMs) were hypomineralized with areas of brown, rough enamel. In addition there were areas of hypoplasia where the enamel had chipped away, exposing the underlying dentine. The maxillary molars were the worst affected by hypoplasia. 6| had a large amalgam restoration. In addition some white and brown hypomineralized areas were visible on the labial surfaces of the newly erupted upper and lower permanent central incisors (**Figs 32.1** and **32.2**).

'Hypomineralized' is the name given to enamel when it has a reduced mineral content.

'Hypoplasia' is the name applied when there is a reduced thickness of enamel.

Upper and lower arches were uncrowded. Space assessed from the distal of 2's to mesial of 6's in each quadrant was 21.5 mm in the lower arch and 22 mm in each upper arch quadrant. On average, 21 mm and 22 mm are required for these distances in the lower and upper arches, respectively. The incisor relationship was just Class I on 1|1; the molar relationship was Class I bilaterally.

■ *Do you think that the enamel hypomineralization and hypoplasia noted on the first permanent molars and the permanent incisors follows a chronological pattern? If so, at what time was the affected enamel formed?*

Yes, it is possible that there is a chronological pattern. The cusp tips of the first permanent molars begin mineralizing from the eighth month of pregnancy. The cusp tips of the incisors and cuspids (canines) from about 3 months of age (the upper lateral incisor slightly later at 10–12 months). Mineralization dates for the permanent dentition are given in **Table 32.1**.

Key point

Mineralization of FPM commences around birth.

Fig. 32.1 Hypomineralized and hypoplastic upper first permanent molars.

Fig. 32.2 Hypomineralized upper and lower permanent incisors.

Table 32.1 Mineralization times for the permanent dentition

Tooth	Mineralization begins (months)
Upper	
Central incisor	3–4
Lateral incisor	10–12
Canine	4–5
First premolar	18–21
Second premolar	24–27
First molar	At birth
Second molar	30–36
Third molar	84–108
Lower	
Central incisor	3–4
Lateral incisor	3–4
Canine	4–5
First premolar	21–24
Second premolar	27–30
First molar	At birth
Second molar	30–36
Third molar	96–120

■ *What specific questions would you like to ask Lisa's mother?*

Pre-natal. Mother's health during pregnancy. Were there any concerns such as high blood pressure and proteinuria – pre-eclampsia?

Peri-natal. Difficult birth. Was the delivery prolonged? Was there a need for assisted delivery by forceps, ventouse or caesarean? All of these could indicate fetal distress.

Post-natal. Did Lisa spend any time in the special care baby unit (SCBU)?

Illnesses in the first 2 years of life, e.g. meningitis, measles, respiratory infections, chickenpox. These disturbances may manifest as enamel defects distributed in the enamel that was forming around birth and in the first 2 years of life.

Further questioning revealed that Lisa was born after a normal pregnancy and delivery but had a significant number of respiratory infections during the first year of life. This confirms your diagnosis of chronological hypoplasia. The correct name for this condition is molar incisor hypomineralization (MIH).

■ *What other differential diagnoses might you consider?*

- *Caries.* Newly erupted teeth are particularly prone to dental caries until their enamel maturation is complete. However, it seems very unlikely, even in the presence of particularly deep fissures, that Lisa, who has no caries in her primary teeth, should develop such caries in her permanent teeth. In addition the overall colour of the permanent molars is not consistent with caries in a tooth of normal morphology. The exposed dentine is slightly softened and does have caries but the overall pattern of destruction of the tooth suggests that caries is secondary to some other predisposing factor such as hypomineralization/hypoplasia. Another factor to consider that is against a diagnosis of caries is the white hypomineralized areas on the incisors. They are neither

the shape nor the distribution of white spot or precarious lesions that one would expect with poor oral hygiene.

- *Amelogenesis imperfecta.* Although the presenting features could be a hypomature form of amelogenesis imperfecta, there are several factors that suggest this is not the case: there is no family history; the primary dentition is not affected; the pattern of the defects is chronological. All of these combined make an inherited abnormality unlikely.

- *Fluorosis.* The defects on the molar teeth could only occur if there was a history of very high endemic fluoride levels, probably in excess of 6 ppm. Such levels do not occur in the UK. Mild fluorosis is seen where children have swallowed toothpaste or have been given supplementation in addition to swallowing toothpaste. However, in such cases there are usually fine opaque white lines following the perikymata and small irregular enamel opacities or flecks that merge into the background enamel colour. Fluorosis does not produce well-demarcated opacities like those seen on the incisors.

Key point

In patients with MIH, your questioning should include:
- Pre-natal period.
- Natal period.
- Post-natal period.
- Systemic illnesses in first 2 years of life.

■ *Is pain from such molar teeth common?*

Yes. There is evidence that these teeth have 5–10 times greater treatment need than normal teeth and are more difficult to anaesthetize. A palatal as well as a buccal infiltration is often required. There is also evidence that children with HFPMs have more behaviour management problems than other children, necessitating adjuncts to treatment such as sedation. In recent years, the prevalence of HFPMs in Europe has been shown to be between 10% and 20% (**Table 32.2**).

Table 32.2 Prevalence of hypomineralized first permanent molars in European studies

Country	Prevalence (%)	Age of children (years)	Year of publication
Finland	19.3	7–13	2001
The Netherlands	10	11	2000
Sweden	15.4	8–16	1987
Sweden	18.5	7–8	2001
UK	14.5	7	2002
Greece	10.2	5.5–12	2008

The histology of extracted HFPMs shows that the yellow/brown areas are more porous and occupy the whole enamel layer. The white/cream areas occupy the inner parts of enamel. The affected areas have a higher carbon, and lower calcium and phosphate content.

Investigations

■ *What investigations are indicated and why?*

Intraoral radiographs are indicated in order to assess the proximity of the coronal defects to the dental pulp. A *panoramic tomogram* is necessary to ascertain the presence and stage of development of the remaining permanent dentition in view of the poor long-term prognosis of the first permanent molars.

A panoramic tomogram revealed all permanent teeth, including third molars, to be present. The furcation of 7's was calcifying. Secondary caries was evident in all first permanent molars but was most pronounced in $\frac{6\ |\ 6}{\ |\ 6}$.

Treatment

■ *What are the main clinical problems in this case?*

Loss of tooth substance: breakdown of enamel tooth wear secondary caries.

Sensitivity.

Appearance.

Key point

Children with MIH:

- Have a higher treatment need.
- Have significantly higher behaviour management problems.

■ *What are the treatment options for the HFPMs in this case?*

Composite/glass ionomer cement (GIC) restorations.

Stainless steel crowns.

Adhesively retained copings.

Extraction.

Composite/GIC restorations

These can be definitive restorations when the area of hypomineralization does not involve a cusp, or temporizing restorations. It is important when restoring these teeth that all the hypomineralized area is removed.

Stainless steel crowns

These are the most durable restoration and can maintain a tooth until a permanent crown can be placed in the teenage years, or until a planned extraction.

Adhesively retained copings

These may be suitable for teeth that are not significantly affected by hypomineralization. When the defect has been removed and replaced by GIC, a coping can be placed on top of the restoration and covering the remainder of the occlusal and cuspal surface.

Extraction

This is the preferred treatment option because:

- HFPMs are of poor long-term prognosis. Although full coverage coronal restorations could be undertaken to retain them, this is an ambitious plan in a 9-year-old child. The restorations undoubtedly would require replacement at some future date due to possible microleakage at the margins and caries. This would incur additional inconvenience and expense to the patient.
- It is the optimal developmental stage to remove $\overline{6}$'s as the furcation of $\overline{7}$'s is calcifying and bodily movement of $\overline{7}$ forward will be encouraged. Timing of $\overline{6}$ removal is more critical than that of $\underline{6}$ as the mesial drift tendency is greater in the upper arch.
- Third molars are also developing and should erupt eventually if the 7's migrate forward to occupy the position of the 6's (**Fig. 32.3**).
- As the molar relationship is Class I bilaterally, removal of $\overline{6}$'s necessitates the removal of $\underline{6}$'s to encourage maintenance of the buccal segment relationship. This is known as compensating (removal of the equivalent opposing tooth) extractions.

Key point

- Ensure all permanent teeth, especially 5's and 8's, are present radiographically before considering FPM extraction.
- Timing of extraction of $\overline{6}$ is more critical than that of $\underline{6}$.
- Consider balancing and/or compensating extractions in patients with FPMs.

Fig. 32.3 (A) Dental panoramic tomogram before removal of all first permanent molars.

Fig. 32.3 (B) Dental panoramic tomogram following removal of all first permanent molars.

■ *What are the treatment options for the incisors in this case?*

Microabrasion.

Localized composite restoration.

Full composite veneer.

Controlled enamel microabrasion may produce a more acceptable result without removing the white areas. This is because the surface enamel layer after microabrasion is relatively prismless and well compacted. The optical properties are changed and a white area may become less perceptible. The technique should not be used if there is a reduced thickness of enamel.

Localized composites can give very acceptable results but are destructive of enamel and may weaken the tooth structure if large areas are removed.

Full composite veneers with a thin layer of a relatively opaque composite may produce an acceptable result without any or very little enamel reduction.

Recommended reading

Beentjes VEVM, Weerheijm KL, Groen HI 2002 Factors involved in the aetiology of molar–incisor hypomineralisation (MIH). Eur J Paediatr Dent 1:9–13.

Jalevik B, Klingberg GA 2002 Dental treatment, dental fear and behaviour management problems in children with severe enamel hypomineralisation of their permanent first molars. Int J Paediatr Dent 12:24–32.

Mackie IC, Blinkhorn AS, Davies PHJ 1989 The extraction of permanent first molars during the mixed dentition period – a guide to treatment planning. J Paediatr Dent 5:85–92.

Zagdwon AM, Toumba KJ, Curzon MEJ 2002 The prevalence of developmental defects in permanent molars in a group of English schoolchildren. Eur J Paediatr Dent 3:91–96.

For revision, see Mind Map 32, page 194.

Tooth discoloration, hypomineralization and hypoplasia

Case 1

SUMMARY

Simon is 8 years old. He has been brought to your surgery by his mother because his teeth are very dark and he is being teased at school. How would you determine the origin of the discoloration?

History

Simon says that the colour of his permanent teeth has remained the same since they erupted (**Fig. 33.1**).

■ *What other questions do you need to ask about the teeth?*

- Do they chip or wear?
- Was the primary dentition affected?
- Has anyone else in the family got, or had, similar teeth?

Positive answers to these questions may suggest an inherited abnormality of the teeth such as amelogenesis or dentinogenesis imperfecta.

■ *Have you also noticed that he has gingival overgrowth?*

Medical history

■ *What specific questions do you need to ask his mother with regard to potential causes of discoloration?*

The pregnancy The health of Simon's mother during her pregnancy and Simon's health during the birth and delivery are important when considering the condition of the first permanent molars (FPMs). The FPMs were the only permanent teeth that had started to mineralize before birth (≈ eighth month of pregnancy). Conditions that may suggest some fetal distress and dysmineralization may be: raised maternal blood pressure; early admission to hospital; premature delivery; prolonged delivery; assisted delivery, e.g. forceps or ventouse, emergency caesarean section; admission to the special care baby unit (SCBU).

Childhood illnesses These may result in a 'chronological hypoplasia' affecting those parts of the teeth that were mineralizing at the time of the illness. Although 'chronological hypoplasia' usually involves some failure of development of enamel matrix giving obvious lines or ridges on the teeth, there may be milder forms that can only be felt with a probe and that present for care because they attract extrinsic stain.

Tablets or medications taken during childhood Tetracycline staining should not occur now in children who have been brought up in developed countries. It is still common in children from developing countries where tetracycline is still used because it is a very effective, cheap, broad-spectrum antibiotic. The only children who may still be affected in developed countries are those with cystic fibrosis who have developed multiple drug resistances as a result of recurrent respiratory infection.

Simon was born with primary biliary atresia. This resulted in progressive liver failure, increasing levels of circulating bilirubin and eventually a liver transplant at the age of 2.5 years. All the permanent teeth developing prior to the transplantation will have intrinsic discoloration as a result of the high circulating bilirubin. The primary dentition will be affected to a lesser extent as a result of staining in secondary dentine. He has gingival overgrowth as a result of immunosuppressive treatment with ciclosporin. **Figure 33.2** shows a photograph taken later at the age of 13. The newly erupted second permanent molars are entirely normal. These teeth started mineralizing about the age of 3 when there was a functioning new liver and normal levels of bilirubin.

Fig. 33.1 Intrinsic discoloration.

Fig. 33.2 Normal colour of second permanent molar.

Dental history

■ *What other lines of questioning do we need to explore if we are considering all the possible causes of intrinsic discoloration?*

■ *Was there a history of infection and/or extraction for decay of any of the primary teeth?*

Localized infection on primary teeth can cause localized abnormalities of enamel formation and mineralization of permanent teeth.

■ *Was there ever any trauma to the primary teeth?*

There is a 50% chance of enamel dysmineralization of permanent successor teeth after primary trauma. These will be localized anomalies.

■ *Fluoride history.*

A full history from birth including areas that the child has lived in, fluoride supplementation and brushing habits is required. Fluorosis will produce a systemic or chronological distribution affecting the teeth that were forming when excess fluoride was taken.

The important categories and questions for a history into intrinsic tooth discoloration and hypoplasia are shown in **Box 33.1**.

Box 33.1 Intrinsic tooth discoloration and hypoplasia

Maternal and neonatal history

- History of pregnancy – maternal problems.
- History of birth – caesarean, forceps, fetal distress.

Family history

- Is anyone in the family similarly affected.

Medical history

- Dates of prolonged illnesses, e.g. the childhood infections, haematological disorders, nutritional diseases etc.
- Medications taken.

Dental history

- Does the discoloration affect all the teeth or just a few teeth.
- Does the discoloration affect both primary and permanent dentitions.
- Has it got worse or did the teeth come through like it.
- History of abscesses of the primary dentition.
- Any pain from teeth.
- Are the teeth chipping or wearing away.

Trauma history

- Has the child any history of an accident to primary or permanent teeth.

Fluoride history

- Where has the child lived.
- History of fluoride supplements.
- Age at commencement of brushing.
- Amount and type of toothpaste.
- Toothpaste eating.

Examination

The important features to note about any intrinsic discoloration or hypoplasia are:

Is it generalized or localized?

Does it affect the primary and permanent dentitions?

■ *In the major categories for questioning shown in Box 33.1, which are likely to cause generalized discoloration and which are likely to cause localized discoloration?*

Generalized: medical; family; fluorosis.

Localized: pregnancy; dental; trauma.

Simon has generalized intrinsic discoloration as a result of biliary atresia causing increased levels of bilirubin.

■ *What is the only method of treatment that will help Simon's appearance?*

Veneering. Composite veneers should be provided until the age of 16 years when they can be replaced with porcelain veneers. Composite veneers may not mask the severe green stain unless opaquing agents are used. Porcelain veneers may be the only realistic alternative and can be provided at a younger age by using a smaller amount of enamel reduction and accepting a slightly thicker final tooth size.

The method of placement of composite veneers is covered in Chapter 34.

Key point

Lines of questioning in discoloration, hypomineralization and hypoplasia:

- Maternal.
- Trauma.
- Medical.
- Fluoride.
- Dental.
- Family.

■ *If a patient came to you with a single discoloured root-filled incisor, what form of treatment should you consider first?*

Non-vital bleaching: this technique has certain advantages, especially in the younger and adolescent patient:

Non-destructive of tooth tissue (already root filled).

No irritation to gingival health that can occur with veneers.

No change in contour of tooth that may make oral hygiene more difficult.

No laboratory assistance required.

The only contraindications to non-vital bleaching would be teeth that already have large composite restorations, teeth that have been stained due to placement of amalgam into an access cavity and poorly obturated teeth.

There are a number of bleaching products available now that can be applied intracoronally. Most of these will contain hydrogen peroxide. However, bleaching can be achieved with sodium perborate alone as the following technique describes.

Materials:

- Rubber dam.
- Glass ionomer cement.
- 37% phosphoric acid.
- Sodium perborate (Bocasan) powder: distilled water.

- Cotton wool.
- Glass ionomer cement.
- White gutta percha.
- Composite resin.

Technique:

1. Take preoperative periapical radiographs; these are essential to check there is an adequate root filling.

2. Clean the teeth with pumice and make a note of the shade of the discoloured tooth.

3. Place rubber dam, isolating the single tooth. Ensure adequate eye protection for the patient, operator and dental nurse.

4. Remove palatal restoration and pulp chamber restoration.

5. Remove root filling to the level of the dentogingival junction – you may need to use adult burs in a miniature contra-angle head.

6. Place 1 mm of glass ionomer cement over the gutta percha.

7. Freshen dentine with a round bur. Do not remove excessively.

8. Etch the pulp chamber with 37% phosphoric acid for 30–60 seconds, wash and dry – this will facilitate the ingress of the bleach.

9. Mix the sodium perborate into a thick paste. This should be done immediately before placement. Place into the tooth, either alone with a flat plastic instrument or on a cotton-wool pledget.

10. Place a dry piece of cotton wool over the perborate mixture.

11. Seal the cavity with glass ionomer cement or Intermediate Restorative Material cement.

12. Repeat the process at weekly intervals until the tooth is slightly overbleached.

13. Place non-setting calcium hydroxide into the pulp chamber for 2 weeks. Seal with glass ionomer cement.

14. Finally, restore the tooth with white gutta percha (to facilitate reopening the pulp chamber again, if necessary, at a later date) and composite resin.

If the colour of a tooth has not significantly improved after three changes of bleach then it is unlikely to do so, and further bleaching should be abandoned. Failure of a tooth to bleach could be due to inadequate removal of filling materials from the pulp chamber.

Slight overbleaching is desirable, but the patient should be instructed to attend the surgery before the next appointment if marked overbleaching has occurred.

Non-vital bleaching has a reputation of causing brittleness of the tooth. This is probably the result of previous injudicious removal of dentine (which only needs to be 'freshened' with a round bur), rather than a direct effect of the bleaching procedure itself.

This method of bleaching has been associated with the later occurrence of external cervical resorption. The exact mechanism of this association is unclear, but it is thought that the bleach diffuses through the dentinal tubules to set up an inflammatory reaction in the periodontal ligament around the cervical region of the tooth. In a small number of teeth there is a gap between enamel and cementum, and in these cases the above explanation is tenable. The purpose of the 1 mm layer of cement is to cover the openings of the dentinal tubules at the level where there may be a communication to the periodontal ligament. In the same way, non-setting calcium hydroxide is placed in the pulp chamber for 2 weeks prior to final restoration in order to eradicate any inflammation in the periodontal ligament that may have been initiated.

Clinical studies have demonstrated that regression can be expected with this technique. The longest study after 8 years gave a 21% failure rate. However, if white gutta percha has been placed within the pulp chamber then it is readily removed and the tooth easily rebleached.

Key point

Restorative techniques in discoloration:
- Microabrasion.
- Bleaching.
- Localized composite.
- Veneers.

Case 2

SUMMARY

Tony is 14 years old. He has come to your surgery because he is concerned by the colour of his teeth and his bad breath (Fig. 33.3).

History

He has noticed his teeth changing colour over the past year. His friends have also commented on his bad breath over this period of time.

The colour of the teeth in **Figure 33.3** is a result of extrinsic staining from chromogenic bacteria due to inadequate oral hygiene. The staining is classically in the gingival and cervical areas of the teeth.

■ *Are there any other causes of extrinsic staining?*

Food and drink. Tea, coffee and dishes such as curry can cause staining of the teeth. Most commonly this occurs in the gingival or cervical areas initially, but if oral hygiene is poor

Fig. 33.3 Extrinsic chromogenic staining.

Fig. 33.4 Extrinsic food staining.

then it can affect a significant part of the whole tooth surface (**Fig. 33.4**).

Arrested caries. This produces a brown stain as a result of chromogenic bacteria.

Medical condition. In biliary atresia and jaundice it is possible for bile pigments in the gingival crevicular fluid to cause extrinsic staining. This is yellow/green in colour.

Drugs. Ferrous sulphate in liquid iron preparations can result in black staining. Rifabutin, an antituberculous drug, is excreted in the crevicular fluid. This results in an orange-red staining.

Chlorhexidine mouthwash when used frequently can cause a brown-black staining.

All these extrinsic stains originate initially around the gingival or cervical area of the tooth but can progress to involve a significant amount of the tooth surface.

■ *How can you confirm your diagnosis of extrinsic discoloration?*

Extrinsic stains can be polished off. Carry out a prophylaxis.

■ *What additional clinical signs are there on* Figure 33.3 **to back up your diagnosis of chromogenic staining secondary to poor oral hygiene?**

Marginal gingivitis.

'White spot' demineralization lesions in the gingival third of the labial enamel are visible on the anterior teeth.

Treatment

■ *How would you treat Tony's bad breath?*

Encourage him. Remember teenagers don't take criticism well! Tell him that he is not alone and lots of 'busy' young people forget twice daily brushing.

Toothbrushing instruction utilizing disclosing tablets or disclosing solution. Brushing twice daily, after breakfast and before school, and then last thing at night with a 1500 ppm paste.

Show him the 'white spot' lesions. Explain that these will progress to decay if the brushing is not corrected.

Daily fluoride mouthwash 0.05% sodium fluoride to encourage enamel remineralization.

■ *What factors in children and adolescents are important in halitosis (bad breath)?*

Plaque index.

Bleeding sites in gingiva.

Food impaction.

Nasal infection.

Tonsillar and adenoidal infection.

Furred tongue especially posterior tongue.

■ *As well as improving his gingival health with improved toothbrushing, what else could be done with the toothbrush?*

Brushing the dorsum of his tongue! Alternative methods can be used to clean the surface of the tongue and various types of 'tongue scrapers' are available commercially. Very occasionally in a child or adolescent the origin of halitosis can be ulceration of oesophageal or gastric origin. If there are symptoms of this then a referral should be made.

Recommended reading

Kilpatrick NM, Welbury RR 2005 Advanced restorative dentistry. In: Welbury RR, Duggal MS, Hosey MT (eds) Paediatric Dentistry, 3rd edn. Oxford University Press, Oxford, pp 205–230.

Wray A, Welbury RR 2001 UK national guidelines in paediatric dentistry: treatment of intrinsic discoloration in permanent anterior teeth in children and adolescents. Int J Paediatr Dent 11:309–315.

For revision, see Mind Map 33, page 195.

Mottled teeth

SUMMARY

Sophie is 8 years old. Her main concern is that all her permanent teeth have white patches, especially the upper central incisors. She is getting teased at school because the upper centrals also have brown patches. What are the causes of the white patches? How may they be treated?

History

Sophie noticed that the permanent teeth came through with the white and brown patches (**Fig. 34.1**). They have not changed in appearance since eruption.

■ *What important questions would you now ask her mother?*

Were the primary teeth normal?

If the answer to this is yes then it is unlikely to be an inherited defect and more likely to have a systemic origin.

■ *Is anyone else in the family affected?*

Unless siblings are subjected to exactly the same systemic diseases and conditions it is likely that an affected sibling will indicate an inherited defect.

Sophie's primary teeth were normal and she had no siblings, but neither her mother's nor her father's family had anyone with a similar problem.

Fig. 34.1 Disfiguring fluorotic mottling affecting upper permanent central incisors.

■ *What childhood illnesses and infections did she have, and when?*

A chronological hypomineralization or hypoplasia would suggest a systemic origin. There were no significant illnesses.

■ *What is Sophie's fluoride history?*

This must include where she has lived, any history of supplements, type of toothpaste used, amount of toothpaste used, any history of eating toothpaste.

It transpired that Sophie had never received any supplements, nor used toothpaste excessively. However, she lived on a farm with its own 'well' water supply. This was subsequently analysed and was found to be over 1 ppm fluoride. The diagnosis was one of fluorosis.

■ *What is the distribution of the mottling that you can see in Figure 34.1?*

White and brown mottling of the incisal half of the labial surface of 1|1 and white mottling of the incisal third of the labial surface of 2|2.

■ *Do you know why the labial surfaces of the upper permanent central incisors are often more affected by mottling?*

Research has shown that these teeth are particularly susceptible to an excess ingestion of fluoride between 24 and 30 months of age.

Mild fluorosis gives a diffuse mottling that may manifest as diffuse lines or patches that merge into the background enamel. When the fluorosis becomes more severe the lines and patches coalesce to produce a confluent white surface. In very severe cases there is also pitting of the enamel. Well-defined or well-demarcated patches that do not follow a systemic or chronological distribution, or are localized, are not likely to be due to fluorosis.

■ *Which part of the enamel does mild fluorosis affect?*

The outer 200–300 μm.

■ *How can you use this knowledge to your advantage during your clinical examination?*

Look for areas of the dentition that are subject to erosion or attrition, e.g. the occlusal surfaces of the first permanent molars. If the mottled enamel has been removed on these surfaces then that confirms that the mottling is in the outer aspect of the enamel and the diagnosis is likely to be one of fluorosis.

Key point

History taking in suspected fluorosis:

- Fluoridated water in places of residence.
- Amount of paste and age brushing started.
- Supplements.
- 'Eating' toothpaste.

■ *In some cases of fluorosis there is, in addition to white mottling, some brown stain. What is the cause of the brown staining?*

This is usually due to extrinsic agents becoming incorporated into the more porous white mottled areas of enamel. The brown mottling tends to get worse with time.

■ *What treatment options for Sophie would you consider for fluorotic mottling?*

Microabrasion.

Composite veneers.

Microabrasion can be done in a variety of ways and is a controlled removal of the surface layer of enamel in order to improve discolorations that are limited to the outer enamel layer. It is not suitable for deep enamel or dentine discoloration. One of the most reliable methods that has been used extensively since 1986 is the hydrochloric acid (HCl)-pumice microabrasion technique. It is achieved by a combination of abrasion and erosion – the term 'abrosion' is sometimes used. In the clinical technique that will be described, no more than 100 μm of enamel is removed. Once completed the procedure should not be repeated again in the future. Too much enamel removal is potentially damaging to the pulp and cosmetically the underlying dentine colour will become more evident.

Indications:

- Fluorosis.
- Idiopathic speckling.
- Post-orthodontic treatment demineralization.
- Prior to veneer placement for well-demarcated stains.
- White/brown surface staining, e.g. secondary to primary predecessor infection or trauma (Turner's teeth).

Materials:

- Bicarbonate of soda/water.
- Copalite varnish/Vaseline.
- Fluoridated toothpaste.
- Non-acidulated fluoride (fluoride drops).
- Pumice.
- Rubber dam.
- Rubber prophylaxis cup.
- Sandpaper polishing discs.
- 18% hydrochloric acid.

Technique:

1. Perform pre-operative vitality tests, take radiographs and photographs.
2. Clean the teeth with pumice and water, wash and dry.
3. Isolate the teeth to be treated with rubber dam, and paint Copalite varnish around the necks of the dam (alternatively place Vaseline around the necks of the teeth under the rubber dam).
4. Place a mixture of sodium bicarbonate and water on the dam behind the teeth, as protection in case of spillage.
5. Mix 18% hydrochloric acid with pumice into a slurry and apply a small amount to the labial surface on either a rubber prophylaxis cup rotating slowly or a wooden stick rubbed over the surface for 5 seconds, before washing for 5 seconds directly into an aspirator tip. Repeat until the stain is reduced, up to a maximum of 10 × 5 seconds

Fig. 34.2 After acid pumice microabrasion.

applications per tooth. Any improvement that is going to occur will have done so by this time.

6. Apply the fluoride drops to the teeth for 3 minutes.
7. Remove the rubber dam.
8. Polish the teeth with the finest sandpaper discs.
9. Polish the teeth with fluoridated toothpaste for 1 minute.
10. Review in 1 month for vitality tests and clinical photographs (**Fig. 34.2**).
11. Review biannually, checking pulpal status.

Critical analysis of the effectiveness of the technique should not be made immediately but delayed for at least 1 month as the appearance of the teeth will continue to improve over this time. Experience has shown that brown mottling is removed more easily than white, but even where white mottling is incompletely removed it nevertheless becomes less perceptible. This phenomenon has been attributed to the relatively prismless layer of compacted surface enamel produced by the 'abrosion' technique, which alters the optical properties of the tooth surface.

Long-term studies of the technique have found no association with pulpal damage, increased caries susceptibility or significant prolonged thermal sensitivity. Patient compliance and satisfaction is good and any dissatisfaction is usually due to inadequate preoperative explanation. The technique is easy to perform for the operator and patient, and is not time consuming. Removal of any mottled area is permanent and achieved with an insignificant loss of surface enamel. Failure to improve appearance by the HCl–pumice microabrasion technique has no harmful effects but may make it easier to mask some lesions with veneers.

Key point

Microabrasion:

- Will improve surface defects, e.g. fluorosis.
- Will not improve deeper defects, e.g. amelogenesis imperfecta.

Figure 34.2 shows the appearance of Sophie's 1|1 1 month after HCl-pumice microabrasion.

■ *Has bleaching of teeth any part to play in the treatment of surface enamel discoloration?*

Yes, external vital bleaching has been used as an initial treatment for fluorotic mottling and as a secondary treatment for residual brown staining after microabrasion. It is, however, more usually associated with the bleaching of the yellow discoloration of ageing – so-called 'nightguard vital bleaching'. This technique involves the daily placement of carbamide peroxide gel into a custom-fitted tray of either the upper or the lower arch. As the name suggests it is carried out by the patient at home and is initially done on a daily basis.

Materials:

- Upper impression and working model.
- Soft mouthguard – avoiding the gingivae.
- 10% carbamide peroxide gel.

Technique:

1. Take an alginate impression of the arch to be treated and cast a working model in stone.
2. Relieve the labial surfaces of the teeth by about 0.5 mm and make a soft, pull-down, vacuum-formed splint as a mouthguard. The splint should be no more than 2 mm in thickness and should not cover the gingivae. It is only a vehicle for the bleaching gel and not intended to protect the gingivae.
3. Instruct the patient on how to floss the teeth thoroughly. Perform a full mouth prophylaxis and instruct them how to apply the gel into the mouthguard.
4. Note that the length of time the guard should be worn depends on the product used.
5. Review about 2 weeks later to check that the patient is not experiencing any sensitivity, and then at 6 weeks, by which time 80% of any colour change should have occurred.

Carbamide peroxide gel (10%) breaks down in the mouth into 3% hydrogen peroxide and 7% urea. Both urea and hydrogen peroxide have low molecular weights, which allow them to diffuse rapidly through enamel and dentine and thus explains the transient pulpal sensitivity occasionally experienced with home bleaching systems.

Pulpal histology with regard to these materials has not been assessed, but no clinical significance has been attributed to the changes seen with 35% hydrogen peroxide over 75 years of usage, except where teeth have been overheated or traumatized. By extrapolation, 3% hydrogen peroxide in the home systems should therefore be safe.

Although most carbamide peroxide materials contain trace amounts of phosphoric and citric acids as stabilizers and preservatives, no indication of etching or a significant change in the surface morphology of enamel has been demonstrated by scanning electron microscopy analysis. There was early concern that bleaching solutions with a low pH would cause demineralization of enamel when the pH fell below the 'critical' pH of 5.2–5.8. However, no evidence of this process has been noted to date in any clinical trials or laboratory tests, and this may be due to the urea (and subsequently the ammonia) and carbon dioxide released on degradation of the carbamide peroxide elevating the pH.

There is an initial decrease in bond strength of enamel to composite resin immediately after home bleaching but this returns to normal within 7 days. This effect has been attributed to the residual oxygen in the bleached tooth surface, which inhibits polymerization of the composite resin. The home bleaching systems do not affect the colour of restorative materials. Any perceived effect is probably due to superficial cleansing.

Minor ulceration or irritation may occur during the initial treatment. It is important to check that the mouthguard does not extend on to the gingivae and that the edges of the guard are smooth. If ulceration persists a decreased exposure time may be necessary. If there is still a problem then allergy is a possibility.

The exact mechanism of bleaching is unknown. Theories of oxidation, photo-oxidation and ion exchange have been suggested. Conversely, the cause of rediscoloration is also unknown. This may be a combination of chemical reduction of the oxidation products previously formed, marginal leakage of restorations allowing ingress of bacterial and chemical byproducts, and salivary or tissue fluid contamination via permeable tooth structure.

Dense fluorotic white plaques and some forms of hypomature amelogenesis imperfecta may be clinically indistinguishable. The microabrasion technique in this situation can be used as a diagnostic aid. Improvement in appearance would support the diagnosis of fluorosis, which affects the outer layer of enamel, whereas amelogenesis commonly affects the whole enamel layer.

Composite veneers may be required to mask dense white fluorotic plaques that are refractory to microabrasion. Most composite veneers placed in children and adolescents are the direct type fashioned at the chairside rather than the indirect or laboratory-made type.

Before proceeding with any veneering technique, the decision must be made whether to reduce the thickness of labial enamel before placing the veneer. Certain factors should be considered:

- Increased labiopalatal bulk makes it harder to maintain good oral hygiene. This may be courting disaster in the adolescent with a dubious oral hygiene technique.
- Composite resin has a better bond strength to enamel when the surface layer of 200–300 μm is removed.
- If a tooth is very discoloured some sort of reduction will be desirable, as a thicker layer of composite will be required to mask the intense stain.
- If a tooth is already instanding or rotated, its appearance can be enhanced by a thicker labial veneer.

New generation, highly polishable, hybrid composite resins can replace relatively large amounts of missing tooth tissue as well as being used in thin sections as a veneer. Combinations of shades can be used to simulate natural colour gradations and hues.

Indications for composite veneers:

- Discoloration.
- Enamel defects.
- Diastemata.
- Malpositioned teeth.
- Large restorations.

Contraindications:

- Insufficient available enamel for bonding.
- Oral habits, e.g. woodwind musicians.

Materials:

- Rubber dam/contoured matrix strips.
- Preparation and finishing burs.

- New generation, highly polishable, hybrid composite resin.
- Sof-Lex polishing discs and interproximal polishing strips.

Technique:

1. Use a tapered diamond bur to reduce labial enamel by 0.3–0.5 mm. Identify the finish line at the gingival margin and also mesially and distally just labial to the contact points.

2. Clean the tooth with a slurry of pumice in water. Wash and dry and select the shade.

3. Isolate the tooth either with rubber dam or a contoured matrix strip. Hold the latter in place by applying unfilled resin to its gingival side against the gingiva and curing for 10 seconds.

4. Etch the enamel for 60 seconds, wash and dry.

5. Where dentine is exposed, apply dentine primer.

6. Apply a thin layer of bonding resin to the labial surface and roughly shape it into all areas with a plastic instrument, then use a brush lubricated with unfilled resin to 'paddle' and smooth it into the desired shape. Cure for 60 seconds gingivally, 60 seconds mesio-incisally, 60 seconds disto-incisally, and 60 seconds from the palatal aspect if incisal coverage has been used. Different shades of composite can be combined to achieve good matches with adjacent teeth and a transition from a relatively dark gingival area to a lighter more translucent incisal region.

7. Flick away the unfilled resin holding the contour strip and remove the strip.

8. Finish the margins with diamond finishing burs and interproximal strips and the labial surface with graded sandpaper discs. Characterization should be added to improve light reflection properties.

The exact design of the composite veneer will depend on each clinical case, but will usually be one of four types: intra-enamel or window preparation; incisal bevel; over-lapped incisal edge; or feathered incisal edge.

Tooth preparation will not usually expose dentine, but this will be unavoidable in some cases of localized hypopla-sia or caries. Sound dentine may need to be covered by glass ionomer cement prior to placement of the composite veneer.

Recommended reading

Croll TP, Cavanaugh RR 1986 Enamel colour modification by controlled hydrochloric acid-pumice abrasion. I. Technique and examples. Quintessence Int 17:81–87.

Heywood VB, Heymann HO 1989 Nightguard vital bleaching. Quintessence Int 20:173–176.

Kilpatrick NM, Welbury RR 2005 Advanced restorative dentistry. In: Welbury RR, Duggal MS, Hosey MT (eds) Paediatric Dentistry, 3rd edn. Oxford University Press, Oxford, pp 205–230.

For revision, see Mind Map 34, page 196.

Dental erosion

SUMMARY

Tom is 9 years old. He is a new patient to your practice. On examination you are concerned by the appearance of the occlusal surfaces of his lower primary molars. What has caused this and how may it be managed?

■ *What do you see (Fig. 35.1)?*

There is erosion of the cusps of Tom's primary molars giving cupping or perimolysis of the cusps with loss of enamel and visible underlying dentine.

■ *How would you define erosion?*

An irreversible loss of tooth substance brought about by a chemical process that does not involve bacterial action.

■ *What foods and drinks have erosive potential?*

See **Box 35.1**. While a wide range of food and drinks is implicated in the problem, the bulk of the damage is done by soft drinks, especially carbonated drinks, which are increasingly available from vending machines in schools and recreational facilities. All carbonated drinks and fruit-based drinks have lowered pH values but the direct relationship between pH and erosion is unclear. Other factors such as titratable acidity, the influence of plaque pH and the

Fig. 35.1 Erosion of cusp tips of primary molars.

buffering capacity of saliva will all influence the erosive potential of a substrate. Three things, however, are clear with erosive loss:

- It is worse if consumption is high.
- It is worse if consumption occurs at bedtime.
- It is worse if brushing occurs directly after consumption.

Box 35.1 Foods and drinks with erosive potential

- Citrus fruits, e.g. lemons, oranges, grapefruits.
- Tart apples.
- Vinegar and pickles.
- Yoghurt.
- All fruit juices including fresh juice and fruit-based squashes.
- Carbonated drinks, including low-calorie varieties, 'sports drinks' and sparkling mineral water.
- Vitamin C tablets.

History

Tom's only complaint was occasional sensitivity on his back teeth as a result of the visible dentine.

■ *What is the best way to find out about Tom's diet?*

A 3- or 4-day written dietary history is the only way to accurately elucidate a constituent of the diet that may be erosive.

■ *Can the pattern of erosion caused by dietary constituents be related to the manner in which the substrate is consumed?*

This is indeed the case. 'Frothing' of a drink between the upper anterior teeth with its retention labially can lead to palatal, interproximal and labial erosion. Retention of a drink specifically on one side of the mouth can lead to erosion on that side only.

■ *You have covered Tom's dietary history. Is your history now complete or are there other questions you need to ask with relation to erosion?*

It is very important to consider gastric acid as a cause of erosion, even in a younger patient. The conditions in children that are associated with chronic regurgitation are shown in **Box 35.2**. The acidity of the stomach contents is below pH 1.0 and therefore any regurgitation or vomiting is damaging to the teeth.

Box 35.2 Conditions associated with chronic regurgitation in children

- Gastro-oesophageal reflux.
- Oesophageal stricture.
- Chronic respiratory disease, e.g. asthma.
- Disease of the liver/pancreas/biliary tree.
- Overfeeding.
- Feeding problems/failure to thrive conditions.
- Mental handicap.
- Cerebral palsy.
- Rumination.

What question would you ask to give you an indication that regurgitation was occurring?

'Do you ever have a bitter taste in your mouth?' There is a group of patients who have gastro-oesophageal reflux disease (GORD). This may be either symptomatic, in which the individual knows what provokes the reflux, or more insidiously, asymptomatic GORD, where the patient is unaware of the problem. The latter case is most likely to occur at night when the horizontal sleeping position makes it more likely that acid will reflux through the lower oesophageal sphincter. In this case the question about a bitter taste in the mouth should have the suffix 'when you wake up'.

What is the common pattern of erosive loss when there is chronic gastric regurgitation?

Initially there is erosion of the palatal surfaces of the upper incisors, canines and premolars. With time this extends to the occlusal and buccal surfaces of the lower molars and premolars.

Whenever there is unexplained erosive loss, an eating disorder should be suspected. There are three such disorders: anorexia nervosa; bulimia nervosa; and rumination. The latter is a condition in which food is voluntarily regurgitated into the oral cavity and either expelled or swallowed again.

Is there a specific pattern of erosive loss in recurrent vomiting?

All tooth surfaces can be affected with the relative exception of the lingual surfaces of the lower teeth, which are protected by the tongue and the saliva from the sublingual papillae.

What would you do if you suspect after questioning Tom and his parents that there may be asymptomatic GORD?

Referral to a paediatrician with an interest in gastrointestinal disease would be appropriate. The paediatrician will seek to eliminate organic disease and then attempt to quantify the problem. The latter may involve 24-hour pH monitoring of the oesophagus with probes in the lower and upper oesophagus. An additional probe could be added to an intraoral appliance to measure mouth pH. Medical and/or surgical treatment may be required to control GORD. Chronic regurgitation can lead to scarring of the oesophagus and dysplastic change, and this is therefore an important condition to diagnose and treat.

Summary of Tom's history

There was no evidence of any gastrointestinal illness but Tom did consume a number of fizzy drinks, especially between meals and when he was at the local sports centre. In addition to these he also drank water and milk.

What advice would you give to Tom regarding his high intake of fizzy drinks?

It is critically important when dealing with children and adolescents not to be too dogmatic in your advice and it is unrealistic to expect youngsters who have been brought up with a high intake of carbonated beverages to stop altogether.

They should be advised to eradicate between-meal fizzy drink consumption but to have the fizzy drink with meals and preferably to drink it with a straw. The presence of food, and the extra saliva that is generated at mealtimes, will help to neutralize the acidity. In addition, a straw will deposit the majority of the carbonated beverage beyond the teeth.

Make sure that the between-meal carbonated drink is not substituted by something with a similar erosive potential, e.g. fresh fruit juice or a juice-based squash.

Milk and water are the most appropriate between-meal drinks. If either of these proves impossible then an extremely well diluted 'no added sugar' squash can be accepted.

No carbonated drinks or fruit drinks should be given last thing at night.

Advocate the consumption of a neutral food immediately after a meal, e.g. cheese.

Management

The most important aspect of the management of Tom's erosion was early diagnosis before there had been damage to the permanent teeth, and subsequently to establish the aetiology and eliminate the cause.

Key point

Management of erosion:
- Early diagnosis.
- Establish aetiology.
- Eliminate cause.

Tom only has occasional sensitivity. What treatment, if any, does he need?

Probably none. The following would be realistic initially:

Daily neutral sodium fluoride mouthwash to try to give maximum resistance to remaining enamel and desensitize the dentine.

High concentration sodium fluoride varnish (Duraphat) to be applied three times a year.

If there is progressive sensitivity then the areas of enamel loss and dentine exposure could be protected by an adhesive restoration. In many cases if erosion is diagnosed early then preventive counselling and the above advice may be sufficient. It is a good idea to make study casts of all patients with signs of erosion or attrition or abrasion to monitor the rate of progression. In more advanced cases than Tom, as in **Figure 35.2A, B** where there is significant sensitivity or

Fig. 35.2 (A) Significant erosive tooth surface loss of labial surfaces of upper permanent incisors.

Fig. 35.2 (B) Significant erosive tooth surface loss of palatal surfaces of upper permanent incisors.

cosmetic problems, then more active intervention is required. **Table 35.1** shows the merits of the different options available.

Table 35.1 Treatment techniques for tooth surface loss

Technique	Advantages	Disadvantages
Cast metal (nickel/chrome or gold)	Fabricated in thin section – requires only 0.5 mm space	May be cosmetically unacceptable due to 'shine through' of metallic grey
	Very accurate fit possible	Cannot be simply repaired or added to intraorally
	Very durable	
	Suitable for posterior restorations in parafunction	
	Does not abrade opposing dentition	
Composite: direct	Least expensive	Technically difficult for palatal veneers
	Can be added to and repaired intraorally	Limited control over occlusal and interproximal contour
	Aesthetically superior to cast metal	Inadequate as a posterior restoration
Composite: indirect	Can be added to and repaired intraorally	Requires more space – minimum of 1.0 mm
	Aesthetically superior to cast metal	Unproven durability
	Control over occlusal contour and vertical dimension	
Porcelain	Best aesthetics	Potentially abrasive to opposing dentition
	Good abrasion resistance	Inferior marginal fit
	Well-tolerated by gingival tissues	Very brittle – has to be used in bulk section
		Hard to repair

Key point

Treatment objectives for erosion:
• Resolve sensitivity.
• Restore missing tooth surface.
• Prevent further tooth tissue loss.
• Maintain a balanced occlusion.

■ *Erosion is only one element of tooth surface loss or wear. What are the other elements?*

Attrition: the wear of the tooth as a result of tooth-to-tooth contact.

Abrasion: physical wear of tooth substance produced by something other than tooth-to-tooth contact.

In children, abrasion is usually due to overzealous toothbrushing, which tends to develop with increasing age. The abnormal brushing technique must be corrected before significant tooth tissue is removed and pulpal exposure occurs. Attrition caused by normal mastication is common especially with the ageing primary dentition. Almost all primary teeth show signs of attrition by the time they exfoliate.

■ *What categories of patient exhibit more attrition than normal?*

Those with significant parafunctional activity, e.g. cerebral palsy and other physical and developmental disorders with intracranial abnormalities. Controlling attritional wear in these patients can be very difficult. Some drugs act to try to reduce such parafunctional activity but even if this is successful in the limbs there is often still residual oral parafunction. This is probably due to the neuronal sensitivity of the mouth and the structures within it.

■ *What restorative materials are the most durable for attritional wear as a result of parafunction?*

Amalgam and stainless steel crowns.

Recommended reading

Kilpatrick NM, Welbury RR 2005 Advanced restorative dentistry. In: Welbury RR, Duggal MS, Hosey MT (eds) Paediatric Dentistry, 3rd edn. Oxford University Press, Oxford, pp 205–230.

Shaw L, O'Sullivan E 2000 UK National Clinical Guidelines in Paediatric Dentistry. Diagnosis and prevention of dental erosion in children. Int J Paediatr Dent 10:356–365.

For revision, see Mind Map 35, page 197.

36

Multiple missing and abnormally shaped teeth

Case 1

SUMMARY

Ellen is almost 11 years old. She is very concerned by the gaps between her upper and lower front teeth. She is hoping to become an actress. She is a new patient to your surgery and has been brought by her mother. What are the causes of the problem and how may it be treated?

History

Ellen is a regular attender with no caries. Her oral hygiene is excellent. There is no history of tooth extraction in either the primary or permanent dentitions.

Medical history

Ellen has no medical problems. She is an active girl who is involved in orienteering with her family as well as being in the local amateur dramatic society.

■ *What question do you need to ask Ellen's mother?*

Is there a family history of missing teeth or gaps?

As you are speaking to Ellen's mother you notice that she has a missing upper right lateral incisor and the canine tooth is prominent. She confirms your question that not only has she got a missing tooth, but her brother and her nephew (son of her brother) have either missing or very small upper lateral incisors.

■ *How prevalent are missing teeth in the population?*

0.1–0.9% in the primary dentition.

3.5–6.5% in the permanent dentition (discounting third molars).

More common in females, than males (1.4–4x). The most common teeth to be absent are the last teeth in each series (i.e. lateral incisor, second premolar, third molar). The presence of a conical (peg) tooth is frequently associated with a missing tooth on the opposite side of the arch. There is frequently a family history.

■ *There are a significant number of syndromes of the head and neck that manifest with missing teeth. Can you name some?*

Ectodermal dysplasia.

Cleft lip and/or palate.

Down syndrome.

Chondro-ectodermal dysplasia (Ellis–van Creveld syndrome).

Reiger syndrome.

Incontinentia pigmenti.

Oro-facial-digital syndrome (types I and II).

Ectodermal dysplasia describes a group of inherited disorders involving ectodermally derived structures, i.e. hair, teeth, nails, skin and sweat glands. The most common form is the hypohidrotic X-linked form. The usual presentation is a male child with:

Multiple congenital absence of teeth.

Fine, sparse hair with shaft abnormalities.

Dry skin.

Frontal bossing.

Maxillary hypoplasia.

Thin lips showing little vermilion margin.

Heterozygous females can be identified dentally with microdontia and hypodontia.

Down syndrome affects 1 in 700 births and is commoner in offspring of older mothers, and is a result of chromosomal translocation. Apart from the morphological features characteristic of the syndrome, there is commonly delayed eruption and generalized microdontia as well as hypodontia of some teeth.

The diagnosis and management of all dental anomalies is extremely important and should not be delayed. Genetic consultation is often desirable to not only confirm the diagnosis but also to help parents understand the risk of future offspring and generations being affected. Conversely, geneticists may require help from paediatric dentists to clarify a diagnosis.

Key point

Hypodontia:

- Prevalence is 3.5–6.5% in permanent dentition (excepting third molar).
- May be associated with a number of syndromes.
- Requires multidisciplinary care.

■ *What factors would you consider important in the management of dental anomalies?*

Reassurance of child and parent.

Elimination of pain.

Genetic counselling.

Restoration of aesthetics.

Provision of adequate function.

Maintenance of vertical dimension of occlusion.

Interdisciplinary formulation of definitive treatment plan.

Examination

Extraoral

Ellen had a normal facial appearance with a Class 1 skeletal pattern.

Intraoral

The following teeth were present:

$$\frac{6\,e\,d\,c\,b\,1\ |\ 1\,b\,c\,d\,e\,6}{6a\ \ 321\ |\ 234\,e\,6}$$ d|d were mobile. The other

primary teeth were firm. The primary molars were infraoccluded.

■ *What special investigations are required?*

A dental panoramic tomogram (**Fig. 36.1**) to check on the present/absence of other permanent teeth.

■ *What is visible from the radiograph?*

Absence of: $\dfrac{8\,7\,5\,3\,2\ |\ 2\,3\,4\,5\,7\,8}{8\,7\,5\,4\ \ |\ 1\ \ \ \ \ \ 5\,7}$

■ *What is the condition known as?*

It is termed severe hypodontia.

■ *What would you do?*

Take impressions and a wax registration for study models. Arrange a joint consultation with paediatric dental/orthodontic/restorative colleagues.

■ *What treatment is likely to be required?*

- Attempt to retain the primary molars for as long as possible.
- Management of infraoccluded molars is dealt with in Chapter 8.
- Fixed appliance to close the upper median diastema; retain with a palatal bonded retainer.
- Assess mesio-distal width 1|1. Probable addition of composite to distal aspect of these teeth to achieve mesiodistal width of 8.5–9 mm.
- Poor prognosis b|b. As the spaces are of concern to Ellen, consider extraction of b|b and replacement with an upper partial denture with prosthetic 2|2.
- In adulthood there will be the option of implants to replace the missing maxillary and mandibular teeth.

Case 2

SUMMARY

Cameron was 3 years old when his mother brought him to the surgery because she was concerned that two of his teeth were joined together (Fig. 36.2). What is the cause and how may it be treated?

Medical and dental history

Cameron is an active child with no medical problems. He has no caries.

■ *What can you see in* Figure 36.2?

The crowns of the upper first and second primary incisors are joined.

A number of different terms have been used to describe the process of the formation of double teeth either on the primary or permanent dentitions: fusion, gemination, dichotomy, synodontia, schizodontia and connation. The mode of development given in older textbooks for the different names are unclear and unproven. The neutral term 'double teeth' is not contentious and describes accurately what the tooth looks like clinically.

■ *How prevalent do you think double teeth are?*

0.5–1.6% in primary dentition.

0.1–0.2% in permanent teeth.

No clear Mendelian trait established.

The clinical manifestation of the anomaly may vary considerably from a minor notch in the incisal edge of an abnormally wide incisor crown to the appearance of two separate crowns. There may be hard tissue continuity between either the crowns or the roots of the two elements or between both. Similarly there may be one unified pulp chamber and radicular pulp or separate ones.

In the primary dentition double teeth more commonly occur in the labial segments of the arches and most frequently in the mandible. Double permanent teeth can occur anywhere in the arch but are probably more frequent when involving incisors.

■ *What are the most important clinical aspects of a double tooth in the primary dentition?*

Fig. 36.1 Severe hypodontia (from Millett and Welbury (2000) with permission).

Fig. 36.2 Double incisor teeth.

Caries may occur in the 'join' between the two coronal elements if it is not easily accessible to a toothbrush.

The presence of a numerical abnormality of the permanent dentition.

Counting a double tooth as one unit in the primary dentition, with relation to the total number of teeth present, may be helpful in predicting the type of numerical abnormality of the permanent dentition. Hypodontia is usually followed by missing permanent teeth. A normal number of teeth in the primary dentition is often associated with permanent supernumeraries. The overall frequency of permanent numerical abnormalities following primary double teeth is between 30% and 50% in Caucasians and is 75% in the Japanese population.

Radiography is therefore important at an appropriate time, so the parent can be advised of future treatment and prognosis and a treatment plan formulated. Extraction of double primary teeth may be necessary if physiological root resorption is significantly retarded. Surgical removal of supernumerary teeth may be required to facilitate eruption of normal units.

> ## Key point
>
> Double primary teeth may:
> - Be associated with numerical abnormalities of the permanent dentition.
> - Be a caries risk.
> - Not undergo normal physiological resorption.

■ *What are the important factors that will dictate whether you retain or extract double permanent teeth?*

Space in the arch.

Aesthetics.

Morphology of pulp chambers and roots.

If the coronal parts of the double teeth are joined but the roots are separate, then it may be feasible to divide the crown and extract one portion of the crown and its root, thereby retaining the other portion of the crown with its root. The retained portion will require root canal treatment and subsequent coronal restoration.

■ *What other types of crown abnormality do you know?*

Accessory cusps.

Invaginations.

Evaginations.

Additional primary cusps are seen on the mesiobuccal aspect of maxillary first molars and the mesiopalatal aspect of maxillary second molars.

The commonest additional cusp in permanent teeth is often on the lingual cingulum, more commonly in the maxilla than the mandible. The name 'talon cusp' is often given to the additional cusp (**Fig. 36.3**). The cusp is composed of enamel, dentine and a horn of pulp tissue. Talons in maxillary anterior teeth such as that shown in **Figure 36.3** can cause a number of problems:

Fig. 36.3 Talon cusp.

Appearance.

Occlusal interference.

Caries in the deep grooves between the cusp and the tooth.

The commonest accessory cusp in the permanent dentition is the mesiopalatal sited tubercle of Carabelli on the maxillary first molar (10–60%).

■ *What are the treatment options for a talon cusp on a maxillary tooth?*

Selective grinding of cusp to encourage obliteration of the pulp horn by secondary dentine.

Aseptic removal of the cusp under rubber dam followed by a limited pulpotomy procedure (immature or mature root).

Aseptic removal of cusp and one-stage endodontic treatment (mature root).

Failure of a pulpotomy technique in an immature tooth will result in the need for induced apical closure with non-setting calcium hydroxide. Many clinicians favour waiting until full root formation has occurred prior to removal of the cusp. Invaginations or invagination of the enamel epithelium into the dental papilla of the underlying tooth germ has been described as 'dens in dente', 'gestant composite odontome' and 'dilated composite odontome'. The correct descriptive term is 'dens invaginatus' or 'invaginated tooth'. The anomaly may vary clinically from a deep cingulum pit in a tooth of normal form (**Fig. 36.4**) to a tooth with grossly distorted crown and root. Invaginated teeth are relatively common, occurring in 1–5% of permanent teeth. Primary invaginations are rare.

The main problem with invaginations is infection. The enamel lining of the invagination is either incomplete or very thin and easily breached, resulting in dentinal caries that quickly progresses to involve the pulp causing a rapidly spreading infection presenting with acute facial cellulitis or acute dentoalveolar abscess. Rarely a large invaginated tooth may cause impaction and non-eruption of an adjacent tooth.

There is an association between invaginated teeth and supernumerary teeth. A full radiographic examination is justified if an invaginated tooth is identified.

Invaginations in crowns of normal morphology should be sealed prophylactically as soon as possible after eruption. If these 'high' invaginations do become pulpally involved then root treatment is possible, because the invaginated portion is accessible and can be removed with a crown bur allowing

Fig. 36.4 Dens in dente of lateral incisor.

access to the normal root canal. All other invaginations usually require extraction.

'Evaginated teeth' or 'dens evaginatus' or 'tuberculated teeth' occurs commonly as a conical tubercular projection arising from the occlusal surface of the central fissure or the lingual plane of the buccal cusp. Premolar teeth are the commonest teeth affected, with permanent molars and canines less commonly affected. The condition is mainly seen in people of Mongolian stock (1–4%), although rarely it is seen in Caucasians.

Evaginations consist of enamel, dentine and a pulpal extension. Evagination should be suspected if a premolar without caries develops a periapical lesion shortly after eruption.

Treatment is the same as 'talon cusp'.

■ *What abnormalities of root form do you know?*

Taurodontism.

Accessory roots.

Pyramidal roots.

Taurodontism (bull-like teeth) applies to multirooted teeth in which the body of the tooth is enlarged corono-apically at the expense of the roots. Radiographs show apparent enlargement of the coronal pulp chamber, usually extending below the level of the alveolar crest before root division. The normal constriction at the level of the amelo-cemental junction is frequently absent in affected teeth. The condition is uncommon in primary teeth but may occur in permanent molars in 6% of the population.

■ *What conditions may taurodontism be associated with?*

Amelogenesis imperfecta.

Trichodento-osseous syndrome.

Ectodermal dysplasia with hypodontia.

Ellis–van Creveld syndrome.

Achondroplasia.

Klinefelter syndrome.

Accessory roots can occur in almost any tooth. Rarely they may be due to early trauma in a forming root. The majority are likely to be due to genetic factors that remain to be specified.

Pyramidal roots describe the reduction in root number in multirooted teeth. Any molar tooth may be affected.

Recommended reading

Cameron A, Widmer R (eds) 2008 Dental anomalies. In: Handbook of Pediatric Dentistry, 3rd edn. Mosby-Wolfe, St Louis, pp 217–277.

Crawford PJM, Aldred MJ 2005 Anomalies of tooth formation and eruption. In: Welbury RR, Duggal MS, Hosey MT (eds) Paediatric Dentistry, 3rd edn. Oxford University Press, Oxford, pp 297–318.

Millett D, Welbury R 2000 Orthodontics and Paediatric Dentistry: Colour Guide. Churchill Livingstone, Edinburgh.

For revision, see Mind Map 36, page 198.

37

Amelogenesis imperfecta

SUMMARY

Mark is 10 years old. He and his parents are concerned because his teeth seem rough. They also stain easily. What is the cause of these problems? What treatment is possible?

■ **What can you see in** *Figure 37.1*?

All erupted teeth have hypoplastic enamel.

History

Mark's mother says that she noticed when the teeth first erupted that they were rough. They pick up stain and are difficult to clean. What key questions do you need to ask?

■ **Was there any systemic illness from birth to early childhood?**

No.

■ **Were the primary teeth similarly affected?**

There was a slight roughening of the primary teeth, although nothing as bad as the permanent teeth.

■ **Is anyone else in the family similarly affected?**

Mark's father and his cousin (father's brother's son) have similar roughness of their teeth.

After having obtained this history it is most likely that Mark has an inherited enamel defect involving enamel – amelogenesis imperfecta. However, defective enamel formation may be caused by genetic or environmental factors. The defective enamel will exhibit either hypoplasia, due to

Fig. 37.1 Hypoplastic amelogenesis imperfecta.

deficient matrix production, or hypomineralization, from imperfect mineralization of the matrix proteins. In hypoplasia the enamel may be thin, grooved or pitted, whereas in hypomineralization it may appear mottled but of normal thickness. The complete range of the causes of developmental abnormalities of enamel are shown in **Box 37.1**.

Box 37.1 Developmental abnormalities of enamel

General factors

- Genetic:
    - Primarily involving enamel – amelogenesis imperfecta.
    - Associated with generalized defects.
- Systemic (chronological):
    - Nutritional deficiencies.
    - Metabolic or biochemical disorder.
    - Toxic substances.
    - Infectious illnesses: pre-natal; peri-natal; neonatal; infancy; early childhood.
- Idiopathic.

Local factors

- Trauma.
- Infection.

Enamel defects of genetic origin may occur either as a phenomenon primarily involving the enamel, with possible secondary effects in other dental tissues and craniofacial structures, or as a component of a more complex syndrome in which defective enamel is only one of a number of more generalized abnormalities.

Medical history

Mark has no medical problems. He is doing very well at school and is a keen basketball player.

Examination

Intraoral examination revealed that all the surfaces of all the erupted permanent teeth are affected by a roughness or 'pitting' (**Fig. 37.1**). The second primary molar teeth that were still present were also affected by a similar roughness that, although not as evident on visual examination, was obvious on tactile examination with a probe. There was no tooth wear.

■ **Why is this pattern of enamel hypoplasia unlikely to be caused by systemic (chronological) influences?**

Primary teeth were affected.

All the enamel surface of the teeth is affected.

Amelogenesis imperfecta (AI) occurs as a result of single gene mutations that follow autosomal-dominant, autosomal-recessive or X-linked patterns of inheritance. The prevalence varies around the world with rates of 1 in 718 in northern Sweden and 1 in 14000 in Michigan, USA. A global quoted figure is often 1 in 10000.

■ **What are the main types of AI?**

- Hypoplastic.
- Hypomineralized: hypocalcified or hypomature.
- 'Mixed'.

Currently there are about 14 different types of AI on the basis of genetic pattern, clinical and radiological features, and histological changes. These are shown in **Table 37.1**.

Table 37.1 Types of amelogenesis imperfecta

Type	Description
Type 1	Hypoplasia
1A	Autosomal-dominant, thin and smooth hypoplasia with eruption defect
1B	Autosomal-dominant, thin and rough hypoplasia
1C	Autosomal-dominant, randomly pitted hypoplasia
1D	Autosomal-dominant, localized hypoplasia
1E	Autosomal-recessive, localized hypoplasia
1F	X-linked hypoplasia
1G	Autosomal-recessive, thin and rough hypoplasia (agenesis)
Type II	Hypocalcification
IIA	Autosomal-dominant, hypocalcification
IIB	Autosomal-recessive, hypocalcification
Type III	Hypomaturation
IIIA	X-linked hypomaturation
IIIB	Autosomal-recessive, pigmented hypomaturation
IIIC	Autosomal-dominant, snow-capped teeth
Type IV	Hypomaturation–hypoplasia with taurodontism
IVA	Autosomal-dominant, hypomaturation with pitted hypoplasia and taurodontism
IVB	Autosomal-dominant, hypomaturation with thin hypoplasia and taurodontism

Genetic enamel defects can be associated with generalized disorders in a number of uncommon or rare genetically determined diseases and clinical syndromes. These diseases and complex syndromes include epidermolysis bullosa, tuberous sclerosis, pseudohypoparathyroidism, trichodento-osseous syndrome, oculodento-osseous dysplasia, vitamin D-dependent rickets, amelo-cerebrohypohidrotic syndrome, amelo-onychohypohidrotic syndrome and some types of mucopolysaccharidosis.

Mark probably has type 1B, autosomal-dominant, thin and rough hypoplasia. An example of a hypomature form of AI is shown in **Figure 37.2**.

Investigations

■ *What investigations are necessary?*

Fig. 37.2 Hypomature amelogenesis imperfecta.

Dental panoramic tomogram

This will confirm the presence of all the permanent dentition. In addition it will diagnose any taurodontism. This is most marked in type IV AI but can affect permanent molars, particularly in the maxilla in other types of AI more frequently than is the norm for the Caucasian population.

Family examination

If it is possible to examine Mark's father's and his cousin's teeth this will help to confirm your diagnosis.

Treatment

The treatment of both amelogenesis and dentinogenesis imperfecta requires early diagnosis in order to improve the long-term prognosis of teeth. Parents need to be educated as to the implications of the condition, and prevention (diet counselling, fluoride supplementation, oral hygiene instruction (OHI)) is a crucial element in the success of any restorative treatment.

There are four main clinical problems associated with inherited enamel and dentine defects:

- Poor aesthetics.
- Chipping and attrition of the enamel.
- Exposure and attrition of the dentine causing sensitivity.
- Poor oral hygiene, gingivitis and caries.

While it is impossible to draw up a definitive treatment plan for all cases, it is possible to define the principles of treatment planning for this group of patients. It is important to realize that not all children with amelogenesis imperfecta or dentinogenesis imperfecta are affected equally. Many will not have marked tooth wear or symptoms, and will not require advanced intervention. **Table 37.2** describes the principles of treatment in terms of the age of the child/adolescent and with regard to the three aspects of care: prevention, restoration and aesthetics.

Table 37.2 Treatment modalities for amelogenesis imperfecta

	Restoration	Aesthetics
Primary dentition: 0–5 years	Adhesive restorations	Minimal intervention
	Stainless steel crowns (SSCs) especially on e's	Compomer/composite veneers
Mixed dentition: 6–16 years	Adhesive restorations/SSCs on primary molars	Composite veneers
	SSCs/adhesive castings on permanent molars	
Permanent dentition: 16+ years	Adhesive castings on premolars	Porcelain veneers
	Full mouth rehabilitation ± crown lengthening	Full crowns

Key point

Main treatment aims for dental anomalies:

- To alleviate symptoms.
- To maintain/restore occlusal height.
- To improve aesthetics.

Mark's major concern was the staining and roughness of his front teeth. Fortunately there was no wear of his posterior teeth and his problem, therefore, was solely a cosmetic one. The pitting or hypoplasia on the upper and lower incisors can be masked by a thin, directly applied composite veneer. This should be extended to include the canines and first premolars when the arches are complete. On occasions, if the smile is a very 'wide' one, it may be necessary to include second premolars. Composite veneers can be replaced by porcelain veneers at age 18 when the gingival contour has achieved adult levels.

If the amelogenesis had been of the hypomineralized variety with more destruction of enamel, it may have been necessary to consider full porcelain crowns for aesthetics in the anterior teeth and either stainless steel crowns or adhesive castings on posterior teeth. The latter may need to be replaced in adolescence/early adulthood by a porcelain bonded full crown (**Table 37.2**).

Recommended reading

Cameron A, Widmer R (eds) 2008 Dental anomalies. In: Handbook of Paediatric Dentistry, 3rd edn. Mosby-Wolfe, St Louis, pp 217–277.

Crawford PJM, Aldred MJ 2005 Anomalies of tooth formation and eruption. In: Welbury RR, Duggal MS, Hosey MT (eds) Paediatric Dentistry, 3rd edn. Oxford Univerty Press, Oxford, pp 297–318.

For revision, see Mind Map 37, page 199.

38

Dentinogenesis imperfecta

SUMMARY

Siobhan is 9 years old. She and her parents are concerned because her permanent teeth are darker than normal and she is getting teased at school. What is the cause of the discoloration? How would you treat it?

History

Siobhan's mother says she noticed that when the permanent teeth erupted they looked darker. Siobhan is very unhappy at school and refuses to smile for any photographs. When she talks she has the habit of covering her mouth with a hand so it is impossible to see her teeth. What can you see in **Figure 38.1A**? What key questions do you need to ask?

■ *Was there any systemic illness from birth until early childhood?*

No. Siobhan had no illness.

■ *Were the primary teeth similarly affected?*

The primary teeth erupted normally but very quickly chipped away becoming worn to gum level.

■ *Is anyone else in the family similarly affected?*

Siobhan's brother and her father have a problem with their teeth. Siobhan's brother is 14 and he has needed crowns on his back teeth and veneers on his front teeth. Siobhan's father needed a lot of treatment when he was younger and has had some teeth crowned. Many of his posterior teeth, however, were extracted.

Even before you have examined the mouth, the history suggests that Siobhan has an inherited defect. **Figure 38.1A** confirms your suspicion that this is dentinogenesis imperfecta (DI).

■ *Why is this DI and not amelogenesis imperfecta (AI)?*

The teeth are translucent.

The enamel is poorly adherent to the underlying dentine and easily chips and wears. The remaining primary canines and molars in **Figures 35.1A, B** are worn to gingival level and have a translucent opalescent appearance.

■ *What investigations do you need to do to confirm your suspicions?*

Dental panoramic tomogram

If this is DI, the dental panoramic radiograph will probably show the following:

- Bulbous crowns with pronounced cervical constriction.
- Shortened roots.
- Progressive pulp chamber and canal obliteration (**Fig. 38.2** (different case)).
- Spontaneous periapical abscess formation.

Family examination

- Family examination of affected members.
- Dentine defects like those of enamel may be subdivided by cause into two main groups based on whether they are of genetic or environmental origin.
- Dentine anomalies that are genetically determined may appear to be limited to the dentition or form part of a more complex generalized disorder (**Box 38.1**).

The most well documented hereditary dentine defects are DI type II (hereditary opalescent dentine), which only affects teeth, and DI type I, in which abnormalities of teeth are associated with osteogenesis imperfecta.

Fig. 38.1 (A) Dentinogenesis imperfecta.

Fig. 38.1 (B) Dentinogenesis imperfecta.

Box 38.1 Hereditary dentine defects

Limited to the dentine

- Dentinogenesis imperfecta type II (hereditary opalescent dentine).
- Dentine dysplasia type I (radicular dentine dysplasia).
- Dentine dysplasia type II (coronal dentine dysplasia).
- Fibrous dysplasia of dentine.

Associated with generalized disorder

- Osteogenesis imperfecta (dentinogenesis imperfecta type I).
- Ehlers-Danlos syndrome.
- Brachioskeletogenital syndrome.
- Vitamin D resistant rickets.
- Vitamin D dependent rickets.
- Hypophosphatasia.

Fig. 38.2 Obliteration of root canals and pulp chambers in dentinogenesis imperfecta.

DI type II

Both dentitions are usually affected. The severity of the defect varies considerably between families and within families. Primary teeth tend to be more severely affected than permanent teeth and the later forming permanent teeth may be the least affected. Enamel tends to chip away from the underlying amelodentinal junction (ADJ), exposing the abnormally soft dentine that undergoes rapid wear. This is most marked in the primary dentition where, within 2 years, the crowns may be worn to the gingival margin and appear as amber-coloured remnants (**Fig. 38.1B**), which may be frequently infected and abscessed. In the permanent dentition following eruption the enamel may look reasonably normal, but histological studies have shown hypomineralized areas in approximately one-third of cases. Radiographic signs are mentioned above. Histologically, the ADJ may appear flattened, and while the subadjacent peripheral dentine may approach normality, the remainder is grossly disordered with an amorphous matrix containing areas of interglobular calcification, abnormally shaped and sized tubules, and cellular inclusions.

■ *Is DI more prevalent than AI?*

Possibly, figures of 1 in 8000 have been estimated (AI 1:10000).

■ *Has DI got as many inheritance patterns as AI?*

No. Invariably it is autosomal dominant with marked expressivity and good penetrance. Two clinical variants of the condition have been described.

- *Shell teeth.* This is rare and seen in the primary dentition. The pulp remains large and the thin enamel and dentine rapidly fragments to cause pulpal infection.
- *DI type III (brandy wine type).* This was first described in Maryland USA and has been traced back to East Anglia in England. It was apparently taken to the USA by one of the sailors who accompanied the Pilgrim Fathers to Maryland. More recently type III defect has been linked to the same locus on chromosome 4q21 as DI type II.

DI type I associated with osteogenesis imperfecta

Osteogenesis imperfecta is a group of connective tissue disorders involving inherited abnormalities of type I collagen. Increased bone fragility is only one aspect of the condition which may include lax joints, blue sclerae, opalescent teeth, hearing loss and a variable degree of bone deformity. The inheritance pattern is either autosomal recessive or dominant. The recessive form is often lethal around birth.

Opalescent teeth are only rarely seen in surviving recessive types. They are commonly a feature of the dominant variety with accompanying bone fragility, bone deformity and blue sclerae.

The primary teeth in DI type I resemble exactly those in DI type II. However, in the permanent dentition the defect is extremely variable. In many cases the upper anterior teeth may have a normal colour and appearance whereas the lower incisors and canines are opalescent, discoloured bluish-brown and wear at the incisal edges. In most cases the enamel does not chip away from underlying dentine as readily as in type II.

Radiographic appearances are as already described with the exception that upper teeth may retain their pulp spaces long after those in the lower jaw. Histological appearances are indistinguishable from type II.

Environmentally determined dentine defects do exist but are less well documented than corresponding anomalies of enamel: trauma, nutritional deficiencies (minerals, proteins and vitamins) and drugs (tetracycline, chemotherapeutic agents – cyclophosphamide) will likely produce increased interglobular dentine, predentine and osteoid.

Key point

Dentinogenesis imperfecta:

- Occurs in 1 in 8000 of the population.
- May be associated with osteogenesis imperfecta.

Treatment

The main clinical problems associated with AI and DI, and the key points of treatment objectives are covered in Chapter 37. The principles of treatment for DI are the same as those for AI with the exception that in the permanent dentition from age 16 crown-lengthening procedures are more common in DI and the provision of overdentures and full dentures is not uncommon. The role of implants in these patients has yet to be defined.

Siobhan's major concern was of the colour of her permanent incisors. There was some wear of first permanent molars. The first permanent molars were treated with adhesive castings with micromechanical retention to luting cement (**Fig. 38.1B**). The upper and lower incisors were veneered with composite resin. This can be extended to include the canines and premolars when the arches are complete. The composite veneers can be replaced by porcelain veneers around the age of 18 years.

Young children with DI often pose the greatest problems. The teeth undergo such excessive wear that they become worn down to gingival level and are unrestorable. Teeth affected by DI are also prone to spontaneous abscesses due to the progressive obliteration of the pulp chambers. In these cases pulp therapy is unsuccessful and extraction of the affected teeth is necessary.

Early consultation with an orthodontist is advisable in inherited abnormalities of enamel and dentine in order to keep the orthodontic requirements simple. Treatment for these patients is possible and in many cases proceeds without problems. The use of removable appliances, where appropriate, and orthodontic bands rather than brackets will minimize the risk of damage to the abnormal enamel. The problem is twofold: there may be frequent bond failure during active treatment or the enamel may be further damaged during debonding. Some orthodontists prefer to use bands even for anterior teeth, while others will use glass ionomer cement as the bonding agent in preference to more conventional resin-based agents. In other instances, cosmetic restorative techniques (veneers and crowns) may be more appropriate than orthodontic treatment.

Recommended reading

Cameron A, Widmer R (eds) 2008 Dental anomalies. In: Handbook of Paediatric Dentistry, 3rd edn. Mosby-Wolfe, St Louis, pp 217–277.

Crawford PJM, Aldred MJ 2005 Anomalies of tooth formation and eruption. In: Welbury RR, Duggal MS, Hosey MT (eds) Paediatric Dentistry, 3rd edn. Oxford Univerty Press, Oxford, pp 297–318.

For revision, see Mind Map 38, page 200.

Gingival bleeding and enlargement

SUMMARY

Kayleigh is 15 years old. She is concerned that her upper gums look abnormal and they bleed whenever she brushes them (Fig. 39.1).

History

Kayleigh has noticed bleeding when she has been brushing for the last year. She is frightened of brushing because of the bleeding and feels that the bleeding is getting worse. She is also very socially conscious of her gums because they look very red and are 'bigger' than normal.

Medical history

Kayleigh has insulin-dependent diabetes. She takes her insulin by subcutaneous injection at 07.30 and 17.30 hours. She has a regulated gram intake of carbohydrate at 07.30, 11.00, 13.00, 15.00, 17.30 and 21.00 hours. Apart from this she is an active girl who plays basketball and hockey at school and has learnt to increase her carbohydrate intake appropriately to cover her sporting activities. Her mum reports that Kayleigh has had the occasional 'rebellion' against her condition and at these times diabetic control has been poor, but generally her control is now good with a stable regimen. She is seen every 2 months by her doctor,

Fig. 39.1 Chronic gingivitis.

and she monitors her blood glucose and urinary glucose at home herself.

Dental history

Kayleigh and her family are regular dental attenders and have just moved to the area with her father's job. This is the first time you have seen her.

Examination

Extraoral examination is normal with no signs of infection. Intraorally there is widespread marginal gingivitis, which is particularly bad in the upper right quadrant anteriorly (**Fig. 39.1**). Clinical and radiographic examination of the teeth reveal a low caries rate with only the need to replace a cracked and deficient restoration in a lower first permanent molar that has recurrent caries.

■ *What factors are contributing to the chronic marginal gingivitis?*

Poor oral hygiene.
Hormonal changes of puberty.
Poorly controlled diabetes mellitus.

Key point

Gingival bleeding can be as a result of:
- Local causes.
- Systemic causes.

The commonest local and systemic causes of gingival bleeding in childhood/adolescence are shown in **Box 39.1**.

Box 39.1 Commonest causes of gingival bleeding in childhood and adolescence

Local causes
- Eruption gingivitis.
- Acute/chronic gingivitis.
- Chronic periodontitis.
- Foreign body entrapment.
- Acute necrotizing ulcerative gingivitis.
- Haemangioma.
- Reactive hyperplasias such as pyogenic granuloma.
- Factitial injury.

Systemic causes
- Hormonal changes such as pregnancy or puberty.
- Diabetes mellitus – poor control.
- Anaemia.
- Leukaemia.
- Any platelet disorder.
- Clotting defects.
- Drugs (e.g. anticoagulants).
- Scurvy.
- HIV-associated periodontal disease.

■ *What do you think may have precipitated the initial gingivitis?*

This is likely to have coincided with one of the periods where diabetic control was poor. Further questioning revealed that about a year ago Kayleigh was struggling to come to terms with her insulin-dependent diabetes. She refused to take her insulin regularly and ended up by being admitted to hospital in coma with ketoacidosis. Her blood sugar at that time was very high and her breath smelt of 'pear drops' due to ketone bodies. This was a hyperglycaemic coma. She was resuscitated with intravenous fluids as she was severely dehydrated, prior to restabilization on an insulin regimen.

■ *What is the other cause of diabetic coma and what are its signs?*

Hypoglycaemic coma occurs due to inadequate carbohydrate (missed meal), exercise or excess insulin. The onset is quicker than the hyperglycaemic coma. The signs of hypoglycaemic coma are very similar to having 'a drink too many', and can be summarized into those caused by adrenaline release and cerebral hypoglycaemia:

Adrenaline release:
- Sweaty warm skin.
- Rapid bounding pulse.
- Dilated (reacting pupils).
- Anxiety, tremor.
- Tingling around mouth.

Cerebral hypoglycaemia:
- Confusion, disorientation.
- Headache.
- Dysarthria.
- Unconsciousness.
- Focal neurological signs, e.g. fits.

If an individual having a hypoglycaemic episode is conscious they should be given sugar orally – 25 g glucose. If comatosed, they require 20 mg of 20% dextrose IV followed by 25 g orally on arousal. Alternatively if intravenous access is difficult, give 1 mg intramuscularly of glucagon. In practical terms, 10 g glucose approximates to:

2 tsp sugar

3 lumps sugar

3 Dextrosol tablets

60 ml Lucozade

15 ml Ribena (full sugar type)

90 ml cola (not diet variety)

one-third pint of milk.

Treatment

Kayleigh's gingivitis probably started as a result of poor diabetic control and unfortunately has been compounded by poor oral hygiene and the hormonal changes of puberty.

■ *Why is the gingivitis worst in the anterior part of the upper right quadrant?*

She is right-handed and this is often the case when a right-handed person changes their brushing action from the left

hand side of the mouth to the right hand side. The opposite would be true for the left-hander.

■ *What other generalized causes of gingival enlargement do you know?*

There are a number of causes, which can be classified into congenital and acquired (**Box 39.2**).

Box 39.2 Systemic causes of gingival enlargement

Congenital
- Hereditary gingival fibromatosis.
- Mucopolysaccharidoses.
- Infantile systemic hyalinosis.

Acquired
- Puberty/pregnancy gingivitis.
- Plasma cell gingivitis.
- Infections – HSV.
- Haematological: acute myeloid leukaemia, preleukaemic leukaemia, aplastic anaemia, vitamin C deficiency (scurvy).
- Drugs: phenytoin, ciclosporin, calcium-channel blockers, vigabatrin.
- Deposits: mucocutaneous amyloidosis.
- Chronic granulomatous disorders: sarcoidosis, Crohn disease, orofacial granulomatosis.

■ *Why is it important to eradicate Kayleigh's gingivitis?*

Poor oral hygiene in combination with diabetes can result in rapid periodontal destruction and attachment loss. An example of this in another subject with diabetes is shown in **Figure 39.2**. There is some evidence that significant periodontitis can upset glycaemic control.

Kayleigh needs reassurance that the bleeding will reduce and stop when her oral hygiene improves. She needs to appreciate the importance of good oral hygiene and the problems that will occur if oral hygiene is poor.

■ *Why is it important not to leave caries in a diabetic?*

Infection of any origin can result in an increased need for insulin. Without an insulin increase there will be a rise in blood sugar resulting in ketosis. Therefore, all infections in a diabetic, including those in the orofacial region, should be treated vigorously with antibiotics. Caries should be treated early to prevent infection.

Fig. 39.2 Gingival and periodontal disease.

Key point

In diabetes:

- Poor oral hygiene will accelerate attachment loss.
- Infection can interfere with diabetic control.

■ *Why is the timing of the appointment to restore Kayleigh's first permanent molar important?*

To not interfere with Kayleigh's carbohydrate intake and precipitate hypoglycaemia, it is probably best to give her an appointment either first thing in the morning, or directly after lunch. For any prolonged surgical procedure in a diabetic person, or any treatment that requires general anaesthesia (GA), a referral to hospital is required. GA will require admission pre-operatively to stabilize insulin and glucose requirements via a drip so that hypoglycaemic coma does not occur with pre-operative GA starvation.

■ *What dietary advice should you give to diabetic patients?*

Do not change your required carbohydrate intakes as these are critical to diabetic control.

Tailor the dental advice to the specific needs of the patient, i.e. take your toothbrush to school if possible. Try to clean your teeth after snacks and at lunchtime. Try to take snacks that provide the necessary sugar but don't remain stuck to the teeth. Use sugar-free gum if it is not possible to brush the teeth during the day.

■ *What other oral manifestations can occur in diabetes?*

Dry mouth.

Swelling of salivary glands (sialosis).

Glossitis.

Burning of tongue.

Oral candidosis if control is poor.

These manifestations are more commonly seen in adults.

Recommended reading

Firatli E, Yilmaz O, Onan U 1996 The relationship between clinical attachment loss and the duration of insulin dependent diabetes mellitus (IDDM) in children and adolescents. J Clin Periodontol 23:362–366.

Karjalainen KM, Knuuttila MLE, Kaar M-L 1997 Relationship between caries and level of metabolic balance in children and adolescents with insulin-dependent diabetes mellitus. Caries Res 31:13–18.

Position paper 1996 Diabetes and periodontal diseases. J Periodontol 67:166–176.

For revision, see Mind Map 39, page 201.

40

Oral ulceration

SUMMARY

Alan is 8 years old. He has been brought to the surgery by his mother because his mouth is so painful he cannot eat (Fig. 40.1). What could cause this problem? How would you treat it?

History

Alan has not been well for a couple of weeks. He had a 'virus' that resulted in his being put to bed and missing school. Just as he was improving from this his mouth became very sore. He has been unable to eat solid food for 3 days and has been on liquids only. He feels hot and lethargic. His gums bleed when he tries to brush them.

Medical history

Alan is generally a healthy boy. He has had a couple of courses of antibiotics for ear infections but has had no real illnesses. He has never been in hospital and is not on any tablets or medicines from his doctor.

■ *Describe the appearance of the upper and lower gingivae in Figure 40.1.*

There is erythematous gingival enlargement with small ulcerations of the gingival margin.

Fig. 40.1 Gingival enlargement and ulceration.

■ *What is the diagnosis?*

Primary herpetic gingivostomatitis.

There are two types of herpes simplex virus: herpes simplex type 1 (HSV-1) and herpes simplex type 2 (HSV-2). Classically HSV-1 causes oral disease and HSV-2 causes genital disease. The viruses, however, are very similar and both can cause both oral and genital disease, although there are differences in recurrence rates. Primary exposure to HSV in the mouth causes acute primary herpetic gingivo-stomatitis (**Fig. 40.1**). The virus causes a viraemia, fever, malaise and lymphadenopathy. All the surfaces of the mouth including the hard palate and attached gingiva can be involved, initially with a vesicular rash that ulcerates and becomes superinfected. The illness lasts for 10–14 days before resolving spontaneously. Diagnosis is usually made on clinical grounds but can be confirmed by a threefold rise in the convalescent antibody titre over that seen in the acute phase or by direct immunofluorescence of vesicular fluid using specific antisera.

Key point
Systemic signs in HSV:
• Fever.
• Malaise.
• Lymphadenopathy.

The primary infection may be mild and subclinical in the majority of young children who are exposed to it, though the condition may be severe and debilitating, and in an immunocompromised individual may lead to severe illness and sometimes herpetic hepatitis or encephalitis, which may be fatal in the absence of treatment.

Oral infection arises from direct contact with secretions from an individual who either has a primary or recurrent HSV infection. Direct inoculation of the fingers or skin with virally contaminated secretions or fluid can lead to local infection, e.g. herpetic whitlow of finger.

HSV is a neurogenic virus, and on recovery from the primary infection the virus may become latent within the trigeminal ganglion or basal ganglia of the brain and may subsequently be reactivated to cause a secondary infection. The secondary infection may cause a 'cold sore' on the lip or Bell's palsy.

Treatment

Alan responded well to rehydration and analgesia such as paracetamol, which is also antipyretic, and an antiseptic mouthwash such as chlorhexidine (Corsodyl) or benzydamine hydrochloride (Difflam). Had Alan not been able to maintain hydration he would have had to be admitted for intravenous fluid therapy. There is no evidence that systemic aciclovir is of any benefit at the relatively late stage of the condition that he presented. If he had been seen within 72 hours of the onset of the infection, aciclovir could have been prescribed, if the clinical severity warranted it. The dose is 200 mg five times daily for 5 days in patients over 2 years of age, and 100 mg five times daily for 2 days in the under 2 year olds. Although aciclovir can shorten the course of the primary infection, there is no evidence that it reduces the incidence of recurrent herpetic lesions.

■ *What are the reasons given for the reactivation of HSV to produce a cold sore (herpes labialis) (Fig. 40.2)?*

See **Box 40.1**.

Box 40.1 Reactivation of HSV

- Trauma.
- Chemicals.
- Heat.
- Hormones.
- Sunlight.
- Emotion.
- Immunosuppression.
- Concurrent infection.

■ *How should herpes labialis be treated?*

Apply aciclovir 5% cream to the lip lesion as soon as tingling or prickling of the prodromal phase is felt. This is usually 24 hours prior to vesiculation and pain.

■ *What other viral infection can occur in the mouths of paediatric patients?*

Varicella zoster virus (VZV) VZV is a neurogenic DNA virus that causes a primary infection in the form of chickenpox. Thereafter it remains dormant until reactivation as shingles.

Epstein–Barr virus (EBV) EBV is a herpes virus with a predilection for infecting B lymphocytes. This infection causes the B lymphocytes to become activated and produce their own antibodies. A primary infection with EBV causes glandular fever or infectious mononucleosis.

Cytomegalovirus This is associated with a glandular fever-like illness in childhood. On occasion it is found in severe atypical oral ulceration in HIV.

Herpes virus type 8 This has been demonstrated in Kaposi sarcoma in HIV infection.

Coxsackie viruses These are RNA viruses and responsible for herpangina or hand, foot and mouth disease.

Herpangina is a Coxsackie A virus that causes a herpes-like oropharyngitis where the ulceration is predominantly on the tonsil, soft palate and uvula. The mild illness is associated with fever and malaise but only persists for a few days.

Fig. 40.2 Recurrent herpes 'cold sore'.

Hand, foot and mouth disease is also Coxsackie A virus and occurs predominantly in children and their families. The condition is characterized by ulceration affecting gingiva, tongue, cheeks and palate. It is associated with vesicles and ulcers on the palms and soles. It may persist for 2 weeks.

Human papilloma virus (HPV) An increasing number of HPV types have been identified. Types 2 and 4, the common wart, occur in children usually due to auto-inoculation by biting fingers or hand warts. Condyloma acuminata or venereal warts can occur on the oral mucosa and are associated with HPV types 6, 11 and 60.

There are a number of other causes of oral ulceration in children and adolescents that are not associated with infections. These are shown in **Box 40.2**.

Box 40.2 Other causes of oral ulceration

- Aphthae.
- Gastrointestinal disease.
- Haematological disease.
- Infections.
- Mucocutaneous disorders.
- Radiotherapy.
- Trauma.
- Carcinoma.

■ *What types of aphthae are there?*

Minor.

Major.

Herpetiform.

Behçet syndrome.

Recurrent aphthae affect up to 20% of the population.

Minor aphthae are commonest and account for 85% of recurrent aphthae. Ulcers are less than 1 cm in diameter, usually only 2–3 mm. They occur singly or in crops of up to 10, last 3 days to 3 weeks and heal without scarring. Ulcers are round or oval with a yellowish-grey base and surrounded by an erythematous halo. They affect only non-keratinized mucosa.

Major aphthae are more severe and usually more than 1 cm in diameter with an irregular outline. They are usually single and often affect the fauces. They are often deeper and bleed, and may last for several weeks or months before healing with scarring. Again, they tend to affect non-keratinized mucosa.

Herpetiform aphthae look similar to primary herpes. The ulcers are 1–2 mm in diameter and large numbers may occur simultaneously. They last from 2 days to 2 weeks before healing without scar formation. Again they affect only non-keratinized mucosa.

Behçet syndrome describes the triad of oral and genital ulceration and anterior uveitis. It is rare in the UK and USA.

■ *What aetiological factors are important in recurrent aphthae?*

See **Box 40.3**. Although only 20% of the population experience recurrent aphthae, there is a positive family history in 50% of fathers and 60% of mothers. There is, in addition, a

Box 40.3 Common aetiological factors in recurrent aphthae in children

Host factors

- Genetic.
- Nutritional.
- Systemic disease.
- Immunity.

Environmental factors

- Trauma.
- Allergy.
- Infection.
- Stress.

Box 40.4 Common dietary allergens in recurrent aphthae

- Cheese.
- Chocolate.
- Nuts.
- Tomatoes.
- Citrus fruits.
- Benzoates.
- Cinnamon aldehyde.

Treatment of recurrent aphthae can be grouped into preventive and symptomatic (**Box 40.5**).

Box 40.5 Therapy for recurrent aphthae

Preventive

- Haematinic replacement.
- Dietary avoidance.
- Tetracycline mouthwash.
- Systemic corticosteroids.
- Colchicine.
- Thalidomide.

Symptomatic

- Chlorhexidine mouthwash.
- Benzydamine mouthwash.
- Topical lidocaine spray.
- Topical lidocaine ice lolly.
- Topical 20% benzocaine to local ulcers.
- Topical steroids.
- Triamcinolone in dental paste.
- Beclomethasone inhaler spray.
- Betamethasone mouthwash.

weak human leucocyte antigen (HLA) association with HLA types A2 and B12.

Nutritional deficiencies of iron, folic acid and B_{12} occur singly or in combination. A lot of these are latent and have a normal peripheral blood picture. It is necessary to assay individual levels of ferritin, folic acid and vitamin B_{12} as well as do a full blood count (FBC).

■ *What systemic diseases in children are commonly associated with aphthae?*

Coeliac disease.

Crohn disease.

Ulcerative colitis.

In older patients and less commonly in children, aphthae may also be associated with pernicious anaemia, HIV infection and malabsorption.

There is an increasing awareness of the role of dietary allergens in recurrent aphthae in children. Common dietary allergens implicated in recurrent aphthae are shown in **Box 40.4**. Patients usually develop fresh ulceration within 12–24 hours of ingesting the suspect food. Foods may be identified more objectively by patch testing. Dietary avoidance is often attended by clinical improvement.

Recommended reading

Scully C, Porter SR 1989 Recurrent aphthous stomatitis: current concepts of etiology, pathogenesis and management. J Oral Pathol Med 18:21–27.

Scully C, Welbury R, Flaitz C, de Almeida OP 2002 A color atlas of orofacial health and disease in children and adolescents, 2nd edn. Martin Dunitz, London.

Wray D, Rees SR, Gibson J, Forsyth A 2000 The role of allergy in oral mucosal diseases. Q J Med 93:507–511.

For revision, see Mind Map 40, page 202.

Key point

Aetiological factors in recurrent aphthae:

- Host related.
- Environment related.

41

Mind Maps

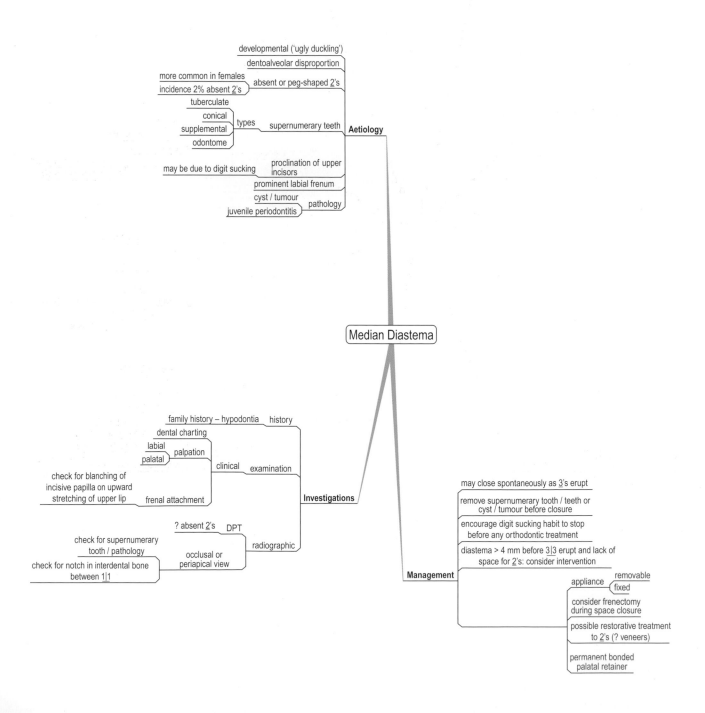

Aetiology

developmental ('ugly duckling')

dentoalveolar disproportion

more common in females

incidence 2% absent 2's — absent or peg-shaped 2's

tuberculate

conical — types — supernumerary teeth

supplemental

odontome

may be due to digit sucking — proclination of upper incisors

prominent labial frenum

cyst / tumour — pathology

juvenile periodontitis

Median Diastema

Investigations

family history – hypodontia — history

dental charting

labial — palpation

palatal

clinical — examination

check for blanching of incisive papilla on upward stretching of upper lip — frenal attachment

? absent 2's — DPT

check for supernumerary tooth / pathology

check for notch in interdental bone between 1|1 — occlusal or periapical view — radiographic

Management

may close spontaneously as 3's erupt

remove supernumerary tooth / teeth or cyst / tumour before closure

encourage digit sucking habit to stop before any orthodontic treatment

diastema > 4 mm before 3|3 erupt and lack of space for 2's: consider intervention

removable — fixed — appliance

consider frenectomy during space closure

possible restorative treatment to 2's (? veneers)

permanent bonded palatal retainer

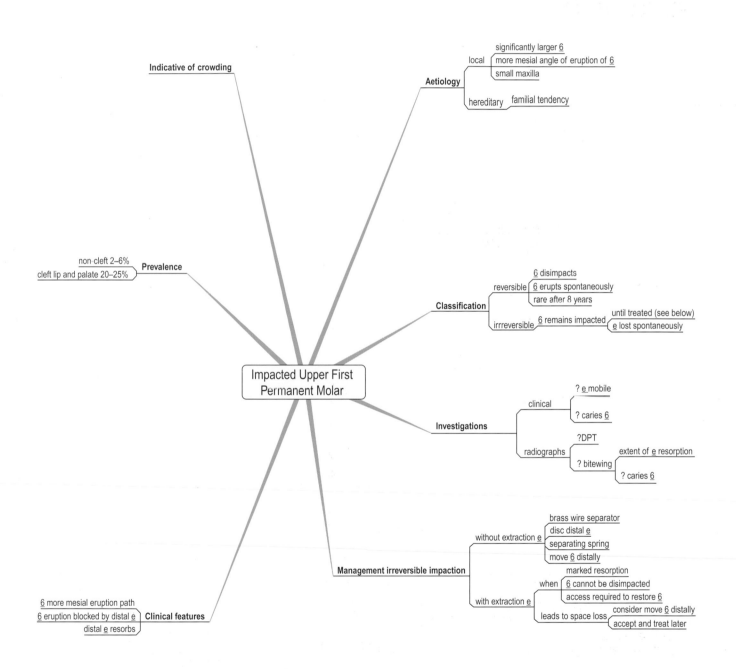

Indicative of crowding

Aetiology — local — significantly larger 6
more mesial angle of eruption of 6
small maxilla
hereditary — familial tendency

Prevalence — non-cleft 2–6%
cleft lip and palate 20–25%

Classification — reversible — 6 disimpacts
6 erupts spontaneously
rare after 8 years
irrreversible — 6 remains impacted — until treated (see below)
e lost spontaneously

Impacted Upper First Permanent Molar

Investigations — clinical — ? e mobile
? caries 6
radiographs — ?DPT
? bitewing — extent of e resorption
? caries 6

Management irreversible impaction — without extraction e — brass wire separator
disc distal e
separating spring
move 6 distally
with extraction e — when — marked resorption
6 cannot be disimpacted
access required to restore 6
leads to space loss — consider move 6 distally
accept and treat later

Clinical features — 6 more mesial eruption path
6 eruption blocked by distal e
distal e resorbs

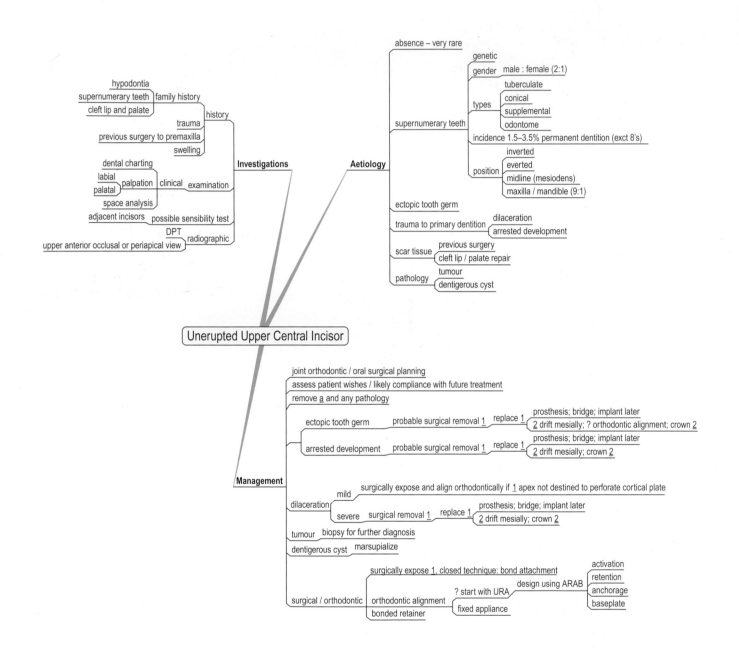

Unerupted Upper Central Incisor

Investigations

history
- family history
  - hypodontia
  - supernumerary teeth
  - cleft lip and palate
- trauma
- previous surgery to premaxilla
- swelling

clinical examination
- dental charting
- palpation
  - labial
  - palatal
- space analysis
- possible sensibility test — adjacent incisors

radiographic
- DPT
- upper anterior occlusal or periapical view

Aetiology

- absence – very rare

supernumerary teeth
- genetic
- gender — male : female (2:1)
- types
  - tuberculate
  - conical
  - supplemental
  - odontome
- incidence 1.5–3.5% permanent dentition (exct 8's)
- position
  - inverted
  - everted
  - midline (mesiodens)
  - maxilla / mandible (9:1)

- ectopic tooth germ

trauma to primary dentition
- dilaceration
- arrested development

scar tissue
- previous surgery
- cleft lip / palate repair

pathology
- tumour
- dentigerous cyst

Management

- joint orthodontic / oral surgical planning
- assess patient wishes / likely compliance with future treatment
- remove <u>a</u> and any pathology

ectopic tooth germ — probable surgical removal <u>1</u> — replace <u>1</u>
- prosthesis; bridge; implant later
- <u>2</u> drift mesially; ? orthodontic alignment; crown <u>2</u>

arrested development — probable surgical removal <u>1</u> — replace <u>1</u>
- prosthesis; bridge; implant later
- <u>2</u> drift mesially; crown <u>2</u>

dilaceration
- mild — surgically expose and align orthodontically if <u>1</u> apex not destined to perforate cortical plate
- severe — surgical removal <u>1</u> — replace <u>1</u>
  - prosthesis; bridge; implant later
  - <u>2</u> drift mesially; crown <u>2</u>

- **tumour** — biopsy for further diagnosis
- **dentigerous cyst** — marsupialize

surgical / orthodontic
- surgically expose 1, closed technique: bond attachment
- orthodontic alignment
  - ? start with URA — design using ARAB
    - activation
    - retention
    - anchorage
    - baseplate
  - fixed appliance
- bonded retainer

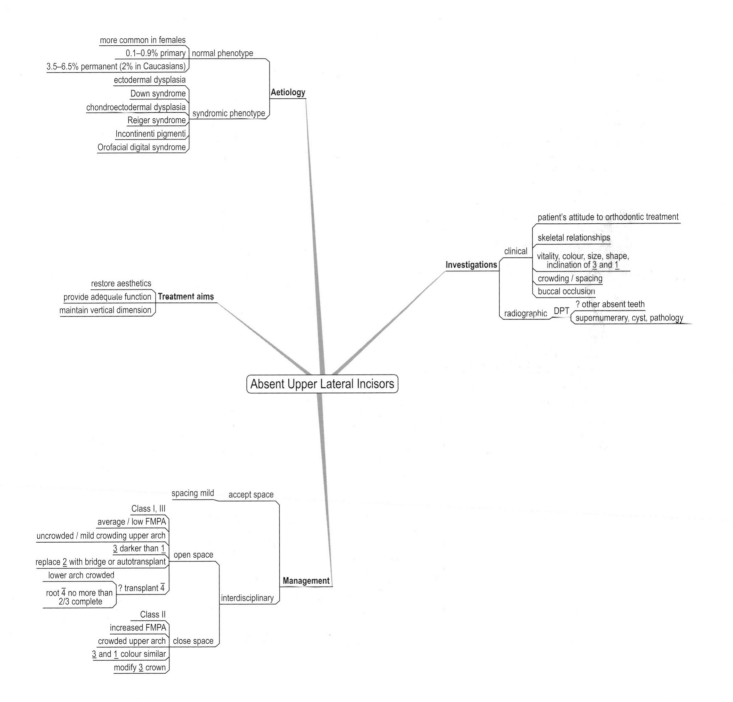

Aetiology

normal phenotype
- more common in females
- 0.1–0.9% primary
- 3.5–6.5% permanent (2% in Caucasians)

syndromic phenotype
- ectodermal dysplasia
- Down syndrome
- chondroectodermal dysplasia
- Reiger syndrome
- Incontinenti pigmenti
- Orofacial digital syndrome

Investigations

clinical
- patient's attitude to orthodontic treatment
- skeletal relationships
- vitality, colour, size, shape, inclination of 3 and 1
- crowding / spacing
- buccal occlusion

radiographic — DPT
- ? other absent teeth
- supernumerary, cyst, pathology

Treatment aims
- restore aesthetics
- provide adequate function
- maintain vertical dimension

Management

accept space
- spacing mild

open space
- Class I, III
- average / low FMPA
- uncrowded / mild crowding upper arch
- 3 darker than 1
- replace 2 with bridge or autotransplant
- lower arch crowded
- ? transplant 4
- root 4 no more than 2/3 complete

interdisciplinary

close space
- Class II
- increased FMPA
- crowded upper arch
- 3 and 1 colour similar
- modify 3 crown

Absent Upper Lateral Incisors

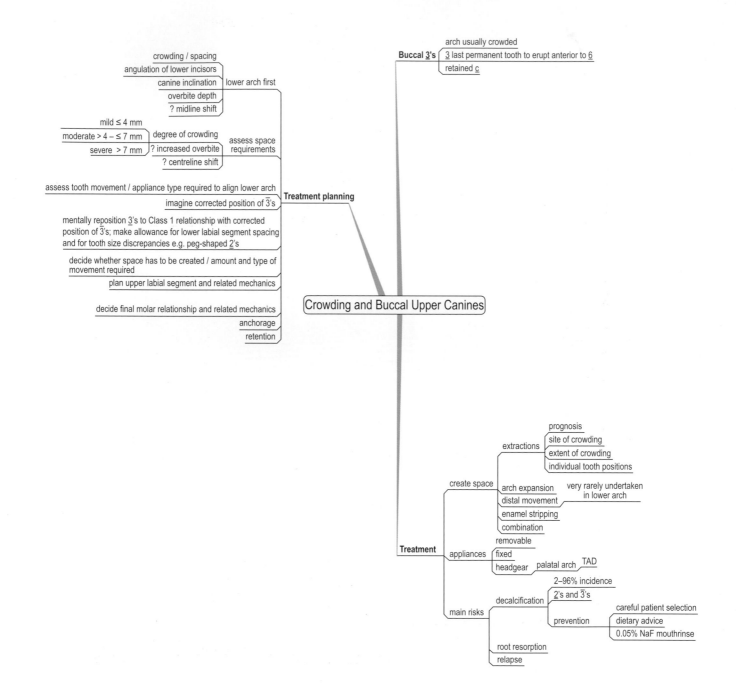

Buccal 3's
- arch usually crowded
- 3 last permanent tooth to erupt anterior to 6
- retained c

Treatment planning

lower arch first
- crowding / spacing
- angulation of lower incisors
- canine inclination
- overbite depth
- ? midline shift

assess space requirements
- degree of crowding
  - mild ≤ 4 mm
  - moderate > 4 – ≤ 7 mm
  - severe > 7 mm
- ? increased overbite
- ? centreline shift

assess tooth movement / appliance type required to align lower arch

imagine corrected position of 3's

mentally reposition 3's to Class 1 relationship with corrected position of 3's; make allowance for lower labial segment spacing and for tooth size discrepancies e.g. peg-shaped 2's

decide whether space has to be created / amount and type of movement required

plan upper labial segment and related mechanics

decide final molar relationship and related mechanics

anchorage

retention

Crowding and Buccal Upper Canines

Treatment

create space
- extractions
  - prognosis
  - site of crowding
  - extent of crowding
  - individual tooth positions
- arch expansion — very rarely undertaken in lower arch
- distal movement
- enamel stripping
- combination

appliances
- removable
- fixed
- headgear — palatal arch — TAD

main risks
- decalcification
  - 2–96% incidence
  - 2's and 3's
  - prevention
    - careful patient selection
    - dietary advice
    - 0.05% NaF mouthrinse
- root resorption
- relapse

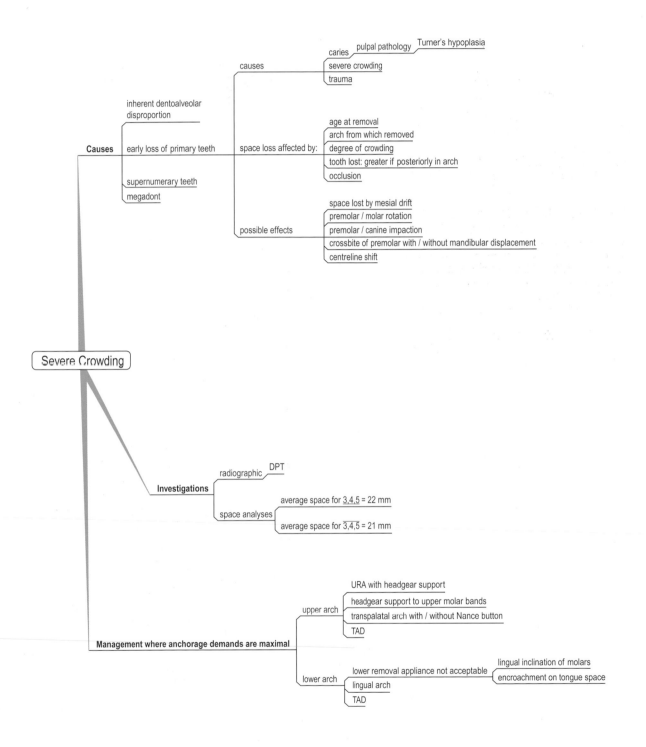

Severe Crowding

Causes

- inherent dentoalveolar disproportion
- early loss of primary teeth
- supernumerary teeth
- megadont

causes
- caries — pulpal pathology — Turner's hypoplasia
- severe crowding
- trauma

space loss affected by:
- age at removal
- arch from which removed
- degree of crowding
- tooth lost: greater if posteriorly in arch
- occlusion

possible effects
- space lost by mesial drift
- premolar / molar rotation
- premolar / canine impaction
- crossbite of premolar with / without mandibular displacement
- centreline shift

Investigations

radiographic — DPT

space analyses
- average space for $\underline{3,4,5}$ = 22 mm
- average space for $\overline{3,4,5}$ = 21 mm

Management where anchorage demands are maximal

upper arch
- URA with headgear support
- headgear support to upper molar bands
- transpalatal arch with / without Nance button
- TAD

lower arch
- lower removal appliance not acceptable
  - lingual inclination of molars
  - encroachment on tongue space
- lingual arch
- TAD

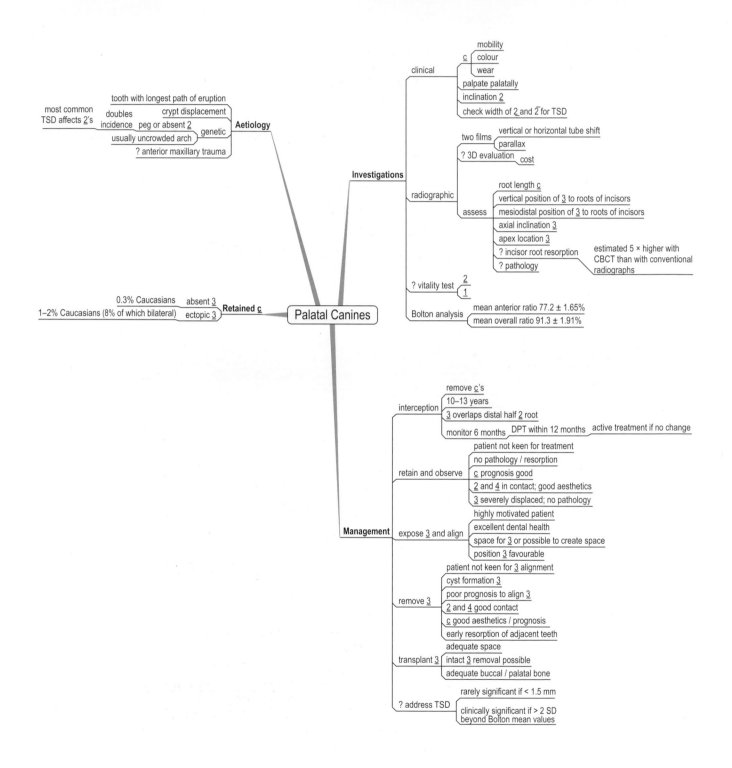

most common
TSD affects 2's

doubles
incidence   peg or absent 2
usually uncrowded arch
? anterior maxillary trauma

tooth with longest path of eruption
crypt displacement
genetic

Aetiology

Investigations

clinical

c { mobility, colour, wear }
palpate palatally
inclination 2
check width of 2 and 2̄ for TSD

radiographic

two films { vertical or horizontal tube shift, parallax }
? 3D evaluation — cost

assess

root length c
vertical position of 3 to roots of incisors
mesiodistal position of 3 to roots of incisors
axial inclination 3
apex location 3
? incisor root resorption
? pathology

estimated 5 × higher with
CBCT than with conventional
radiographs

? vitality test 2/1

Bolton analysis

mean anterior ratio 77.2 ± 1.65%
mean overall ratio 91.3 ± 1.91%

0.3% Caucasians   absent 3
1–2% Caucasians (8% of which bilateral)   ectopic 3   **Retained c**

Palatal Canines

Management

interception

remove c's
10–13 years
3 overlaps distal half 2 root
monitor 6 months   DPT within 12 months   active treatment if no change

retain and observe

patient not keen for treatment
no pathology / resorption
c prognosis good
2 and 4 in contact; good aesthetics
3 severely displaced; no pathology

expose 3 and align

highly motivated patient
excellent dental health
space for 3 or possible to create space
position 3 favourable

remove 3

patient not keen for 3 alignment
cyst formation 3
poor prognosis to align 3
2 and 4 good contact
c good aesthetics / prognosis
early resorption of adjacent teeth

transplant 3

adequate space
intact 3 removal possible
adequate buccal / palatal bone

? address TSD

rarely significant if < 1.5 mm
clinically significant if > 2 SD
beyond Bolton mean values

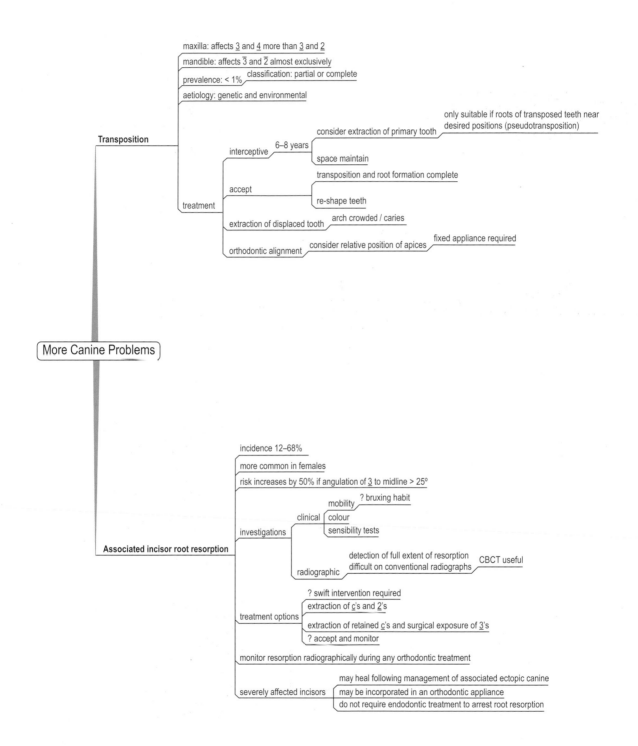

Transposition

maxilla: affects 3 and 4 more than 3 and 2

mandible: affects 3̄ and 2̄ almost exclusively

prevalence: < 1% — classification: partial or complete

aetiology: genetic and environmental

treatment
- interceptive — 6–8 years
  - consider extraction of primary tooth — only suitable if roots of transposed teeth near desired positions (pseudotransposition)
  - space maintain
- accept
  - transposition and root formation complete
  - re-shape teeth
- extraction of displaced tooth — arch crowded / caries
- orthodontic alignment — consider relative position of apices — fixed appliance required

Associated incisor root resorption

incidence 12–68%

more common in females

risk increases by 50% if angulation of 3 to midline > 25º

investigations
- clinical
  - mobility — ? bruxing habit
  - colour
  - sensibility tests
- radiographic — detection of full extent of resorption difficult on conventional radiographs — CBCT useful

treatment options
- ? swift intervention required
- extraction of c's and 2's
- extraction of retained c's and surgical exposure of 3's
- ? accept and monitor

monitor resorption radiographically during any orthodontic treatment

severely affected incisors
- may heal following management of associated ectopic canine
- may be incorporated in an orthodontic appliance
- do not require endodontic treatment to arrest root resorption

More Canine Problems

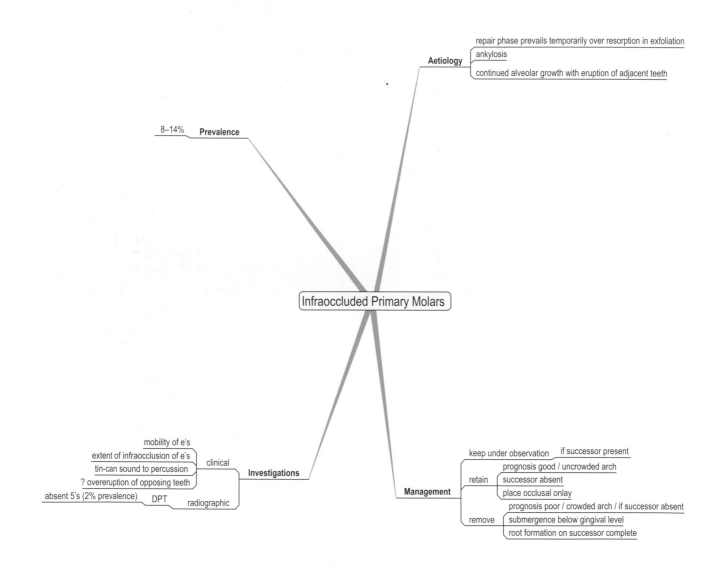

Aetiology
repair phase prevails temporarily over resorption in exfoliation
ankylosis
continued alveolar growth with eruption of adjacent teeth

8–14% **Prevalence**

Infraoccluded Primary Molars

mobility of e's
extent of infraocclusion of e's
tin-can sound to percussion   clinical
? overeruption of opposing teeth
absent 5's (2% prevalence) DPT   radiographic

Investigations

Management
keep under observation   if successor present
                    prognosis good / uncrowded arch
retain   successor absent
             place occlusal onlay
             prognosis poor / crowded arch / if successor absent
remove   submergence below gingival level
             root formation on successor complete

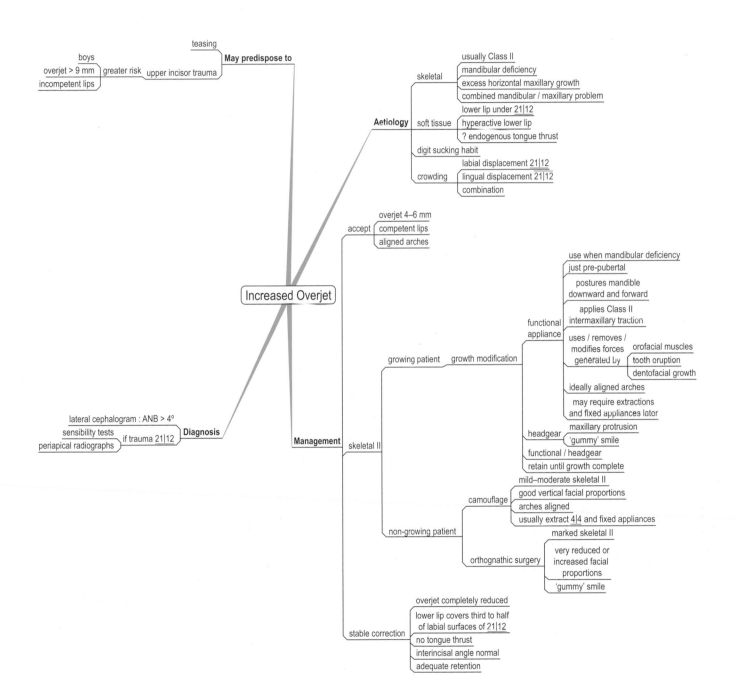

May predispose to

teasing

upper incisor trauma

greater risk

boys
overjet > 9 mm
incompetent lips

Aetiology

skeletal
- usually Class II
- mandibular deficiency
- excess horizontal maxillary growth
- combined mandibular / maxillary problem

soft tissue
- lower lip under 21|12
- hyperactive lower lip
- ? endogenous tongue thrust

digit sucking habit

crowding
- labial displacement 21|12
- lingual displacement 21|12
- combination

Increased Overjet

Diagnosis

lateral cephalogram : ANB > 4°

sensibility tests
periapical radiographs
if trauma 21|12

Management

accept
- overjet 4–6 mm
- competent lips
- aligned arches

skeletal II

growing patient — growth modification

functional appliance
- use when mandibular deficiency
- just pre-pubertal
- postures mandible downward and forward
- applies Class II intermaxillary traction
- uses / removes / modifies forces generated by
  - orofacial muscles
  - tooth eruption
  - dentofacial growth

- ideally aligned arches
- may require extractions and fixed appliances later

headgear
- maxillary protrusion
- 'gummy' smile

functional / headgear

retain until growth complete

non-growing patient

camouflage
- mild–moderate skeletal II
- good vertical facial proportions
- arches aligned
- usually extract 4|4 and fixed appliances

orthognathic surgery
- marked skeletal II
- very reduced or increased facial proportions
- 'gummy' smile

stable correction
- overjet completely reduced
- lower lip covers third to half of labial surfaces of 21|12
- no tongue thrust
- interincisal angle normal
- adequate retention

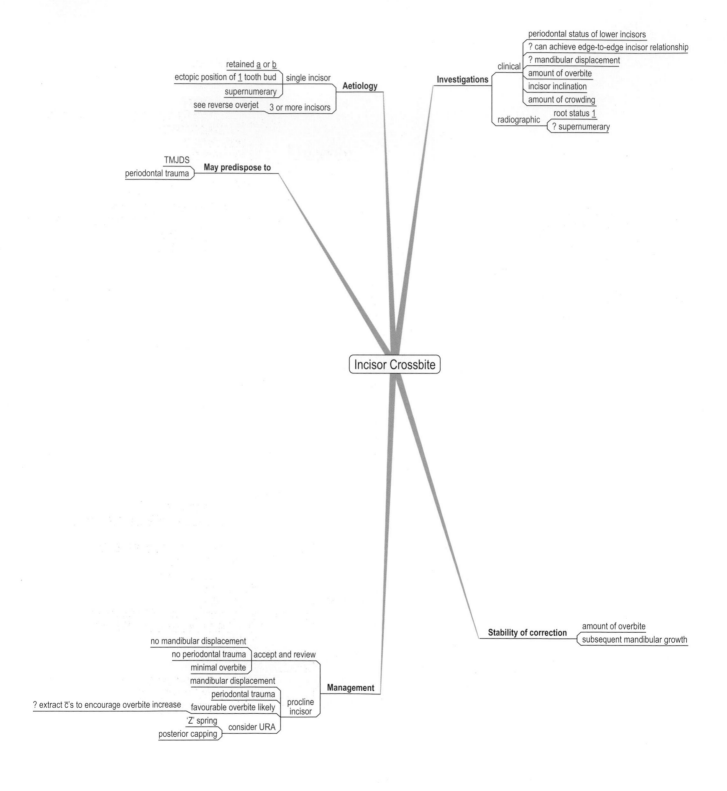

retained <u>a</u> or <u>b</u>
ectopic position of <u>1</u> tooth bud ⎤ single incisor
supernumerary
see reverse overjet ⎦ 3 or more incisors
Aetiology

Investigations

clinical
periodontal status of lower incisors
? can achieve edge-to-edge incisor relationship
? mandibular displacement
amount of overbite
incisor inclination
amount of crowding

radiographic
root status <u>1</u>
? supernumerary

TMJDS
periodontal trauma ⎤ **May predispose to**

Incisor Crossbite

Stability of correction
amount of overbite
subsequent mandibular growth

no mandibular displacement
no periodontal trauma ⎤ accept and review
minimal overbite
mandibular displacement
periodontal trauma
? extract c̄'s to encourage overbite increase — favourable overbite likely ⎤ procline incisor
'Z' spring
posterior capping ⎤ consider URA

Management

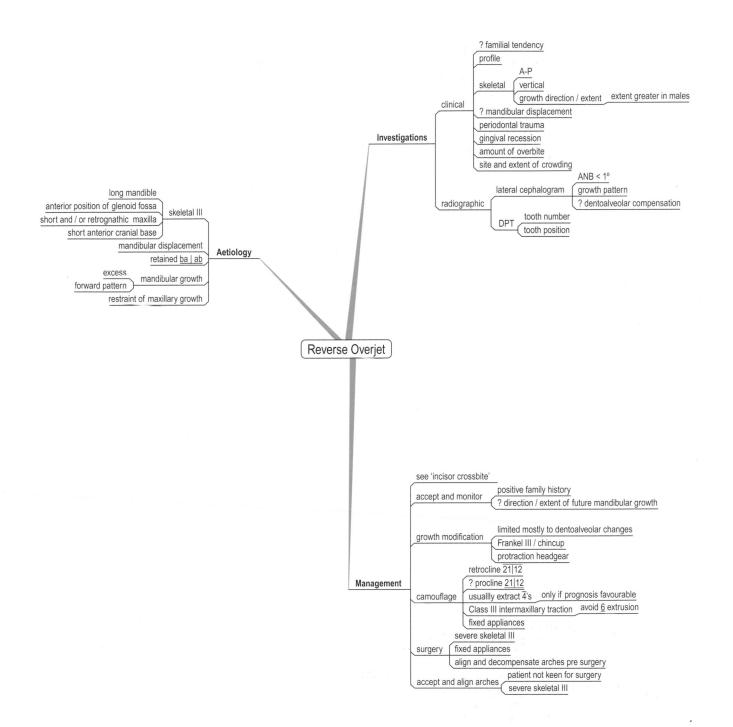

Investigations

clinical
- ? familial tendency
- profile
- skeletal
  - A-P
  - vertical
  - growth direction / extent — extent greater in males
- ? mandibular displacement
- periodontal trauma
- gingival recession
- amount of overbite
- site and extent of crowding

radiographic
- lateral cephalogram
  - ANB < 1°
  - growth pattern
  - ? dentoalveolar compensation
- DPT
  - tooth number
  - tooth position

Aetiology

skeletal III
- long mandible
- anterior position of glenoid fossa
- short and / or retrognathic maxilla
- short anterior cranial base

- mandibular displacement
- retained ba | ab

mandibular growth
- excess
- forward pattern
- restraint of maxillary growth

Reverse Overjet

Management

accept and monitor
- see 'incisor crossbite'
- positive family history
- ? direction / extent of future mandibular growth

growth modification
- limited mostly to dentoalveolar changes
- Frankel III / chincup
- protraction headgear

camouflage
- retrocline 21|12
- ? procline 21|12
- usuallly extract 4's — only if prognosis favourable
- Class III intermaxillary traction — avoid 6 extrusion
- fixed appliances

surgery
- severe skeletal III
- fixed appliances
- align and decompensate arches pre surgery

accept and align arches
- patient not keen for surgery
- severe skeletal III

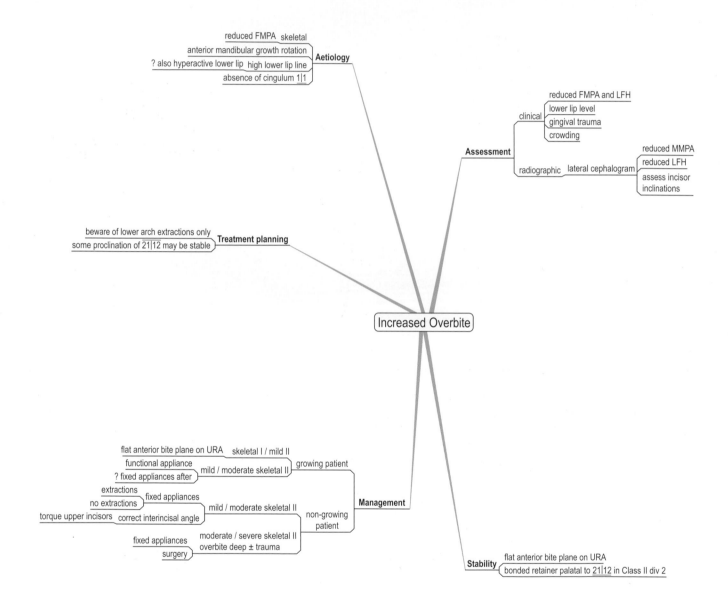

reduced FMPA skeletal
anterior mandibular growth rotation
? also hyperactive lower lip high lower lip line
absence of cingulum 1|1

Aetiology

reduced FMPA and LFH
clinical lower lip level
gingival trauma
crowding

Assessment

reduced MMPA
radiographic lateral cephalogram reduced LFH
assess incisor
inclinations

beware of lower arch extractions only
some proclination of 21|12 may be stable

Treatment planning

Increased Overbite

flat anterior bite plane on URA skeletal I / mild II
functional appliance mild / moderate skeletal II growing patient
? fixed appliances after

extractions
no extractions fixed appliances
torque upper incisors correct interincisal angle mild / moderate skeletal II non-growing patient

fixed appliances moderate / severe skeletal II
surgery overbite deep ± trauma

Management

Stability flat anterior bite plane on URA
bonded retainer palatal to 21|12 in Class II div 2

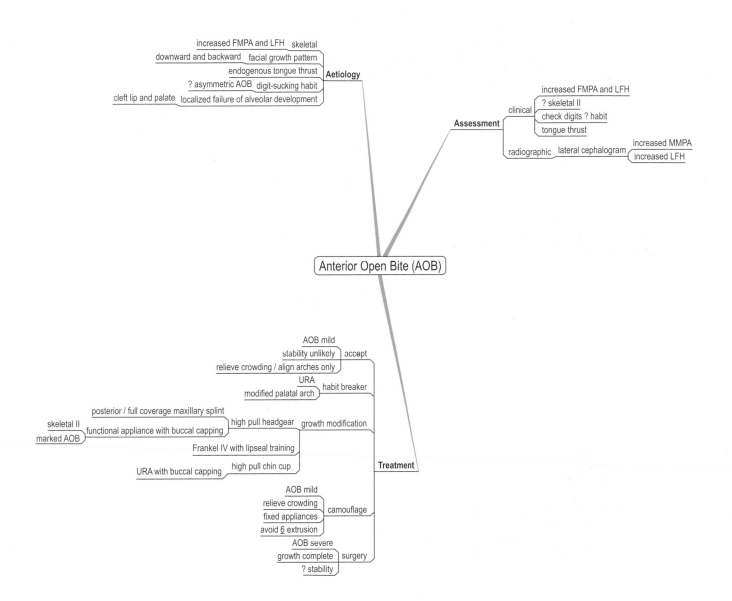

Aetiology

increased FMPA and LFH   skeletal

downward and backward   facial growth pattern

endogenous tongue thrust

? asymmetric AOB   digit-sucking habit

cleft lip and palate   localized failure of alveolar development

Assessment

clinical

increased FMPA and LFH

? skeletal II

check digits ? habit

tongue thrust

radiographic   lateral cephalogram

increased MMPA

increased LFH

Anterior Open Bite (AOB)

Treatment

AOB mild

stability unlikely   accept

relieve crowding / align arches only

URA

modified palatal arch   habit breaker

posterior / full coverage maxillary splint

skeletal II

functional appliance with buccal capping   high pull headgear   growth modification

marked AOB

Frankel IV with lipseal training

URA with buccal capping   high pull chin cup

AOB mild

relieve crowding   camouflage

fixed appliances

avoid 6 extrusion

AOB severe

growth complete   surgery

? stability

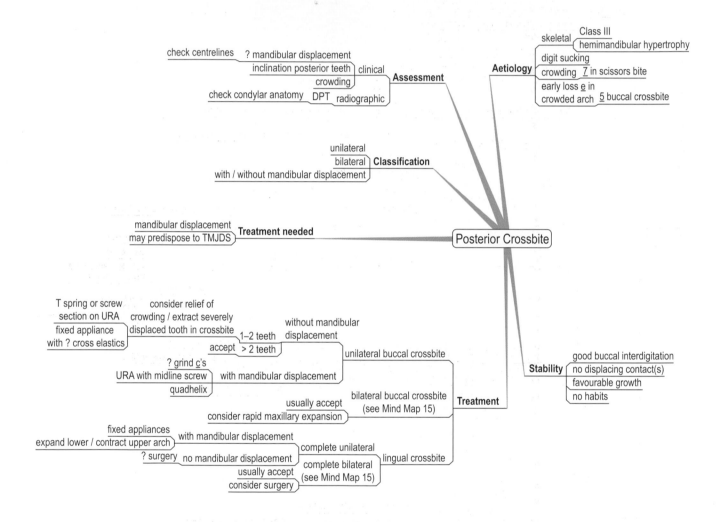

check centrelines   ? mandibular displacement
inclination posterior teeth   clinical
crowding
check condylar anatomy   DPT   radiographic   **Assessment**

skeletal   Class III
hemimandibular hypertrophy
digit sucking
crowding   7 in scissors bite
early loss e in
crowded arch   5 buccal crossbite   **Aetiology**

unilateral
bilateral   **Classification**
with / without mandibular displacement

mandibular displacement   **Treatment needed**
may predispose to TMJDS

Posterior Crossbite

T spring or screw   consider relief of
section on URA   crowding / extract severely
fixed appliance   displaced tooth in crossbite   1–2 teeth   without mandibular
with ? cross elastics   accept   > 2 teeth   displacement

? grind c's   unilateral buccal crossbite
URA with midline screw   with mandibular displacement
quadhelix
usually accept   bilateral buccal crossbite
consider rapid maxillary expansion   (see Mind Map 15)   **Treatment**

fixed appliances   with mandibular displacement
expand lower / contract upper arch   complete unilateral
? surgery   no mandibular displacement   lingual crossbite
usually accept   complete bilateral
consider surgery   (see Mind Map 15)

good buccal interdigitation
no displacing contact(s)
favourable growth   **Stability**
no habits

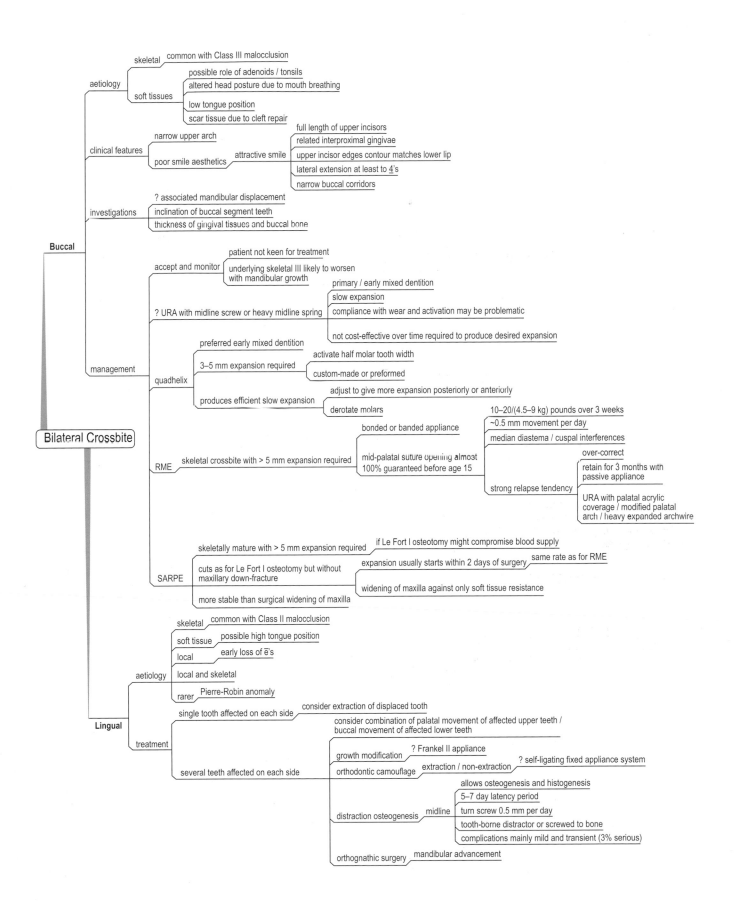

Bilateral Crossbite

Buccal

- aetiology
  - skeletal — common with Class III malocclusion
  - soft tissues
    - possible role of adenoids / tonsils
    - altered head posture due to mouth breathing
    - low tongue position
    - scar tissue due to cleft repair
- clinical features
  - narrow upper arch
  - poor smile aesthetics — attractive smile
    - full length of upper incisors
    - related interproximal gingivae
    - upper incisor edges contour matches lower lip
    - lateral extension at least to 4's
    - narrow buccal corridors
- investigations
  - ? associated mandibular displacement
  - inclination of buccal segment teeth
  - thickness of gingival tissues and buccal bone
- management
  - accept and monitor
    - patient not keen for treatment
    - underlying skeletal III likely to worsen with mandibular growth
  - ? URA with midline screw or heavy midline spring
    - primary / early mixed dentition
    - slow expansion
    - compliance with wear and activation may be problematic
    - not cost-effective over time required to produce desired expansion
  - quadhelix
    - preferred early mixed dentition
    - 3–5 mm expansion required
      - activate half molar tooth width
      - custom-made or preformed
    - produces efficient slow expansion
      - adjust to give more expansion posteriorly or anteriorly
      - derotate molars
  - RME
    - skeletal crossbite with > 5 mm expansion required
      - bonded or banded appliance
      - mid-palatal suture opening almost 100% guaranteed before age 15
        - 10–20/(4.5–9 kg) pounds over 3 weeks
        - ~0.5 mm movement per day
        - median diastema / cuspal interferences
        - strong relapse tendency
          - over-correct
          - retain for 3 months with passive appliance
          - URA with palatal acrylic coverage / modified palatal arch / heavy expanded archwire
  - SARPE
    - skeletally mature with > 5 mm expansion required
      - if Le Fort I osteotomy might compromise blood supply
    - cuts as for Le Fort I osteotomy but without maxillary down-fracture
      - expansion usually starts within 2 days of surgery — same rate as for RME
      - widening of maxilla against only soft tissue resistance
    - more stable than surgical widening of maxilla

Lingual

- aetiology
  - skeletal — common with Class II malocclusion
  - soft tissue — possible high tongue position
  - local — early loss of e̅'s
  - local and skeletal
  - rarer — Pierre-Robin anomaly
- treatment
  - single tooth affected on each side
    - consider extraction of displaced tooth
    - consider combination of palatal movement of affected upper teeth / buccal movement of affected lower teeth
  - several teeth affected on each side
    - growth modification — ? Frankel II appliance
    - orthodontic camouflage — extraction / non-extraction — ? self-ligating fixed appliance system
    - distraction osteogenesis — midline
      - allows osteogenesis and histogenesis
      - 5–7 day latency period
      - turn screw 0.5 mm per day
      - tooth-borne distractor or screwed to bone
      - complications mainly mild and transient (3% serious)
    - orthognathic surgery — mandibular advancement

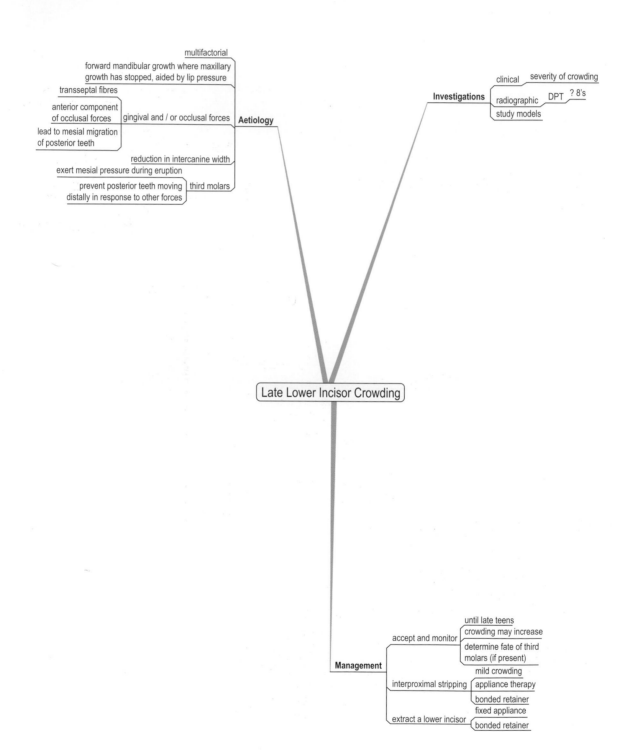

multifactorial

forward mandibular growth where maxillary
growth has stopped, aided by lip pressure

transseptal fibres

anterior component
of occlusal forces   gingival and / or occlusal forces   **Aetiology**

lead to mesial migration
of posterior teeth

reduction in intercanine width

exert mesial pressure during eruption

prevent posterior teeth moving   third molars
distally in response to other forces

Investigations   clinical   severity of crowding

radiographic   DPT   ? 8's

study models

Late Lower Incisor Crowding

Management

until late teens

accept and monitor   crowding may increase

determine fate of third
molars (if present)

mild crowding

interproximal stripping   appliance therapy

bonded retainer

fixed appliance

extract a lower incisor   bonded retainer

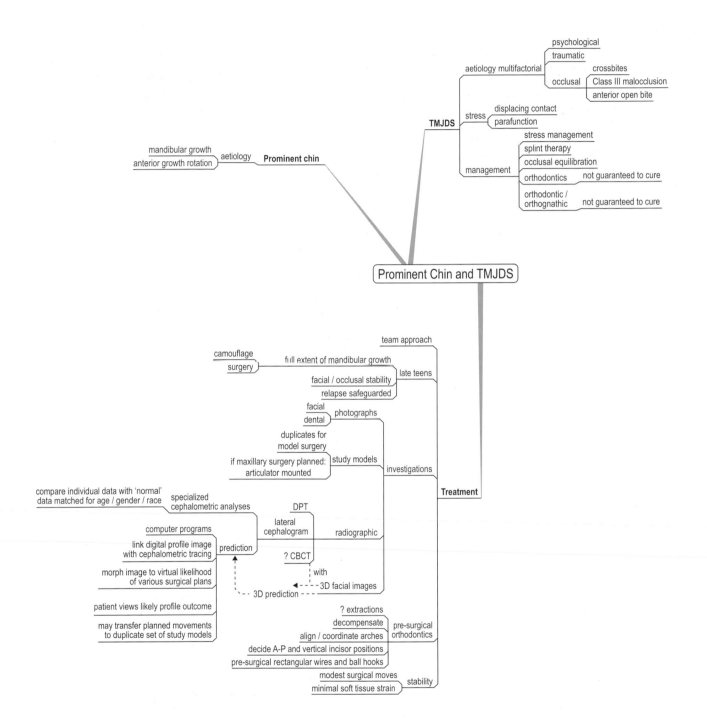

Prominent Chin and TMJDS

TMJDS

aetiology multifactorial
- psychological
- traumatic
- occlusal
  - crossbites
  - Class III malocclusion
  - anterior open bite

stress
- displacing contact
- parafunction

management
- stress management
- splint therapy
- occlusal equilibration
- orthodontics — not guaranteed to cure
- orthodontic / orthognathic — not guaranteed to cure

Prominent chin

aetiology
- mandibular growth
- anterior growth rotation

Treatment

camouflage

surgery — full extent of mandibular growth

team approach

late teens
- facial / occlusal stability
- relapse safeguarded

investigations

photographs
- facial
- dental

study models
- duplicates for model surgery
- if maxillary surgery planned: articulator mounted

radiographic
- DPT
- lateral cephalogram
- ? CBCT — with
  - 3D facial images

prediction
- specialized cephalometric analyses — compare individual data with 'normal' data matched for age / gender / race
- computer programs
- link digital profile image with cephalometric tracing
- morph image to virtual likelihood of various surgical plans
- patient views likely profile outcome
- may transfer planned movements to duplicate set of study models

3D prediction

pre-surgical orthodontics
- ? extractions
- decompensate
- align / coordinate arches
- decide A-P and vertical incisor positions
- pre-surgical rectangular wires and ball hooks

stability
- modest surgical moves
- minimal soft tissue strain

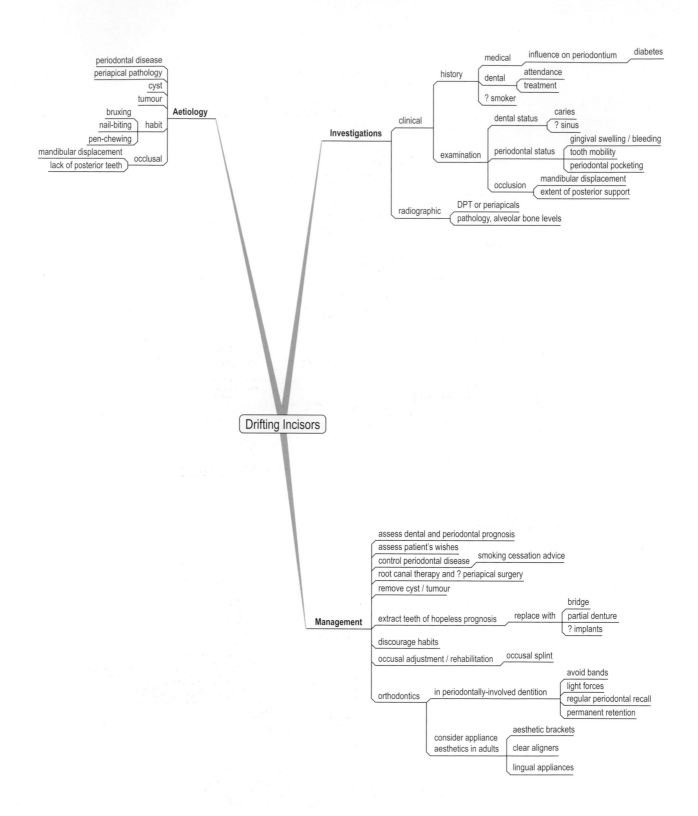

Aetiology

- periodontal disease
- periapical pathology
- cyst
- tumour
- habit
  - bruxing
  - nail-biting
  - pen-chewing
- occlusal
  - mandibular displacement
  - lack of posterior teeth

Investigations

- clinical
  - history
    - medical — influence on periodontium — diabetes
    - dental
      - attendance
      - treatment
    - ? smoker
  - examination
    - dental status
      - caries
      - ? sinus
    - periodontal status
      - gingival swelling / bleeding
      - tooth mobility
      - periodontal pocketing
    - occlusion
      - mandibular displacement
      - extent of posterior support
- radiographic
  - DPT or periapicals
  - pathology, alveolar bone levels

Drifting Incisors

Management

- assess dental and periodontal prognosis
- assess patient's wishes
- control periodontal disease — smoking cessation advice
- root canal therapy and ? periapical surgery
- remove cyst / tumour
- extract teeth of hopeless prognosis — replace with
  - bridge
  - partial denture
  - ? implants
- discourage habits
- occusal adjustment / rehabilitation — occusal splint
- orthodontics
  - in periodontally-involved dentition
    - avoid bands
    - light forces
    - regular periodontal recall
    - permanent retention
  - consider appliance aesthetics in adults
    - aesthetic brackets
    - clear aligners
    - lingual appliances

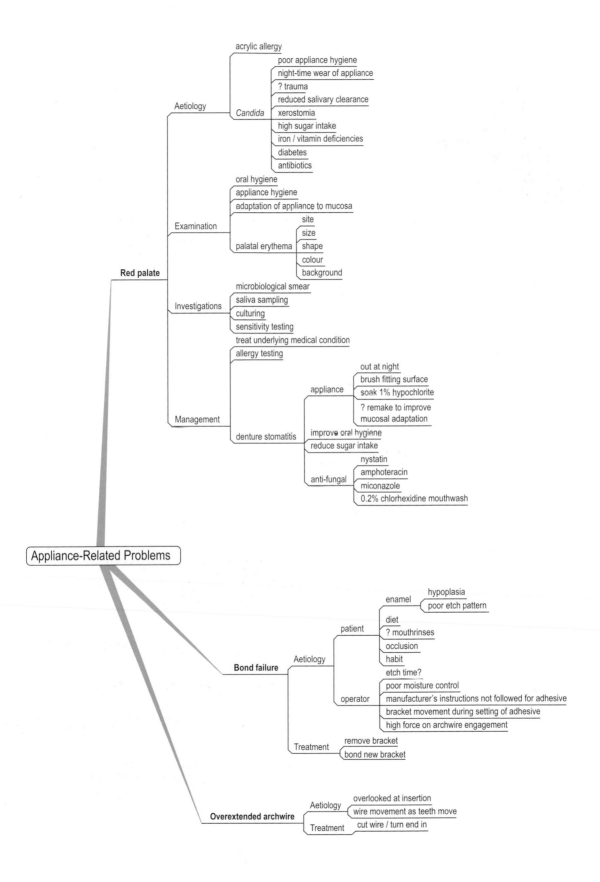

Red palate

Aetiology
- acrylic allergy
- *Candida*
  - poor appliance hygiene
  - night-time wear of appliance
  - ? trauma
  - reduced salivary clearance
  - xerostomia
  - high sugar intake
  - iron / vitamin deficiencies
  - diabetes
  - antibiotics

Examination
- oral hygiene
- appliance hygiene
- adaptation of appliance to mucosa
- palatal erythema
  - site
  - size
  - shape
  - colour
  - background

Investigations
- microbiological smear
- saliva sampling
- culturing
- sensitivity testing

Management
- treat underlying medical condition
- allergy testing
- denture stomatitis
  - appliance
    - out at night
    - brush fitting surface
    - soak 1% hypochlorite
    - ? remake to improve mucosal adaptation
  - improve oral hygiene
  - reduce sugar intake
  - anti-fungal
    - nystatin
    - amphoteracin
    - miconazole
    - 0.2% chlorhexidine mouthwash

Appliance-Related Problems

Bond failure

Aetiology
- patient
  - enamel
    - hypoplasia
    - poor etch pattern
  - diet
  - ? mouthrinses
  - occlusion
  - habit
- operator
  - etch time?
  - poor moisture control
  - manufacturer's instructions not followed for adhesive
  - bracket movement during setting of adhesive
  - high force on archwire engagement

Treatment
- remove bracket
- bond new bracket

Overextended archwire

Aetiology
- overlooked at insertion
- wire movement as teeth move

Treatment
- cut wire / turn end in

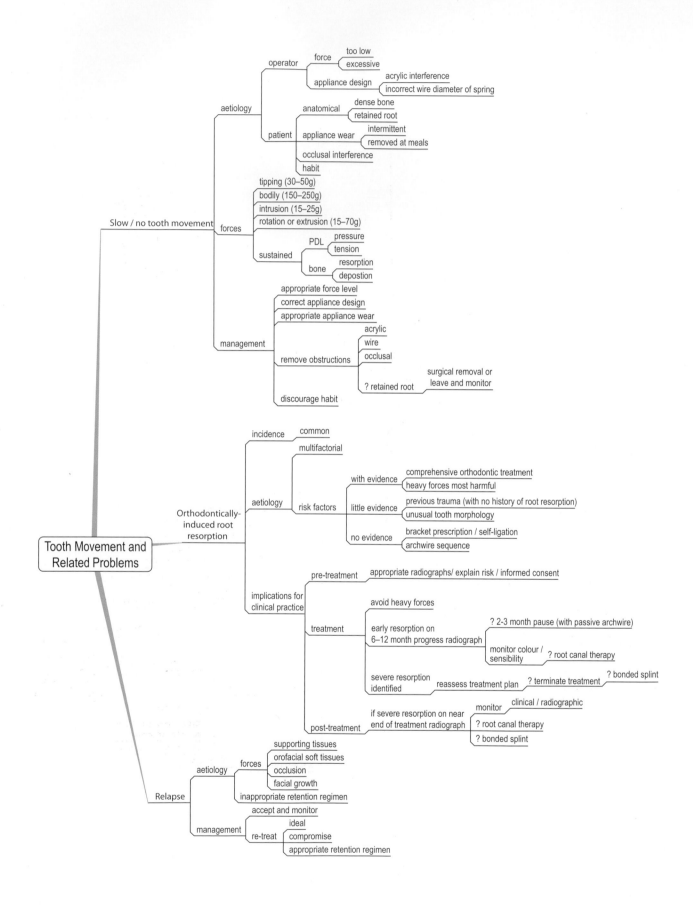

Tooth Movement and Related Problems

Slow / no tooth movement

aetiology
operator
force
too low
excessive
appliance design
acrylic interference
incorrect wire diameter of spring

patient
anatomical
dense bone
retained root
appliance wear
intermittent
removed at meals
occlusal interference
habit

forces
tipping (30–50g)
bodily (150–250g)
intrusion (15–25g)
rotation or extrusion (15–70g)
sustained
PDL
pressure
tension
bone
resorption
depostion

management
appropriate force level
correct appliance design
appropriate appliance wear
remove obstructions
acrylic
wire
occlusal
? retained root
surgical removal or leave and monitor
discourage habit

Orthodontically-induced root resorption

incidence
common

aetiology
multifactorial
risk factors
with evidence
comprehensive orthodontic treatment
heavy forces most harmful
little evidence
previous trauma (with no history of root resorption)
unusual tooth morphology
no evidence
bracket prescription / self-ligation
archwire sequence

implications for clinical practice
pre-treatment
appropriate radiographs/ explain risk / informed consent

treatment
avoid heavy forces
early resorption on 6–12 month progress radiograph
? 2-3 month pause (with passive archwire)
monitor colour / sensibility
? root canal therapy
severe resorption identified
reassess treatment plan
? terminate treatment
? bonded splint

post-treatment
if severe resorption on near end of treatment radiograph
monitor
clinical / radiographic
? root canal therapy
? bonded splint

Relapse

aetiology
forces
supporting tissues
orofacial soft tissues
occlusion
facial growth
inappropriate retention regimen

management
accept and monitor
re-treat
ideal
compromise
appropriate retention regimen

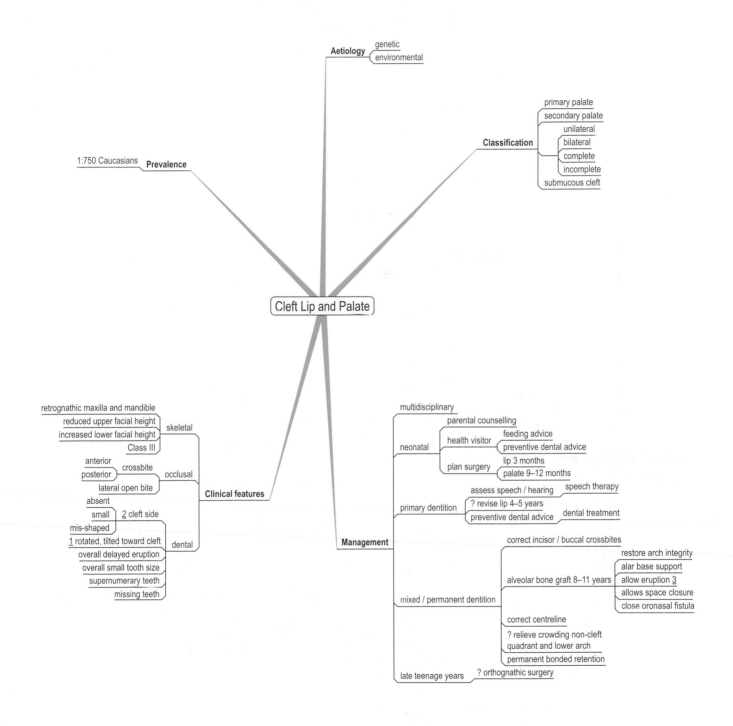

Aetiology
genetic
environmental

Classification
primary palate
secondary palate
unilateral
bilateral
complete
incomplete
submucous cleft

1:750 Caucasians **Prevalence**

Cleft Lip and Palate

Clinical features

retrognathic maxilla and mandible
reduced upper facial height
increased lower facial height   skeletal
Class III

anterior
posterior crossbite   occlusal
lateral open bite

absent
small   2 cleft side
mis-shaped
1 rotated, tilted toward cleft   dental
overall delayed eruption
overall small tooth size
supernumerary teeth
missing teeth

Management

multidisciplinary
parental counselling
health visitor   feeding advice
neonatal   preventive dental advice
plan surgery   lip 3 months
palate 9–12 months

assess speech / hearing   speech therapy
primary dentition   ? revise lip 4–5 years
preventive dental advice   dental treatment

correct incisor / buccal crossbites
restore arch integrity
alar base support
alveolar bone graft 8–11 years   allow eruption 3
mixed / permanent dentition   allows space closure
close oronasal fistula

correct centreline
? relieve crowding non-cleft
quadrant and lower arch
permanent bonded retention

late teenage years   ? orthognathic surgery

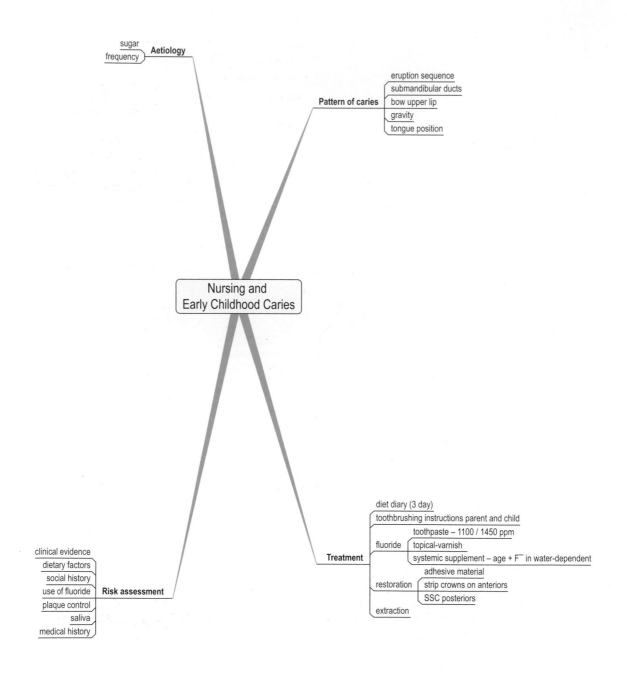

sugar
frequency **Aetiology**

Pattern of caries
- eruption sequence
- submandibular ducts
- bow upper lip
- gravity
- tongue position

Nursing and
Early Childhood Caries

Treatment
- diet diary (3 day)
- toothbrushing instructions parent and child
- fluoride
  - toothpaste – 1100 / 1450 ppm
  - topical-varnish
  - systemic supplement – age + F⁻ in water-dependent
- restoration
  - adhesive material
  - strip crowns on anteriors
  - SSC posteriors
- extraction

clinical evidence
dietary factors
social history
use of fluoride **Risk assessment**
plaque control
saliva
medical history

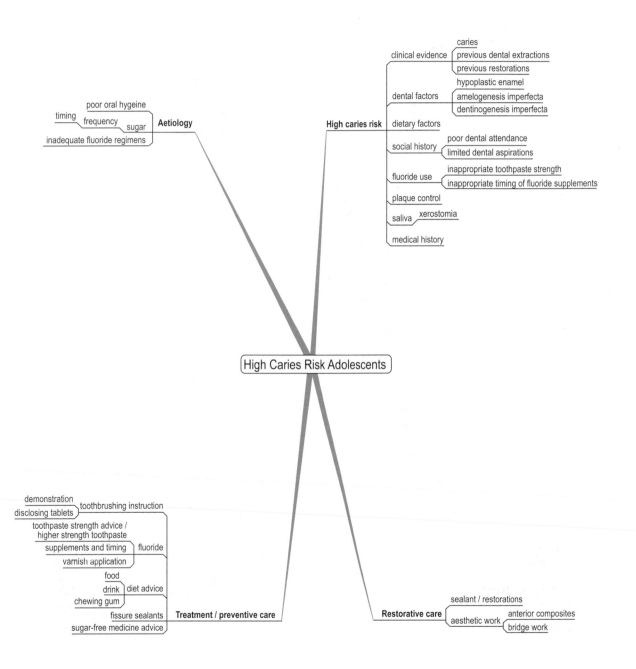

Aetiology

poor oral hygeine
timing
frequency sugar
inadequate fluoride regimens

High caries risk

clinical evidence
  caries
  previous dental extractions
  previous restorations
dental factors
  hypoplastic enamel
  amelogenesis imperfecta
  dentinogenesis imperfecta
dietary factors
social history
  poor dental attendance
  limited dental aspirations
fluoride use
  inappropriate toothpaste strength
  inappropriate timing of fluoride supplements
plaque control
saliva xerostomia
medical history

High Caries Risk Adolescents

Treatment / preventive care

demonstration
disclosing tablets toothbrushing instruction
toothpaste strength advice /
higher strength toothpaste
supplements and timing fluoride
varnish application
food
drink diet advice
chewing gum
fissure sealants
sugar-free medicine advice

Restorative care

sealant / restorations
aesthetic work anterior composites
  bridge work

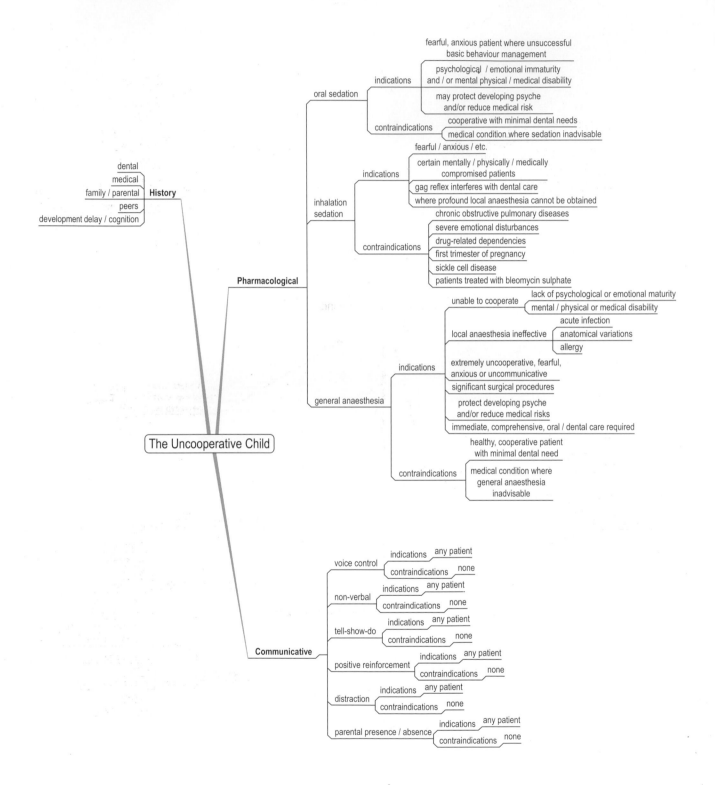

The Uncooperative Child

History
- dental
- medical
- family / parental
- peers
- development delay / cognition

Pharmacological

oral sedation
- indications
  - fearful, anxious patient where unsuccessful basic behaviour management
  - psychological / emotional immaturity and / or mental physical / medical disability
  - may protect developing psyche and/or reduce medical risk
- contraindications
  - cooperative with minimal dental needs
  - medical condition where sedation inadvisable

inhalation sedation
- indications
  - fearful / anxious / etc.
  - certain mentally / physically / medically compromised patients
  - gag reflex interferes with dental care
  - where profound local anaesthesia cannot be obtained
- contraindications
  - chronic obstructive pulmonary diseases
  - severe emotional disturbances
  - drug-related dependencies
  - first trimester of pregnancy
  - sickle cell disease
  - patients treated with bleomycin sulphate

general anaesthesia
- indications
  - unable to cooperate
    - lack of psychological or emotional maturity
    - mental / physical or medical disability
  - local anaesthesia ineffective
    - acute infection
    - anatomical variations
    - allergy
  - extremely uncooperative, fearful, anxious or uncommunicative
  - significant surgical procedures
  - protect developing psyche and/or reduce medical risks
  - immediate, comprehensive, oral / dental care required
- contraindications
  - healthy, cooperative patient with minimal dental need
  - medical condition where general anaesthesia inadvisable

Communicative

voice control
- indications — any patient
- contraindications — none

non-verbal
- indications — any patient
- contraindications — none

tell-show-do
- indications — any patient
- contraindications — none

positive reinforcement
- indications — any patient
- contraindications — none

distraction
- indications — any patient
- contraindications — none

parental presence / absence
- indications — any patient
- contraindications — none

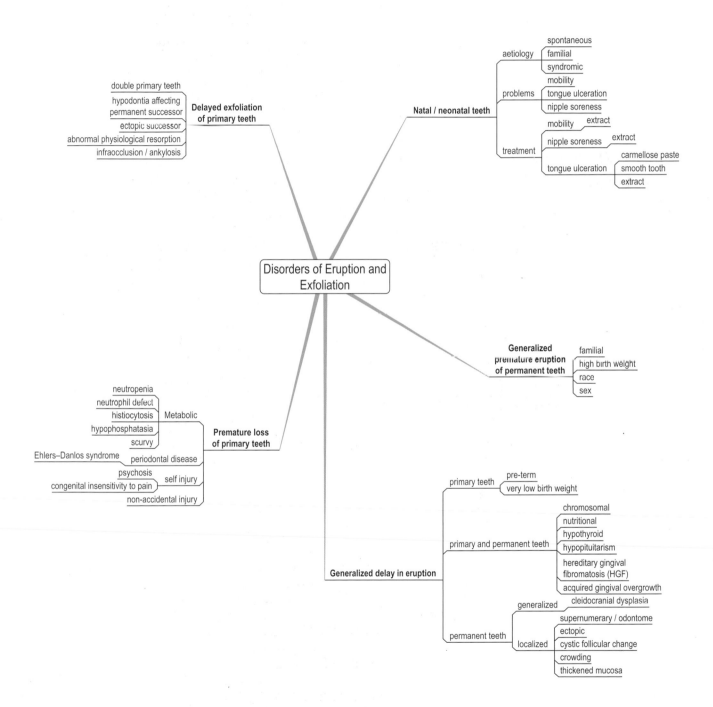

double primary teeth

hypodontia affecting
permanent successor

ectopic successor

abnormal physiological resorption

infraocclusion / ankylosis

**Delayed exfoliation
of primary teeth**

Natal / neonatal teeth

aetiology
- spontaneous
- familial
- syndromic

problems
- mobility
- tongue ulceration
- nipple soreness

treatment
- mobility — extract
- nipple soreness — extract
- tongue ulceration
  - carmellose paste
  - smooth tooth
  - extract

Disorders of Eruption and
Exfoliation

**Generalized
premature eruption
of permanent teeth**
- familial
- high birth weight
- race
- sex

neutropenia

neutrophil defect

histiocytosis

hypophosphatasia

scurvy

Metabolic

Ehlers–Danlos syndrome — periodontal disease

psychosis

congenital insensitivity to pain

self injury

non-accidental injury

**Premature loss
of primary teeth**

Generalized delay in eruption

primary teeth
- pre-term
- very low birth weight

primary and permanent teeth
- chromosomal
- nutritional
- hypothyroid
- hypopituitarism
- hereditary gingival fibromatosis (HGF)
- acquired gingival overgrowth

permanent teeth
- generalized — cleidocranial dysplasia
- localized
  - supernumerary / odontome
  - ectopic
  - cystic follicular change
  - crowding
  - thickened mucosa

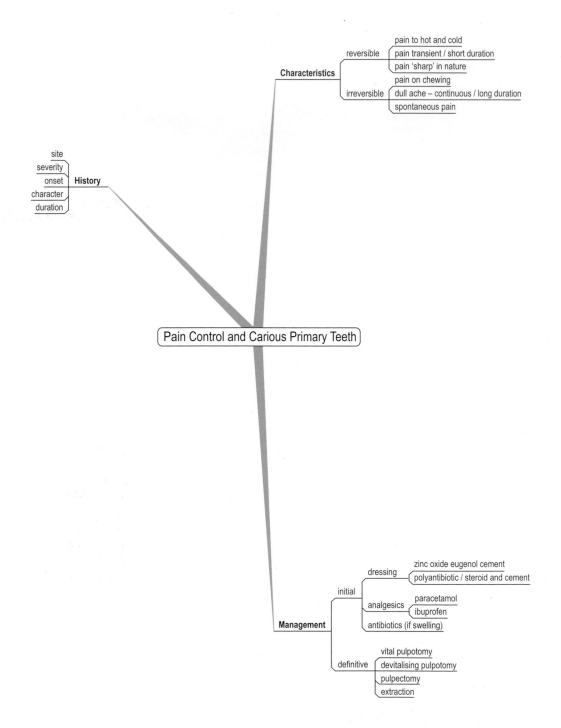

Characteristics

reversible
- pain to hot and cold
- pain transient / short duration
- pain 'sharp' in nature

irreversible
- pain on chewing
- dull ache – continuous / long duration
- spontaneous pain

History
- site
- severity
- onset
- character
- duration

Pain Control and Carious Primary Teeth

Management

initial
- dressing
  - zinc oxide eugenol cement
  - polyantibiotic / steroid and cement
- analgesics
  - paracetamol
  - ibuprofen
- antibiotics (if swelling)

definitive
- vital pulpotomy
- devitalising pulpotomy
- pulpectomy
- extraction

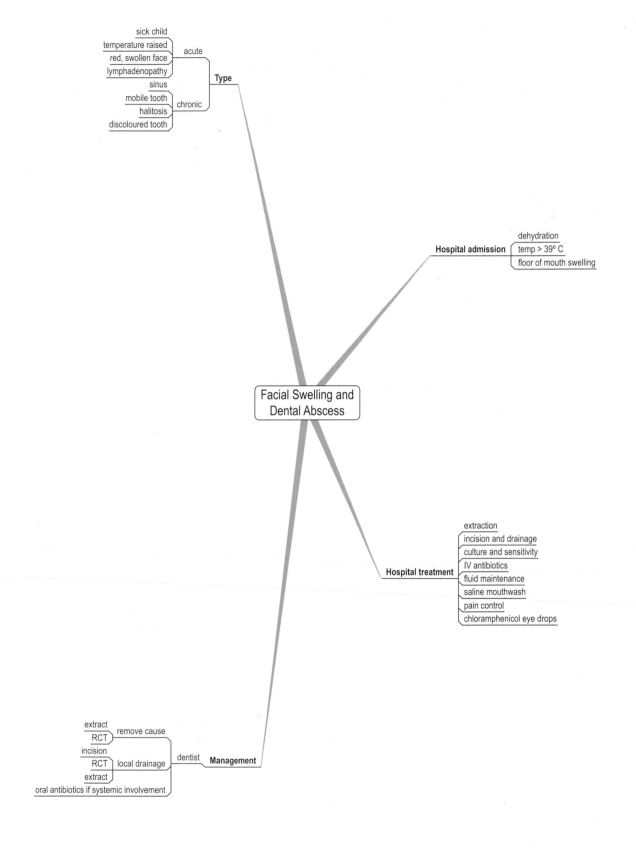

sick child
temperature raised
red, swollen face   acute
lymphadenopathy
sinus   **Type**
mobile tooth   chronic
halitosis
discoloured tooth

                                                                    dehydration
                                        Hospital admission   temp > 39º C
                                                                    floor of mouth swelling

Facial Swelling and
Dental Abscess

                                                                    extraction
                                                                    incision and drainage
                                                                    culture and sensitivity
                                          Hospital treatment   IV antibiotics
                                                                    fluid maintenance
                                                                    saline mouthwash
                                                                    pain control
                                                                    chloramphenicol eye drops

extract
            remove cause
RCT
incision   dentist   **Management**
RCT   local drainage
extract
oral antibiotics if systemic involvement

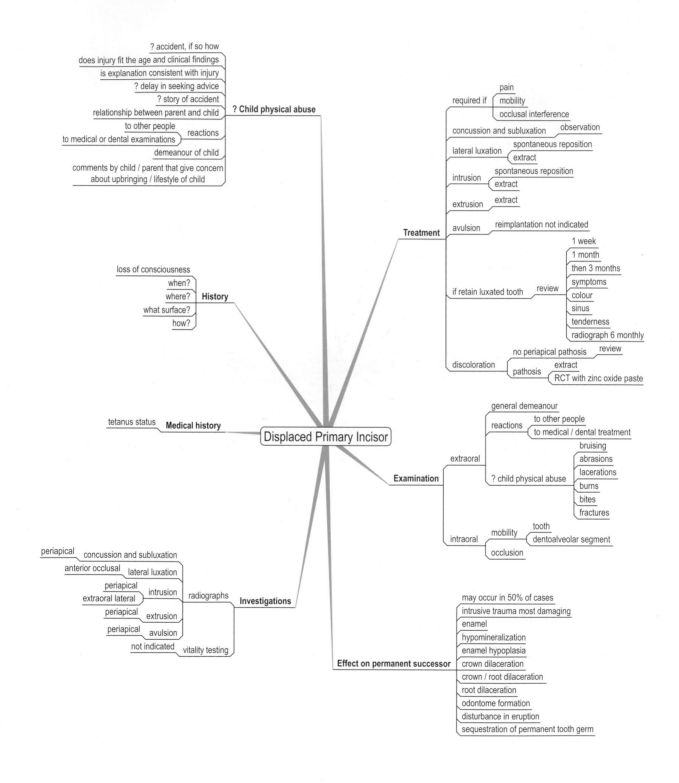

? accident, if so how
does injury fit the age and clinical findings
is explanation consistent with injury
? delay in seeking advice
? story of accident
relationship between parent and child
to other people
to medical or dental examinations } reactions
demeanour of child
comments by child / parent that give concern
about upbringing / lifestyle of child

? Child physical abuse

Treatment

required if
pain
mobility
occlusal interference

concussion and subluxation — observation

lateral luxation
spontaneous reposition
extract

intrusion
spontaneous reposition
extract

extrusion — extract

avulsion — reimplantation not indicated

if retain luxated tooth — review
1 week
1 month
then 3 months
symptoms
colour
sinus
tenderness
radiograph 6 monthly

discoloration
no periapical pathosis — review
pathosis
extract
RCT with zinc oxide paste

loss of consciousness
when?
where?
what surface?
how?

History

Displaced Primary Incisor

tetanus status **Medical history**

Examination

extraoral
reactions
general demeanour
to other people
to medical / dental treatment

? child physical abuse
bruising
abrasions
lacerations
burns
bites
fractures

intraoral
mobility
tooth
dentoalveolar segment
occlusion

periapical — concussion and subluxation
anterior occlusal — lateral luxation
periapical
extraoral lateral } intrusion
periapical
extrusion
periapical
avulsion
not indicated — vitality testing

radiographs

Investigations

Effect on permanent successor
may occur in 50% of cases
intrusive trauma most damaging
enamel
hypomineralization
enamel hypoplasia
crown dilaceration
crown / root dilaceration
root dilaceration
odontome formation
disturbance in eruption
sequestration of permanent tooth germ

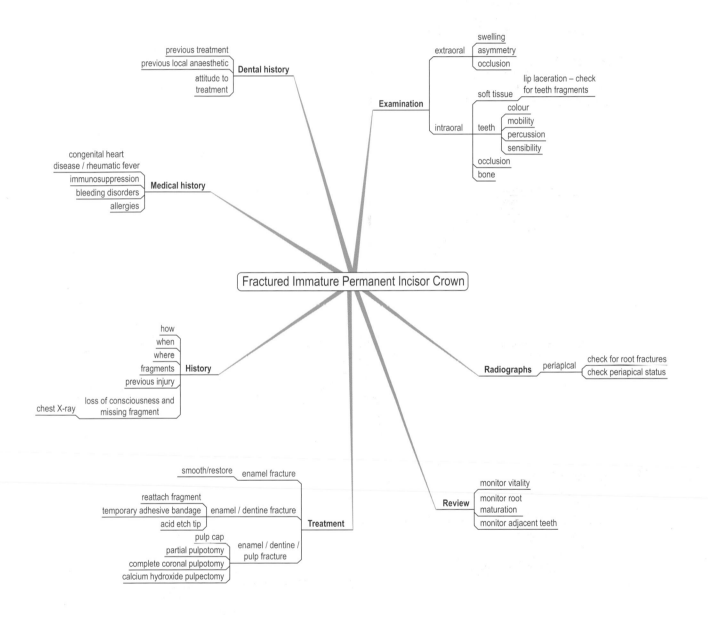

Dental history
- previous treatment
- previous local anaesthetic
- attitude to treatment

Medical history
- congenital heart disease / rheumatic fever
- immunosuppression
- bleeding disorders
- allergies

History
- how
- when
- where
- fragments
- previous injury
- loss of consciousness and missing fragment
  - chest X-ray

Examination
- extraoral
  - swelling
  - asymmetry
  - occlusion
- intraoral
  - soft tissue
    - lip laceration – check for teeth fragments
  - teeth
    - colour
    - mobility
    - percussion
    - sensibility
  - occlusion
  - bone

Fractured Immature Permanent Incisor Crown

Radiographs
- periapical
  - check for root fractures
  - check periapical status

Review
- monitor vitality
- monitor root maturation
- monitor adjacent teeth

Treatment
- enamel fracture
  - smooth/restore
- enamel / dentine fracture
  - reattach fragment
  - temporary adhesive bandage
  - acid etch tip
- enamel / dentine / pulp fracture
  - pulp cap
  - partial pulpotomy
  - complete coronal pulpotomy
  - calcium hydroxide pulpectomy

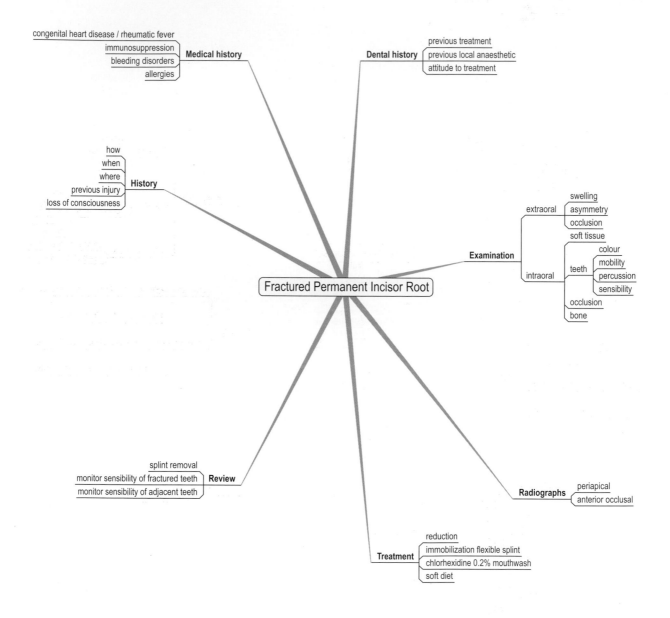

congenital heart disease / rheumatic fever
immunosuppression
bleeding disorders
allergies

Medical history

previous treatment
previous local anaesthetic
attitude to treatment

Dental history

how
when
where
previous injury
loss of consciousness

History

Fractured Permanent Incisor Root

Examination

extraoral
swelling
asymmetry
occlusion

intraoral
soft tissue
teeth
colour
mobility
percussion
sensibility
occlusion
bone

splint removal
monitor sensibility of fractured teeth
monitor sensibility of adjacent teeth

Review

Radiographs
periapical
anterior occlusal

Treatment
reduction
immobilization flexible splint
chlorhexidine 0.2% mouthwash
soft diet

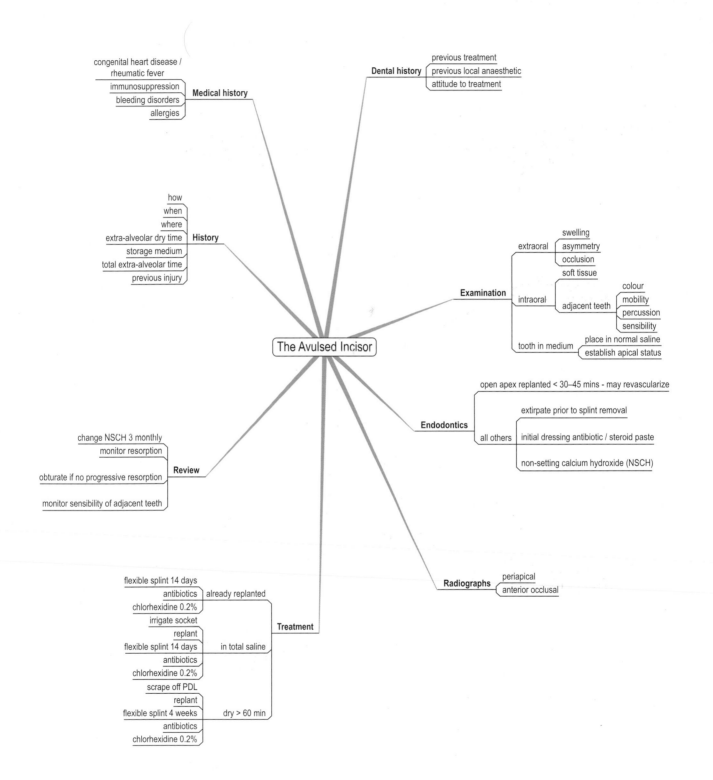

Medical history
- congenital heart disease / rheumatic fever
- immunosuppression
- bleeding disorders
- allergies

Dental history
- previous treatment
- previous local anaesthetic
- attitude to treatment

History
- how
- when
- where
- extra-alveolar dry time
- storage medium
- total extra-alveolar time
- previous injury

Examination
- extraoral
  - swelling
  - asymmetry
  - occlusion
- intraoral
  - soft tissue
  - adjacent teeth
    - colour
    - mobility
    - percussion
    - sensibility
- tooth in medium
  - place in normal saline
  - establish apical status

Endodontics
- open apex replanted < 30–45 mins - may revascularize
- all others
  - extirpate prior to splint removal
  - initial dressing antibiotic / steroid paste
  - non-setting calcium hydroxide (NSCH)

Review
- change NSCH 3 monthly
- monitor resorption
- obturate if no progressive resorption
- monitor sensibility of adjacent teeth

Radiographs
- periapical
- anterior occlusal

Treatment
- already replanted
  - flexible splint 14 days
  - antibiotics
  - chlorhexidine 0.2%
- in total saline
  - irrigate socket
  - replant
  - flexible splint 14 days
  - antibiotics
  - chlorhexidine 0.2%
- dry > 60 min
  - scrape off PDL
  - replant
  - flexible splint 4 weeks
  - antibiotics
  - chlorhexidine 0.2%

The Avulsed Incisor

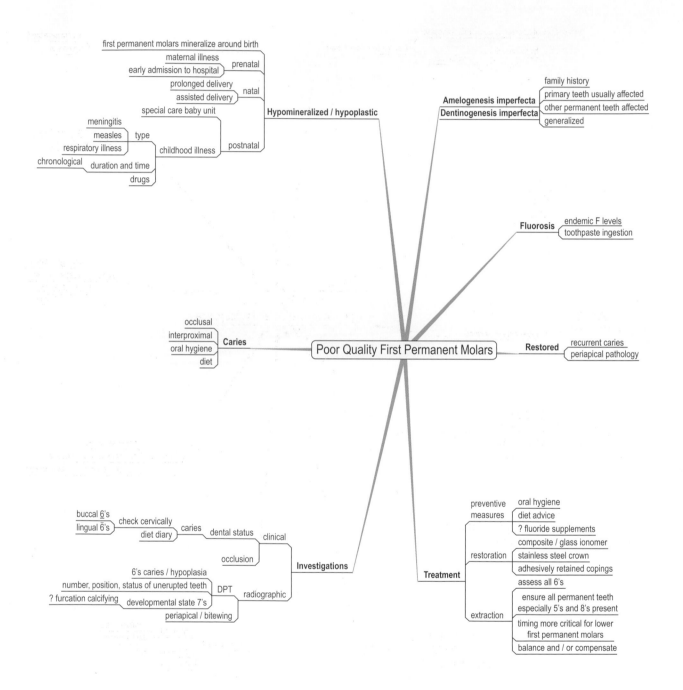

first permanent molars mineralize around birth

maternal illness
early admission to hospital ⟩ prenatal

prolonged delivery
assisted delivery ⟩ natal

special care baby unit

meningitis
measles   type
respiratory illness
chronological   duration and time   childhood illness   postnatal
drugs

Hypomineralized / hypoplastic

Amelogenesis imperfecta
Dentinogenesis imperfecta

family history
primary teeth usually affected
other permanent teeth affected
generalized

Fluorosis   endemic F levels
toothpaste ingestion

occlusal
interproximal
oral hygiene   Caries
diet

Poor Quality First Permanent Molars

Restored   recurrent caries
periapical pathology

buccal 6's
lingual 6's   check cervically
diet diary   caries   dental status   clinical
occlusion

6's caries / hypoplasia
number, position, status of unerupted teeth   DPT   radiographic
? furcation calcifying   developmental state 7's
periapical / bitewing

Investigations

Treatment

preventive
measures   oral hygiene
diet advice
? fluoride supplements

restoration   composite / glass ionomer
stainless steel crown
adhesively retained copings

extraction   assess all 6's
ensure all permanent teeth
especially 5's and 8's present
timing more critical for lower
first permanent molars
balance and / or compensate

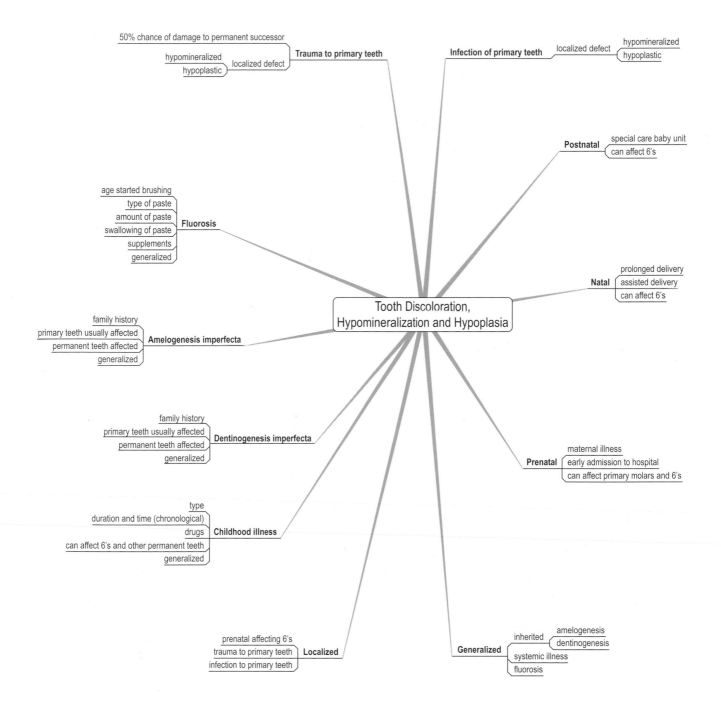

50% chance of damage to permanent successor

hypomineralized
hypoplastic — localized defect — **Trauma to primary teeth**

Infection of primary teeth — localized defect — hypomineralized
hypoplastic

Postnatal — special care baby unit
can affect 6's

age started brushing
type of paste
amount of paste
swallowing of paste — **Fluorosis**
supplements
generalized

Natal — prolonged delivery
assisted delivery
can affect 6's

family history
primary teeth usually affected
permanent teeth affected — **Amelogenesis imperfecta**
generalized

Tooth Discoloration,
Hypomineralization and Hypoplasia

family history
primary teeth usually affected
permanent teeth affected — **Dentinogenesis imperfecta**
generalized

Prenatal — maternal illness
early admission to hospital
can affect primary molars and 6's

type
duration and time (chronological)
drugs — **Childhood illness**
can affect 6's and other permanent teeth
generalized

prenatal affecting 6's
trauma to primary teeth — **Localized**
infection to primary teeth

Generalized — inherited — amelogenesis
dentinogenesis
systemic illness
fluorosis

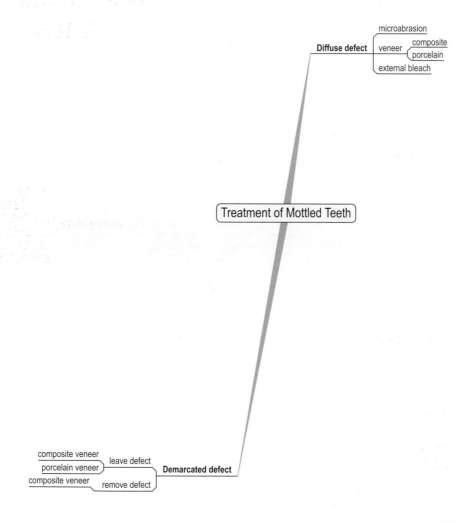

microabrasion

Diffuse defect

veneer

composite

porcelain

external bleach

Treatment of Mottled Teeth

composite veneer

leave defect

porcelain veneer

Demarcated defect

composite veneer

remove defect

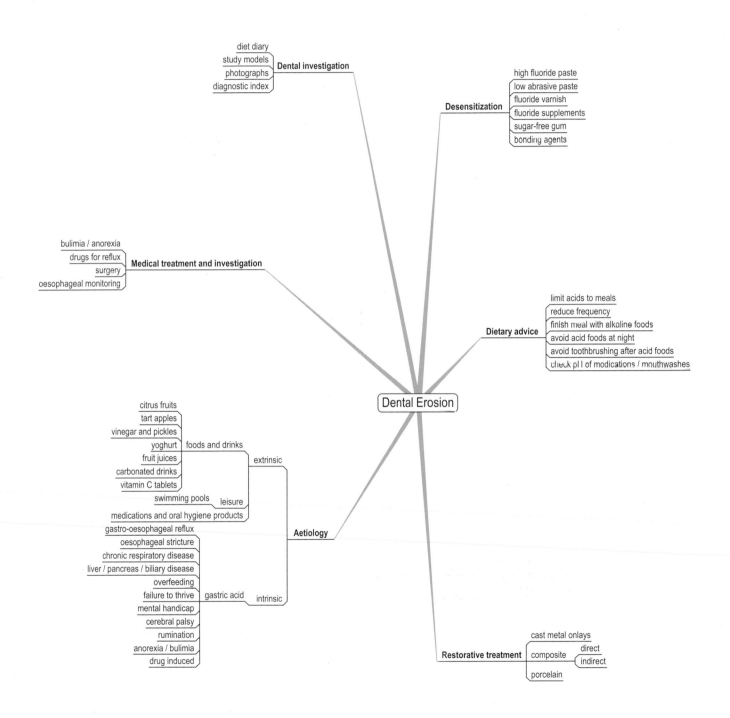

Dental investigation
- diet diary
- study models
- photographs
- diagnostic index

Desensitization
- high fluoride paste
- low abrasive paste
- fluoride varnish
- fluoride supplements
- sugar-free gum
- bonding agents

Medical treatment and investigation
- bulimia / anorexia
- drugs for reflux
- surgery
- oesophageal monitoring

Dietary advice
- limit acids to meals
- reduce frequency
- finish meal with alkaline foods
- avoid acid foods at night
- avoid toothbrushing after acid foods
- check pH of medications / mouthwashes

Dental Erosion

Aetiology

extrinsic
- foods and drinks
  - citrus fruits
  - tart apples
  - vinegar and pickles
  - yoghurt
  - fruit juices
  - carbonated drinks
  - vitamin C tablets
- leisure
  - swimming pools
- medications and oral hygiene products

intrinsic
- gastric acid
  - gastro-oesophageal reflux
  - oesophageal stricture
  - chronic respiratory disease
  - liver / pancreas / biliary disease
  - overfeeding
  - failure to thrive
  - mental handicap
  - cerebral palsy
  - rumination
  - anorexia / bulimia
  - drug induced

Restorative treatment
- cast metal onlays
- composite
  - direct
  - indirect
- porcelain

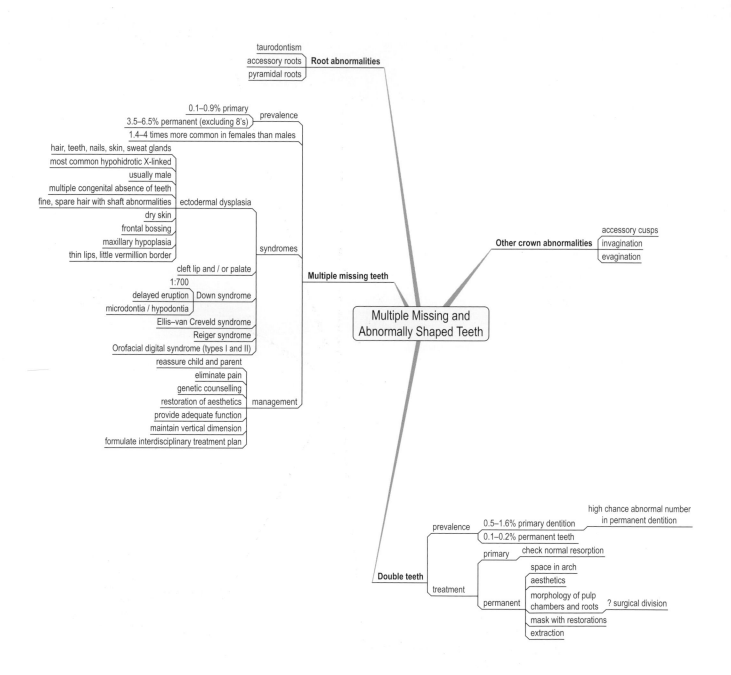

taurodontism
accessory roots   **Root abnormalities**
pyramidal roots

0.1–0.9% primary
3.5–6.5% permanent (excluding 8's)   prevalence
1.4–4 times more common in females than males

hair, teeth, nails, skin, sweat glands
most common hypohidrotic X-linked
usually male
multiple congenital absence of teeth
fine, spare hair with shaft abnormalities   ectodermal dysplasia
dry skin
frontal bossing
maxillary hypoplasia
thin lips, little vermillion border

cleft lip and / or palate
1:700
delayed eruption   Down syndrome
microdontia / hypodontia
Ellis–van Creveld syndrome
Reiger syndrome
Orofacial digital syndrome (types I and II)

reassure child and parent
eliminate pain
genetic counselling
restoration of aesthetics   management
provide adequate function
maintain vertical dimension
formulate interdisciplinary treatment plan

syndromes

Multiple missing teeth

Multiple Missing and
Abnormally Shaped Teeth

Other crown abnormalities
accessory cusps
invagination
evagination

Double teeth

prevalence
0.5–1.6% primary dentition   high chance abnormal number in permanent dentition
0.1–0.2% permanent teeth

primary   check normal resorption

treatment

permanent
space in arch
aesthetics
morphology of pulp chambers and roots   ? surgical division
mask with restorations
extraction

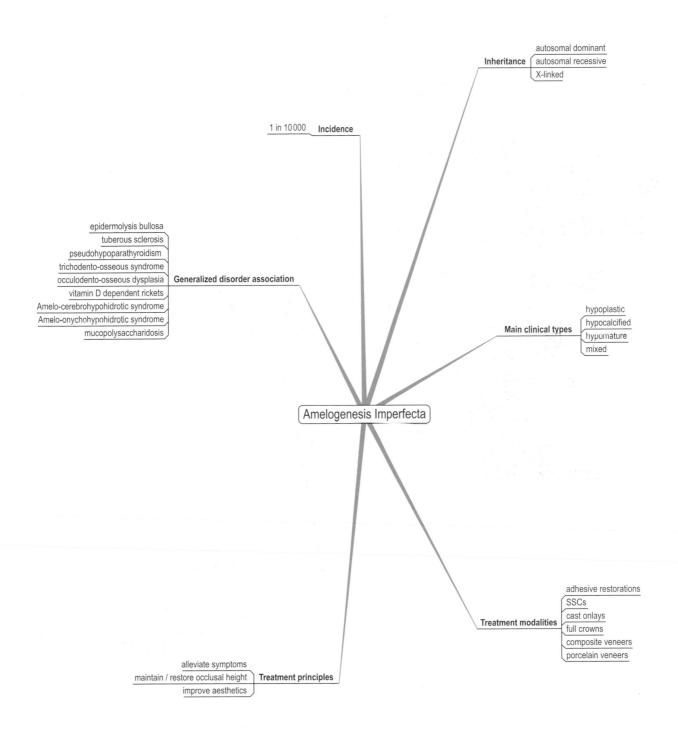

Inheritance
- autosomal dominant
- autosomal recessive
- X-linked

Incidence
- 1 in 10 000

Generalized disorder association
- epidermolysis bullosa
- tuberous sclerosis
- pseudohypoparathyroidism
- trichodento-osseous syndrome
- occulodento-osseous dysplasia
- vitamin D dependent rickets
- Amelo-cerebrohypohidrotic syndrome
- Amelo-onychohypohidrotic syndrome
- mucopolysaccharidosis

Main clinical types
- hypoplastic
- hypocalcified
- hypomature
- mixed

Amelogenesis Imperfecta

Treatment modalities
- adhesive restorations
- SSCs
- cast onlays
- full crowns
- composite veneers
- porcelain veneers

Treatment principles
- alleviate symptoms
- maintain / restore occlusal height
- improve aesthetics

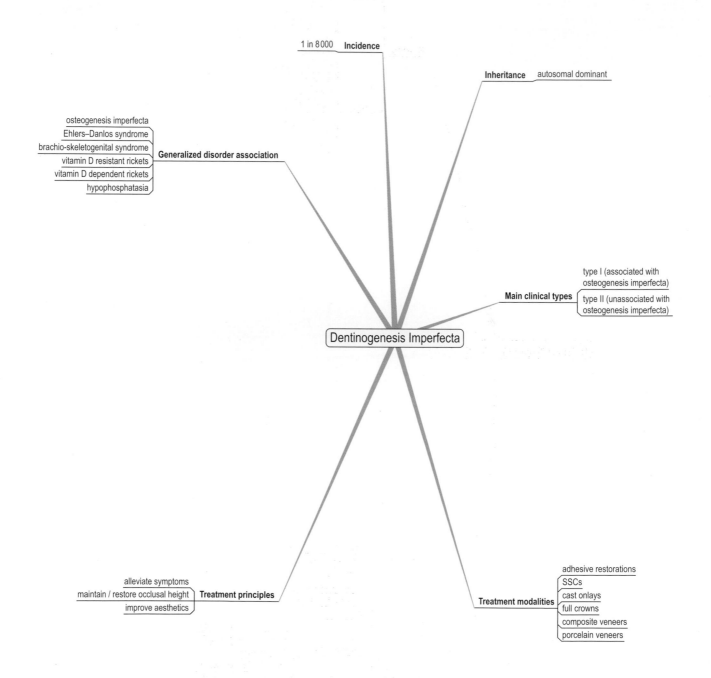

1 in 8 000 **Incidence**

Inheritance autosomal dominant

osteogenesis imperfecta
Ehlers–Danlos syndrome
brachio-skeletogenital syndrome
vitamin D resistant rickets
vitamin D dependent rickets
hypophosphatasia
Generalized disorder association

Main clinical types
type I (associated with osteogenesis imperfecta)
type II (unassociated with osteogenesis imperfecta)

Dentinogenesis Imperfecta

alleviate symptoms
maintain / restore occlusal height
improve aesthetics
Treatment principles

Treatment modalities
adhesive restorations
SSCs
cast onlays
full crowns
composite veneers
porcelain veneers

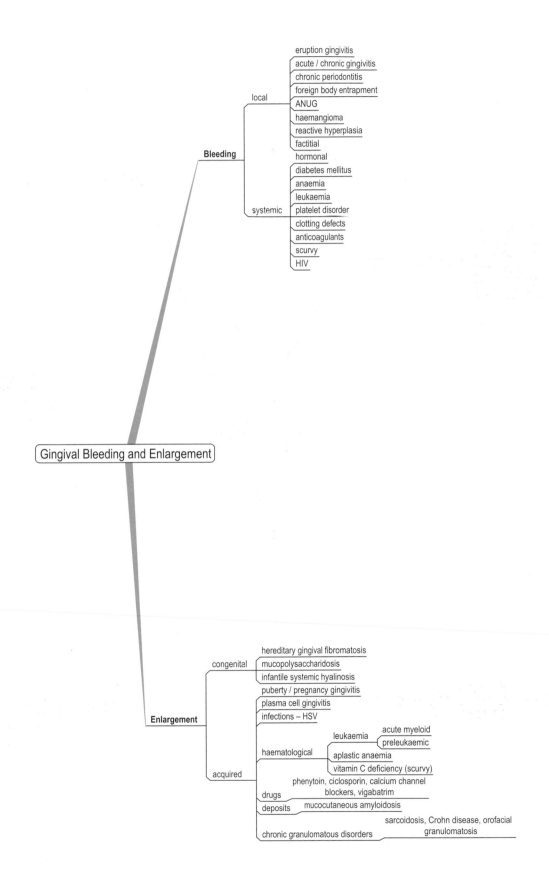

Gingival Bleeding and Enlargement

Bleeding

local
- eruption gingivitis
- acute / chronic gingivitis
- chronic periodontitis
- foreign body entrapment
- ANUG
- haemangioma
- reactive hyperplasia
- factitial

systemic
- hormonal
- diabetes mellitus
- anaemia
- leukaemia
- platelet disorder
- clotting defects
- anticoagulants
- scurvy
- HIV

Enlargement

congenital
- hereditary gingival fibromatosis
- mucopolysaccharidosis
- infantile systemic hyalinosis

acquired
- puberty / pregnancy gingivitis
- plasma cell gingivitis
- infections – HSV
- haematological
  - leukaemia
    - acute myeloid
    - preleukaemic
  - aplastic anaemia
  - vitamin C deficiency (scurvy)
- drugs
  - phenytoin, ciclosporin, calcium channel blockers, vigabatrim
- deposits
  - mucocutaneous amyloidosis
- chronic granulomatous disorders
  - sarcoidosis, Crohn disease, orofacial granulomatosis

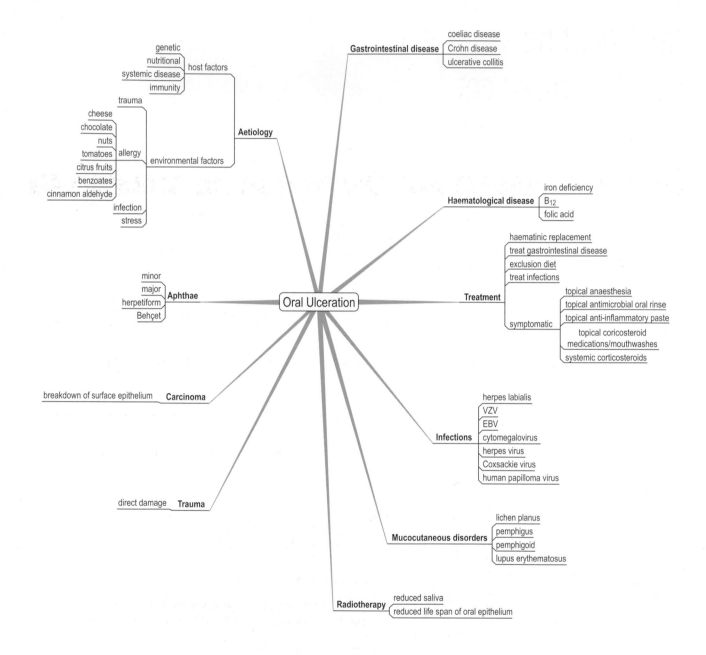

Aetiology

host factors
- genetic
- nutritional
- systemic disease
- immunity

environmental factors
- trauma
- allergy
  - cheese
  - chocolate
  - nuts
  - tomatoes
  - citrus fruits
  - benzoates
  - cinnamon aldehyde
- infection
- stress

Gastrointestinal disease
- coeliac disease
- Crohn disease
- ulcerative collitis

Haematological disease
- iron deficiency
- B_{12}
- folic acid

Treatment
- haematinic replacement
- treat gastrointestinal disease
- exclusion diet
- treat infections
- symptomatic
  - topical anaesthesia
  - topical antimicrobial oral rinse
  - topical anti-inflammatory paste
  - topical coricosteroid medications/mouthwashes
  - systemic corticosteroids

Aphthae
- minor
- major
- herpetiform
- Behçet

Oral Ulceration

Carcinoma
- breakdown of surface epithelium

Infections
- herpes labialis
- VZV
- EBV
- cytomegalovirus
- herpes virus
- Coxsackie virus
- human papilloma virus

Trauma
- direct damage

Mucocutaneous disorders
- lichen planus
- pemphigus
- pemphigoid
- lupus erythematosus

Radiotherapy
- reduced saliva
- reduced life span of oral epithelium

The index of orthodontic treatment need: dental health component

Grade	Characteristics
1 None	Extremely minor malocclusions including displacements <1 mm
2 Little	a. Increased overjet >3.5 mm but ≤6 mm with competent lips
	b. Reverse overjet >0 mm but ≤1 mm
	c. Anterior or posterior crossbite with ≤1 mm discrepancy between retruded contact position and intercuspal position
	d. Displacement of teeth >1 mm but ≤2 mm
	e. Anterior or posterior open bite >1 mm but ≤2 mm
	f. Increased overbite ≥3.5 mm without gingival contact
	g. Prenormal or postnormal occlusions with no other anomalies; includes up to half a unit discrepancy
3 Moderate	a. Increased overjet >3.5 mm but ≤6 mm with incompetent lips
	b. Reverse overjet >1 mm but ≤3.5 mm
	c. Anterior or posterior crossbites with >1 mm but ≤2 mm discrepancy between retruded contact position and intercuspal position
	d. Displacement of teeth >2 mm but ≤4 mm
	e. Lateral or anterior open bite >2 mm but ≤4 mm
	f. Increased and complete overbite without gingival or palatal trauma
4 Great	a. Increased overjet >6 mm but ≤9 mm
	b. Reverse overjet >3.5 mm with no masticatory or speech difficulties
	c. Anterior or posterior crossbite with >2 mm discrepancy between retruded contact position and intercuspal position
	d. Severe displacements of teeth >4 mm
	e. Extreme lateral or anterior open bites >4 mm
	f. Increased and complete overbite with gingival or palatal trauma
	h. Less extensive hypodontia, requiring prerestorative orthodontics or orthodontic space closure to obviate the need for a prosthesis
	i. Posterior lingual crossbite with no functional occlusal contact in one or both buccal segments
	m. Reverse overjet >1 mm but <3.5 mm, with recorded masticatory and speech difficulties
	t. Partially erupted teeth, tipped and impacted against adjacent teeth
	x. Supplemental teeth
5 Very great	a. Increased overjet >9 mm
	h. Extensive hypodontia with restorative implications (more than one tooth missing in any quadrant) requiring prerestorative orthodontics
	i. Impeded eruption of teeth (with the exception of third molars) owing to crowding, displacement, the presence of supernumerary teeth, retained deciduous teeth and any pathological cause
	m. Reverse overjet >3.5 mm with reported masticatory and speech difficulties
	p. Defects of cleft lip and palate
	s. Submerged deciduous teeth

From Heasman P 2008 Master Dentistry Vol. 2, Restorative Dentistry, Paediatric Dentistry and Orthodontics, 2nd edn. Churchill Livingstone, Edinburgh, with permission.

Lateral cephalometric analysis

Aim and objective of cephalometric analysis

Aim: To assess the anteroposterior and vertical relationships of the upper and lower teeth with supporting alveolar bone to their respective maxillary and mandibular bases and to the cranial base.

Objective: To compare the patient to normal population standards appropriate to their racial group, identifying any differences between the two.

Practice of cephalometric analysis

Ensure that teeth are in occlusion and that the patient is not postured forward.

In a darkened room, by tracing or digitizing, identify the points and planes listed in **Table A2.1** (**Fig. A2.1**); always trace the most prominent image. For bilateral landmarks, unless directly superimposed, take the average. Calculate angular and linear measurements.

Cephalometric interpretation

For Caucasians, compare individual values with Eastman norms (**Table A2.2**).

Skeletal relationships

- *A-P.* If SNA < or >81° and S–N/maxillary plane within 8° ± 3°, correct ANB as follows: for every °SNA > 81°, subtract 0.5° from ANB value and vice versa.
- *Vertical.* MMPA and facial % should lend support to each other usually.

Tooth position

- To assess if overjet reduction is possible by tipping movement, do a prognosis tracing (**Fig. A2.2**), or for every 1 mm of overjet reduction subtract 2.5° from $\underline{1}$ angulation. If the final angulation is not <95° to maxillary plane, tipping is acceptable.

- Check $\overline{1}$ angulation to mandibular plane in conjunction with ANB and MMPA. There is an inverse relationship between $\overline{1}$ angulation and MMPA.
- Interincisal angle: as this increases, overbite deepens.

Table A2.1 Definition of commonly used cephalometric points and planes

Points and planes	Definition
S	sella: midpoint of sella turcica
N	nasion: most anterior point of the frontonasal suture (may use the deepest point at the junction of the frontal and nasal bones instead)
P	porion: uppermost, outermost point on the bony external auditory meatus (upper border of the condylar head is at the same level, which helps location)
O	orbitale: most inferior anterior point on the margin of the orbit (use average of the left and right orbital shadows)
ANS	tip of the anterior nasal spine
PNS	tip of the posterior nasal spine (pterygomaxillary fissure is directly above, which helps location)
A	A point: most posterior point of the concavity on the anterior surface of the premaxilla in the midline below ANS
B	B point: most posterior point of the concavity on the anterior surface of the mandible in the midline above pogonion
Pog	pogonion: most anterior point on the bony chin
Me	menton: lowermost point on the mandibular symphysis in the midline
Go	gonion: most posterior-inferior point at the angle of the mandible (bisect the angle between tangent to the posterior ramus and inferior body of the mandible to locate)
Planes S–N line	line drawn through S and N
Frankfort plane	line connecting porion and orbitale
Maxillary plane	line joining PNS and ANS
Mandibular plane	line joining Go and Me
Functional occlusal plane	line drawn between the cusp tips of the first permanent molars and premolars/primary molars

From Heasman P 2008 Master Dentistry Vol. 2, Restorative Dentistry, Paediatric Dentistry and Orthodontics, 2nd edn. Churchill Livingstone, Edinburgh, with permission.

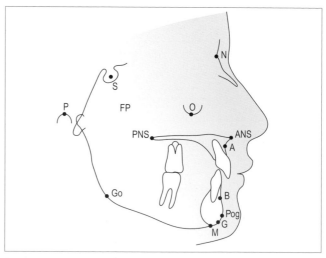

Fig. A2.1 Standard cephalometric points (from Heasman P 2008 Master Dentistry Vol. 2, Restorative Dentistry, Paediatric Dentistry and Orthodontics, 2nd edn. Churchill Livingstone, Edinburgh, with permission).

Table A2.2 Normal Eastman cephalometric values for Caucasians

Parameter	Value (± SD)
SNA	81 ± 3°
SNB	78 ± 3°
ANB	3 ± 2°
S–N/Max	8 ± 3°
$\overline{1}$ to maxillary plane	109 ± 6°
$\overline{1}$ to mandibular plane	93 ± 6°
Interincisal angle	135 ± 10°
MMPA	27 ± 4°
Facial proportion	55 ± 2%

From Heasman P 2008 Master Dentistry Vol. 2, Restorative Dentistry, Paediatric Dentistry and Orthodontics, 2nd edn. Churchill Livingstone, Edinburgh, with permission.

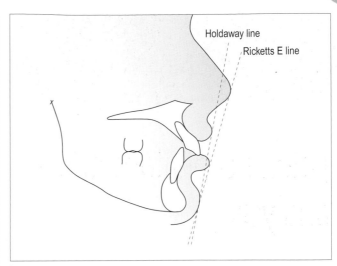

Fig. A2.3 Soft tissue lines.

- $\overline{1}$ to APo: this is an aesthetic reference line but it is unwise to use for treatment planning purposes.

Soft tissue analysis

- *Holdaway line.* Lower lip should be ± 1 mm to this line.
- *Ricketts' E-line.* Lower lip should be 0 mm (± 2 mm) in front of this with the upper lip slightly behind (**Fig. A2.3**).

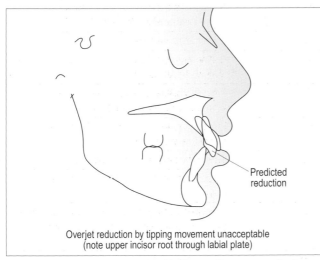

Overjet reduction by tipping movement unacceptable
(note upper incisor root through labial plate)

Fig. A2.2 Prognosis tracing.

Note: Page numbers followed by *b* indicate boxes, *f* indicate figures and *t* indicate tables

A

abrasion (technique) and microabrasion
  enamel defects in incisors, 134
  fluorotic mottling, 140
  white-spot lesions with fixed appliances,
    18
abscess, 116–118
absent teeth *see* hypodontia
accessory cusps, 148–149
accessory roots, 149
aciclovir (acyclovir), herpetic
    gingivostomatitis, 159–161
acid causing erosion
  dietary, 143–144
  gastric, 143
acid–pumice abrasion/microabrasion
  fluorotic mottling, 140
  white-spot lesions with fixed appliances,
    18
acrylated labial bow, lower incisor
    crowding (late presentation),
    75–76
acrylic allergy, 88
acrylic splints, TMJ pain and prominent
    chin, 80
activator–type functional appliances for
    increased overbite, 56
acyclovir, herpetic gingivostomatitis,
    159–161
adherence (compliance) problems,
    functional appliances for increased
    overjet, 45
adhesive restorations, 114
adhesively-retained copings, poor-quality
    first permanent molars, 133
adolescence (teens)
  caries prevention, 103–106
  gingival bleeding and overgrowth,
    156–158
  late
    lower incisor crowding presenting in,
      74–76
    prominent chin and TMJ pain
      reassessed in, 78–79
aesthetics
  amelogenesis imperfecta, 151t
  appliances, drifting incisors, 85
alignment
  upper canine, 91–92
    space creation for, 29–31, 30t
    in transposition, 33
  upper incisor, 9
allergy
  acrylic, 88
  dietary substances, recurrent aphthae
    with, 161, 161b
alveolar bone
  grafts in cleft lip and palate,
    99
  injury, splinting, 126

maldevelopment causing anterior open
    bite, 59t
  see also extra-alveolar dry time
amalgam, 114
amelogenesis imperfecta, 132, 150–152
  dentinogenesis imperfecta compared
    with, 153
  types, 151t
anaesthesia, general *see* general anaesthesia
analgesics, 117t
  commonly used, 113t, 117t
  dosages, 113t, 117t
  see also pain relief
anchorage
  with bilateral crossbite, 69
  with crowding, 23–24
    and buccal upper canines, after first
      premolar extraction, 17–18
    temporary (TAD), 23–24
  with incisor crossbite, 49
  with incisor drifting, 86
  with incisor overbite, 56
  with palatal upper canines, 30
angulation
  canines, with absent upper lateral
    incisors, 12
  incisors
    with absent upper lateral incisors,
      12
    with reverse overjet, 51t
ankylosis, primary molars, 38–40, 38b
  see also infraocclusion
anodontia, partial *see* hypodontia
anterior open bite, 58–61
antibiotics, 117
  commonly used, 117t
  intravenous, 117, 117t
  oral/per oral, 116, 117t
antifungals, palatal stomatitis, 88
antiviral agents, herpetic gingivostomatitis,
    159–161
aphthae, recurrent, 160–161
apices of traumatised central incisor roots,
    123
appliances
  anchorage *see* anchorage
  with anterior open bite, 60–61
  with buccal segment (posterior) crossbite,
    64
    bilateral crossbite, 68t, 69
    lingual crossbite (bilateral), 72–73
  with canine transposition, 33
  with crowding, 22–23
    and buccal upper canines, 16, 18
  with incisor absence (upper lateral), 10,
    12–13
  with incisor crossbite, 49
  with incisor drift, 85
  with increased crowding (lowers - late
    presentation), 75–76
  with increased overbite, 54, 56

with increased overjet, 43–44
  design problem, 45
with infraoccluded primary molars, 39
problems with, 87–95
with reversed overjet, 52
with TMJ pain and prominent chin, 81
with unerupted upper central incisor, 8
see also fixed appliances; functional
    appliances; quadhelix; removable
    appliances
arches
  crowding *see* crowding
  impressions *see* impressions
  lower, with buccal upper canines and
    crowding, 17
    expansion, 17
  lower, with infra-occluded primary
    molars, 39–40
  occlusal anomaly following overjet
    correction, 44
  spaced, in management of absent upper
    lateral incisors, 12
  upper
    with absent upper lateral incisors,
      spacing, 12
    with infra-occluded primary molars,
      39
arches, upper, severe crowding, 21
  see also transpalatal arch
attrition
  in late lower incisor crowding,
    approximal, lack in modern diet, 75
  wear due to, 145
avulsed central incisors, 128–130

B

bacteria, chromogenic, 137–138
bad breath, 138
bands
  avoidance with periodontal disease, 86
  dentinogenesis imperfecta, 155
baseplate
  in bilateral crossbite, 69
  in incisor crossbite, 49
  in incisor overbite, 56
  palatal upper canines, 30
behaviour management, 107–109
Behçet's syndrome, 160
bilateral crossbite, 66–73
bilirubin causing staining, 135
bite *see* crossbite; open bite; overbite
biteplane, flat anterior, with absent upper
    lateral incisors, 13
bitewing radiograph
  caries (primaries), 113–114
  caries prevention, adolescent, 104
bleaching, 136–137
  fluorotic mottling, 140–142
  root-filled incisor, 136–137
bone, alveolar *see* alveolar bone

brackets
  bond failure, 89–90
  drifting incisors, 85t
brandy wine type dentinogenesis
    imperfecta, 154
breastfeeding and caries, 100
breath, bad, 138
bridge, resin-retained (for replacement of
    upper lateral incisors), 13
brown staining
  arrested caries, 138
  fluorosis, 140
buccal blocks, 44
buccal eruption of upper permanent
    canines, 15–19
buccal segment
  with absent upper lateral incisors,
      movement distally, 12–13
  crossbite see crossbite

C

camouflage, orthodontic, with increased
    overjet, 45
Candida and palatal stomatitis, 88
canine(s)
  eruption
    buccal, of upper permanent canines,
        15–19
    dates, 2t
    failure, 20–25
    palatal, of upper permanent canines,
        26–31
  permanent
    mineralization dates, 132t
    palatal eruption, 26–31
  primary
    with absent upper lateral incisors,
        management, 12
    retention of upper canines, 26–31
  removal, 23
  retraction (upper), 91–92
  transposition, 32–34
  see also intercanine width
canine fossa infection, maxillary, 116,
    116f
carbamide peroxide gel, 140–141
carbonated drinks causing erosion, 143–144
caries (decay), 100–102, 113–115
  adolescent, prevention, 103–106
  arrested, brown stain, 138
  diabetic patient, 156
    treatment, 157–158
  extraction see extraction
  first permanent molars, 132
  with incisor crossbite, management, 49
  nursing and early childhood, 100–102
  pain control see pain relief
  restorations see restorations
Carisolv, 102
cast metal with tooth surface loss, 145t
cavernous sinus thrombosis, 116
cellulitis, facial, 116
central diastema, 1–4
central incisors see incisors
centreline shift/displacement
  with incisor crossbite, assessment, 49
  with posterior crossbite
    assessment, 63
    causes, 63
  with unerupted upper central incisors, 6
    correction, 8
    prevention, 6

cephalometry, 204–205
  aim and objective, 204
  anterior open bite, 59
  bilateral crossbite, 67
  increased overbite, 55–56
  increased overjet, 43–44
  infra-occluded primary molars, 38
  practice, 204
  reverse overjet, 51
  TMJ pain and prominent chin, 77, 79t
chewing gum, sugar-free, adolescent, 106
child physical abuse, 119–120
chin, prominent, and TMJ pain, 77–82
chin cup therapy, reverse overjet, 52
chromogenic bacteria, 137–138
chronological (enamel) hypoplasia (=molar
    incisor hypomineralization; MIH), 132,
    135
cleft lip and palate, 96–99
cleidocranial dysplasia, unerupted
    permanent teeth, 110
CMV, 160
cold sores, 160–161
colour, anterior teeth (canine/incisors), 12
  traumatized teeth, 121, 123
  see also discolouration
coma, diabetic, 157
  hypoglycaemic, 157–158
communicative management, 107
compliance problems, functional appliances
    for increased overjet, 45
compomer restoration, primary upper
    incisors, 102
composite coverage
  dentinogenesis imperfecta, 155
  enamel defects, 136
  fluorotic mottling, 141
  poor-quality and discoloured permanent
      teeth, 133, 136
  surface loss/wear, 145t
  see also veneers
computed tomography, palatal canines, 28
congenital structural abnormalities see
    developmental abnormalities
consent, informed, 109
copings, poor-quality first permanent
    molars, 133
coronal portion of tooth see crown
coxsackie viruses, 160
CPP-ACP gum, 106
CPP-ACP mouse and CPP-ACFP tooth
    mousse, 106
crossbite
  bilateral, 66–73
  buccal segment/posterior, 62–65
    bilateral, 66
    in cleft lip and palate, 98–99, 99f
  incisor, 47–49
  with palatal upper canines, correction,
      30
  with reverse overjet, profile and occlusion
      following correction, 53
crowding, 15–19
  in absent upper lateral incisor
      management, 12
  in increased overbite, assessment, 55
  in increased overjet aetiology, 42t
  lower incisor, late presentation, 74–76
  in reverse overjet, assessment, 51t
  severe, 20–25
crown (coronal portion), incisor
  fracture, in permanent central incisor,
      122–124

non-vital, with root fracture, 126–127
  shape abnormalities, 147
crown (restoration), poor-quality first
    permanent molars, 133
cusps, accessory, 148–149
cyclical neutropenia, premature exfoliation,
    111, 111f
cytomegalovirus, 160

D

decalcification with fixed appliance
    therapy, 18, 18b
deciduous teeth see primary teeth
deglutition (swallowing) pattern, anterior
    open bite, 58
dens evaginatus, 149
dens invaginatus, 148–149
dental panoramic tomogram see panoramic
    radiograph
dentine defects
  environmentally determined, 154
  hereditary (other than dentinogenesis
      imperfecta), 154
dentinoenamel fracture, central incisor
    crown, 123
dentinogenesis imperfecta, 153–155
  treatment, 151, 154–155
dentoalveolar injury, splinting, 126
'denture' stomatitis with fixed appliances,
    87–88
desensitization
  pulp therapy, 114
  with surface loss, 144–145
developmental abnormalities/
    malformations/anomalies
  enamel, 150–152
  lip and palate, 96–99
  misshapen teeth, 146
  missing teeth, 146
  upper lateral incisor absence, 11, 11b
  upper premolar rotations, 22
developmental delay, 107
diabetes
  gingival bleeding and enlargement,
      156–158
  periodontal pathology and drifting
      incisors, 85
diastema (gaps), median/central, 1–4
dietary analysis and advice
  caries prevention
    adolescent, 105
    infant/early childhood, 101–102
  cleft lip and palate, 97
  diabetic patients, 158
  erosion, 143–144
dietary causes (food and drink)
  aphthae, 161
  erosion, 143
  infant/early childhood caries,
      100
  late lower incisor crowding, 75
  staining, 137–138
dietary history, and adolescent caries
    prevention, 104
digit (thumb) sucking, 94
  anterior open bite with, 59–60,
      59t
  increased overjet with, 42t
  persuasion to discontinue, 60
  posterior/buccal crossbite segment with,
      63, 63b, 63t
    bilateral, 66

discolouration/staining, 131–138
  bleaching see bleaching
  extrinsic, 137
  traumatized teeth, 121
  see also mottling
distraction (diverting attention), 108
distraction osteogenesis, bilateral lingual
    crossbite, 72, 72t
double teeth, 147
Down's syndrome, 146
drainage of pus, 117
dressings, pulpitis, 113
drifting
  of lower second premolars into contact
    with second molars, 78
  of upper incisors, 83–86
drink see entries under dietary
drug-induced conditions
  dentine defects, 154
  staining, 135, 138
drug therapy see specific (types of) drugs
dry times with avulsed incisor, 128–130
dysmineralization see hypomineralization

E

Eastman cephalometric values for
    Caucasians, 205t
eating disorder, 144
EBV (Epstein–Barr virus), 160
ectodermal dysplasia, 146
ectopic eruption
  upper permanent canines
    buccal, 15–19
    palatal eruption, 26–31
  upper permanent first molars, 3–4, 3t
edge-to-edge incisor contact
  crossbite, 48
  reverse overjet, 51t
electric pulp testing, fractured permanent
    incisor root, 126
emergency care with bracket bond failure,
    90
enamel defects
  developmental causes, 150–152
  first permanent molars, 131–134
  fluorosis-related, 139
  incisors see incisors (permanent)
  see also amelogenesis imperfecta;
    hypomineralization; hypoplasia
enamel–dentine fracture, central incisor
    crown, 123
endocarditis, infective, risk, 20
endodontics, luxated primary incisor, 121f
environmental causes
  dentine defects, 154
  recurrent aphthae, 161
Epstein–Barr virus, 160
erosion see surface, wear/loss/erosion
eruption
  dates, primary/permanent teeth, 2t
  early/premature, 110–112
  ectopic see ectopic eruption
  excessive, opposing teeth, 38
  failure/delay see unerupted teeth
Essix retainers, 23, 25
evaginated teeth, 149
examination (in behaviour management),
    108–109
exfoliation (natural loss of primary teeth)
  delayed, upper canines, 26–31
  premature, 111–112
expansion see arches; maxillary expansion

extra-alveolar dry time (EADT), avulsed
    incisor, 128–130
extraction/removal
  abscessed teeth, 116–118
  with canine transposition (of most
    displaced tooth), 33
  with carious/decayed primary teeth,
    molars, 114
  with crowding, 16, 23
    of first premolars, 16–18, 23
    of lower incisors, 76
    of lower premolars, 76
    of lower third molars, 76
    of upper canines, 23
  doubled permanent teeth, 148
  with ectopic eruption
    of canines and root resorption of lateral
      incisors, 35–36
    of permanent upper first molars, of
      deciduous second (e) upper molars,
      4
  with poor-quality first permanent molars,
    133
  with reverse overjet, 51t
  with unerupted upper permanent central
    incisor (of supernumerary tooth), 8
eye swelling
  and dental abscess, 116–118
  and fractured permanent incisor root, 125

F

facial features and photography
  with anterior open bite, 58
  with buccal upper canines and crowding,
    15
  with increased overjet, 42
  with prominent chin and TMJ pain, 79t
facial growth
  post-treatment, 95
  in reverse overjet, assessment of direction
    and extent, 51t
facial soft tissues see soft tissues
facial swelling see swelling
fetal problems see pregnancy-related
    problems
fissure sealants, adolescent, 105–106
fixation with TMJ pain and prominent
    chin, 81
fixed appliances
  absent upper lateral incisors, 12–13
  anterior open bite, 60–61, 60f
  buccal crossbite (bilateral), 68–69
  buccal upper canines and crowding, 16,
    18
  drifting incisors, 85
  increased overbite, 56
  infra-occluded primary molars, 39
  lingual crossbite (bilateral), 72
  problems, 89–90
  TMJ pain and prominent chin, 81
  tooth movements with, 94–95
  transposition of canines, 33
fizzy (carbonated) drinks causing erosion,
    143–144
fluoride history, 136, 139
  adolescent, 104
  mottling, 139
  preschool child (with caries), 101t
fluoride mouthwash
  adolescent, 104
  sensitive (eroded) teeth, 144
  under-6s, contraindicated, 101

fluoride supplementation/therapy
  adolescent, 104–105
  preschool caries, 100
fluoride toothpaste
  adolescent, 104, 106
  infant/early childhood, 101
fluoride varnish
  adolescent, 104–105
  infant/early childhood, 101
  sensitive (eroded) teeth, 144
fluorosis (excess fluoride intake), 132,
    139–142
food see entries under dietary
forces
  causing late lower incisor crowding, 75
  destabilizing orthodontic result, 94
formocresol, pulpotomy, 114
fracture
  incisor root, 84, 125
  incisor tooth, 122–124
Fränkel II appliance for bilateral lingual
    crossbite, 72–73, 72f
Fränkel III appliance for reversed overjet,
    52, 52f
Frankfort–mandibular plane angle (FMPA),
    with increased overjet, 42
functional appliances
  for anterior open bite, 60
  for increased overbite, 54, 56
  for increased overjet, 43–44
    compliance problems, 45
    design problems, 45
    results, 45f
  for reversed overjet, 52, 52f
fungal infections with fixed appliances, 88

G

gastro-oesophageal reflux and gastric
    regurgitation, 143
gender and(sex) cleft lip and palate, 96
general anaesthesia, 109
  carious primary molar extraction, 158
  contraindications, 109
  indications, 107
genetic disorders
  dentine (other than dentinogenesis
    imperfecta), 154b
  enamel, 150
  see also amelogenesis imperfecta
genetic factors, maxillary canine ectopia,
    27
gingiva
  bleeding, 156–158
  health improvement, 138
  overgrowth/enlargement, 135, 156–158
    oral ulceration and, 159, 159f
  pressure from, causing late lower incisor
    crowding, 75
  ulceration, 159, 159f
gingival third root fractures (central
    incisor), 127
gingivitis, 156–158
gingivoplasty, labial, 9
gingivostomatitis, primary herpetic,
    159–161
glass ionomer cement, poor-quality first
    permanent molars, 133
grafting, alveolar bone, in cleft lip and
    palate, 99
growth see facial growth; mandibular
    growth; maxillary growth
gums see gingiva

H

habitual digit-sucking sucking *see* digit
   sucking
halitosis, 138
hand, foot and mouth disease, 160
Hawley retainer, severe crowding, 25
head and neck syndromes associated with
   missing teeth, 146
headgear wear (with appliances)
  with absent upper lateral incisors, 13
  with severe crowding, 23–24
heredity *see* genetic disorders; genetic
   factors
herpangina, 160
herpes labialis, 160–161
herpes virus type-8, 160
herpetic gingivostomatitis, primary,
   159–161
herpetiform aphthae, 160
HHV-8 (herpes virus type 8), 160
Holdaway line, 205
hospital admission, orofacial infection, 117,
   118b
HPV, 160
HSV, 159–161
human papilloma virus, 160
hydrochloric acid–pumice microabrasion
   see acid–pumice abrasion
hyperglycaemic coma, 157
hypodontia (absent/missing teeth), 146
  epidemiology, 38–39, 39b
  multiple/severe, 146
  upper incisors, 10–14
hypoglycaemic coma, 157–158
hypomature amelogenesis imperfecta, 151,
   151f, 151t
hypomineralization/dysmineralization
   (enamel), 132, 135–138
  first permanent molars, 132
  hypoplasia and, distinction, 131
hypomineralized amelogenesis imperfecta,
   152
hypoplasia, enamel, 135–138
  causes (other than chronological), 21
   inherited, 150, 151t
  chronological (=molar incisor
    hypomineralization; MIH), 132
    hypomineralization and, distinction,
     131

I

ibuprofen, dosage, 113t
illness *see* medical conditions
impacted upper first molars
  causes, 3
  frequency/prevalence, 3
  treatment, 4
impressions, dental arch
  late lower incisor crowding, 75
  posterior crossbite, 63
incisors (permanent)
  central
   absence, 6b
   eruption dates, 2t
   mineralization dates, 132t
   mottling, 139
   root fracture, 125–127
   rotations, 1
   sensibility testing, 6
   trauma, 122–130
   unerupted upper, 5–9

colour/size/shape/angulation, 12
  hypomineralization, 131
   treatment, 134
  lateral
   absence, 10–14
   eruption dates, 2t
   pulp extirpation, 118
   root resorption by ectopic canines,
    35–36
   rotations, with increased overbite,
    56–57
  lower, crowding, late presentation,
   74–76
  prominent *see* overjet
  root-filled *see* root canal treatment
  upper
   absence, 10–14
   crossbite, 47–49
   drifting, 83–86
   mottling, 139
   space creation, 2
   trauma *see* trauma
incisors (primary)
  central
   displacement, 119–121
   eruption dates, 2t
  doubled (joined at crown), 147
  lateral, eruption dates, 2t
  premature exfoliation, 111–112
  rotations, median diastema and, 1
  space creation in development, 2
  upper, caries, 100
   restoration, 102
inclination, incisors, 17
  with crossbite, 48
Index of Orthodontic Treatment Need:
  dental health component, 203
infants
  caries, 100–102
  cleft lip and palate management,
   96
infection
  diabetic patient, 157–158
  enamel defects/discolouration due to,
   132, 136
  endocardial, risk, 20
  fungal, with fixed appliances, 88
  oral ulcers due to, 159–161
  orofacial, 116–118
inflammatory resorption with avulsed
   incisor, 128–129
informed consent, 109
infraocclusion (primary teeth), 112
  molars, 37–40
  see also ankylosis
infraorbital nerve injury, 125
inhalational sedation, 108
inheritance *see* genetic disorders; genetic
   factors
injury *see* trauma
insulin-dependent diabetes, gingival
   bleeding and enlargement, 156–158
intercanine width, reduced, causing late
   lower incisor crowding, 75
intermaxillary fixation with TMJ pain and
   prominent chin, 81
interproximal stripping, late lower incisor
   crowding, 75–76
invaginations, 148–149
Invisalign
  drifting incisors, 83
  lower incisor crowding (late
   presentation), 79

K

Kaposi sarcoma-associated virus (herpes
   virus type 8), 160
Kim mechanics, anterior open bite, 61

L

labial bow
  with absent upper permanent central
    incisor, 8, 13
  with increased overbite, 56
  with lower incisor crowding (late
    presentation), 75–76
labial gingivoplasty, 9
labial herpes, 160–161
labial recession related to lower central
   incisor, 49
labial segment problems (crowding etc.),
   21, 23–24
  buccal upper canines, treatment planning,
   17
  drifting incisors, 84–85
labial surface of upper central incisors,
   mottling, 139
lateral incisors *see* incisors
lateral radiograph, cephalometric *see*
   cephalometry
Le Fort I advancement, TMJ pain and
   prominent chin, 81
lingual crossbite, bilateral, 70–73
lip(s)
  cephalometric analysis, 205
  cleft, and palate, 96–99
  tooth fragment in, 122
  see also entries under labial
luxated primary incisor, 119–121

M

malformations *see* developmental
   abnormalities
mandibular displacement on closure
  incisor crossbite, 48
  increased overbite, 55t
  posterior crossbite, 63–64, 63b
  prominent chin and TMJ pain, 78
  reverse overjet, 51, 51t
mandibular distraction osteogenesis,
   bilateral lingual crossbite, 72, 72t
mandibular growth
  in late lower incisor crowding causation,
   75
  in posterior crossbite causation, 63t
  in reverse overjet
   in causation, 51t
   modification, 52
mandibular infection, 116–118
mandibular path of closure, prominent
   chin and TMJ pain, 78
mandibular prominence and TMJ pain,
   77–82
mandibular setback osteotomy with TMJ
   pain and prominent chin, 81
maternally-related problems *see* pregnancy
maxillary advancement, Le Fort I, TMJ
   pain and prominent chin, 81
maxillary canine fossa infection, 116, 116f
maxillary expansion (palatal expansion) in
   bilateral crossbite, rapid (RME; RPE),
   68f, 68t, 69
  surgically-assisted, 68t, 70
  unfeasible, 70

maxillary growth in reverse overjet causation, restraint, 51t
maxillary tooth, talon cusp, 148–149
median diastema, 1–4
medical conditions/illness, childhood (incl. systemic disease)
  congenital/developmental *see* developmental abnormalities
  dentinogenesis imperfecta, 154
  discolouration due to, 135, 138
  enamel abnormalities, 150b
  gingival bleeding due to, 156
  gingival enlargement due to, 157b
  oral ulceration/aphthae due to, 161
  poor quality first permanent molars, 132
  see also syndromes
medications *see* drug-induced conditions *and specific (types of) drugs*
mental repositioning of buccal upper canines, 17
microabrasion *see* abrasion
midline mandibular distraction osteogenesis, bilateral lingual crossbite, 72, 72t
mid-palatal suture, bilateral crossbite, 68–69
milk
  adolescent consumption, 104
milk teeth *see* primary teeth
Millard repair, 97
mineralization
  dates, 132t
  reduced levels *see* hypomineralization
misshapen teeth, 147
missing teeth *see* hypodontia
mobility *see* movement
molars (permanent)
  with absent upper lateral incisors, achieving a Class I relationship, 12–13
  with buccal upper canines, deciding on final relationships, 17
  eruption dates, 2t
  first (6)
    poor quality/discoloured, 131–134
    restoration *see* restorations
  first (6) upper
    ectopic eruption, 3–4, 3t
    impacted *see* impacted upper first molars
  mineralization dates, 132t
  second (7) lower, lower second premolars drifting into contact with, 78
  with severe crowding, deciding on final relationships, 23
  third (8), in late lower incisor crowding
    as causative factor, 75
    lower, extraction, 76
molars (primary)
  ankylosis, 38–40, 38b
  caries and pulp treatment, 113–115
  early loss, space loss following, 21–22
  eruption dates, 2t
  first (d)
    infraocclusion of upper, 112
    restoration with cavities, 102
  second (e) lower, infra-occluded, 32–34
  second (e) upper, management with ectopic eruption of permanent upper first molars, 4
  surface loss, 143–145
mother *see* parents; pregnancy
mottling, 139–142

movement/mobility, tooth
  of anterior teeth in trauma, assessment, 123
  of natal teeth, 110
  orthodontic
    with absent upper lateral incisors, 13
    problems relating to, 91–92
    with unerupted upper central incisor, 8
  see also drifting

N

natal teeth, 110–112
neonates
  cleft lip and palate management, 96
  teeth, 110–112
neutropenia, cyclic, premature exfoliation, 111, 111f
nightguard vital bleaching, 140–141
night-time feeding and infant/early childhood caries, 101
nitrous oxide, 108
non-verbal communication, 107
numerical abnormalities *see* hypodontia; supernumerary teeth
nursing caries, 100–102

O

occlusal radiograph
  cleft lip and palate, 99
  palatal upper permanent canines, 28
  unerupted upper permanent central incisor, 7
occlusion
  buccal segment *see* buccal segment
  cleft lip and palate, 97
  digit sucking affecting *see* digit sucking
  forces, causing late lower incisor crowding, 75
  post-treatment
    with bilateral (buccal segment) crossbite, 69–70
    with buccal segment (posterior) crossbite, 64, 65f
    with drifting incisors, 86f
    with incisor crossbite, 49
    with increased overbite, relapse and its prevention/minimization, 56–57
    with increased overbite, result, 57
    with increased overjet, 45f
    with lingual segment crossbite, 66
    with reverse overjet, 53
    with TMJ pain and prominent chin, 82f
  in TMJ joint dysfunction aetiology/predisposition, 78
  see also infraocclusion
opalescent dentine, hereditary (dentinogenesis imperfecta type II), 153
open bite
  anterior, 58–61
  posterior, 44–45
oral cavity (mouth)
  diabetic manifestations, 158
  in increased overbite, appearance, 54
  ulceration, 159–161
oral hygiene
  bilateral crossbite, 68
  cleft lip and palate, 97–98
  diabetes and, 157
  discoloration/staining due to poor levels, 138
  improving hygiene, 138

incisor crossbite, 49
infant/early childhood caries prevention, 101
severe crowding, 20
oral sedation, 107
orbital fracture, 125
orofacial infection, 116–118
orofacial soft tissues *see* soft tissues
orofacial swelling *see* swelling
orthognathic surgery, TMJ pain and prominent chin, 78–81
osteogenesis imperfecta, dentinogenesis imperfecta type I associated with, 154
osteotomy, mandibular setback, with TMJ pain and prominent chin, 81
overbite
  increased, 54–57
  with reverse overjet, amount, 51t
  traumatic, 54–57
  upper central incisor, amount, 48
overeruption, opposing teeth, 38
overjet
  increased, 41–46
  reverse, 50–53

P

pain
  poor-quality permanent molars and, 132
  TMJ, and prominent chin, 77–82
  uncooperative child with, 107–109
pain relief/control, 113–115
  caries, 113–115
  nursing, 102
  see also analgesics
palatal expansion *see* maxillary expansion
palatally-erupting upper canines, 26–31
palate
  cleft lip and, 96–99
  red (palatal stomatitis), with fixed appliances, 87–88
panoramic radiograph/tomogram
  absent/missing teeth, 147
    upper permanent lateral incisors, 11–12
  amelogenesis imperfecta, 151
  anterior open bite, 59
  buccal segment (posterior) crossbite, 63–64
    bilateral, 67
  buccal upper permanent canines and crowding, 16
  cleft lip and palate, 98–99
  dentinogenesis imperfecta, 153
  incisor crossbite, 48
  incisor crowding (lowers - late presentation), 75
  increased overbite, 55
  increased overjet, 43
  infra-occluded primary molars, 38
  median diastema, 3
  palatal upper permanent canines, 28
  poor-quality first permanent molars, 133
  reverse overjet, 51
  severe crowding, 22
  of tooth movements with removable appliance, 92–94
  unerupted upper permanent central incisor, 7
paracetamol, dosage, 113t
parafunctional activity, attrition with, 145

parents
  physical abuse by, 119–120
  presence/absence in behavioural
      management, 108
percussion of anterior teeth, post-trauma,
    123
periapical periodontitis, drifting incisors, 84
periapical radiograph
  canine transposition, 33
  drifting incisors, 84
  root fracture (incisor), 125
  tooth movements with removable
      appliances, 92, 94
  traumatized incisors
    permanent tooth fracture, 123
    primary tooth, 120
periodontal ligament (PL) damage with
    avulsed incisor, 128
  survival of PL related to extra alveolar
      dry time, 129–130
periodontal pathology with drifting
    incisors, 84–85
  treatment considerations in, 86
  treatment of, 85
periodontal probing depths with increased
    overbite, 55
periodontal status of lower central incisor
    with crossbite, 48
periodontitis, periapical, drifting incisors, 84
permanent teeth, 125–127
  in amelogenesis imperfecta, treatment
      modalities, 151t
  double, 147–148
    extraction, 148
  eruption
    dates, 2t
    delay/failure see unerupted teeth
  mineralization see mineralization
  premature exfoliation, 111b
  trauma, 122–127
  trauma of primary incisor affecting, 120
  see also specific teeth
physical abuse, 119–120
plaque control, 101t, 103
porcelain for tooth surface loss, 145t
position, tooth, cephalometric analysis,
    204–205
positive reinforcement, 107–108
posterior crossbite see crossbite
posterior open bite, 44–45
pregnancy-related problems (maternal/
    intrauterine/fetal)
  discolouration, 135
  poor quality first permanent molars, 132
premaxilla, anterior, vertical parallax for
    determining position of unerupted
    objects in, 7
premolars (permanent)
  drifting of lower second premolars into
      contact with second molars, 78
  eruption dates, 2t
  extraction/removal
    in crowding and buccal upper canines,
        17–18
    in crowding of lower incisors, 76
  fissure sealants, adolescent, 105–106
  mineralization dates, 132t
  root fragment, 92
  rotations (upper), causes, 22
premolars (primary), eruption dates, 2t
preschool children, caries, 100–102
pressure zones in retraction of upper
    canines by tipping force, 91

primary (deciduous/milk) teeth
  amelogenesis imperfecta affecting, 150
    treatment modalities, 151t
  caries, 100, 113–115
    restorations see restorations
  in cleft lip and palate, 97
  dentinogenesis imperfecta affecting,
      153–154
  in discoloration of permanent teeth,
      history-taking relating to, 136
  double, 147
  eruption
    dates, 2t
    premature, 110–112
  exfoliation see exfoliation
  infraocclusion see infraocclusion
  surface loss, 143–145
  trauma, 119–121
  see also specific teeth
procline with incisor crossbite
  appliance to achieve, 49
  space required to, 48
pulp capping, permanent incisors, 123
pulp chamber obliteration in
    dentinogenesis imperfecta, 153, 154f
pulp testing, electric, fractured permanent
    incisor root, 126
pulp treatment (in general)
  permanent incisors, 123–124
  primary molars, 114
pulpectomy/pulp extirpation
  permanent incisor, 118
  primary molar, 114
pulpitis, 113, 113t
pulpotomy
  partial, permanent incisor, 123–124
  primary molar, 114
pus, drainage and culture, 117
pyramidal roots, 149

Q

quadhelix, posterior (buccal segment)
    crossbite, 64
  bilateral, 68t
  in cleft lip and palate, 99

R

radiography
  absent/missing teeth, 147
    upper permanent lateral incisors, 11–12
  adolescent, and caries prevention, 104
  amelogenesis imperfecta, 151
  anterior open bite, 59–60
  buccal segment (posterior) crossbite, 63–64
    bilateral, 67
  carious primaries, 113–114
  cleft lip and palate, 98–99
  dentinogenesis imperfecta, 153–154, 154f
  double teeth, 148
  ectopic canines (permanent), 35
    buccal upper canines and crowding, 16
    palatal upper canines, 28–29
  incisor crossbite, 48
  incisor drift, 84
  incisor fragment in lip, 122
  incisor root fracture, 125
  increased overbite, 55–56
  increased overjet, 43
  infra-occluded primary molars, 38–39
  lower incisor crowding (late
      presentation), 75

median diastema, 6–7
poor quality first permanent molars, 133
posterior crossbite, 63–64
reverse overjet, 51
severe crowding, 22
TMJ pain and prominent chin, 79, 79t
of tooth movements, with removable
    appliance, 92–94
transposition of canines, 33
traumatized incisors
  permanent tooth fracture, 122–123
  primary teeth, 120
unerupted upper permanent central
    incisor, 7
rapid maxillary expansion see maxillary
    expansion
reduction, incisor root fracture, 126
regurgitation, gastric, 143
reimplantation see replantation
reinforcement, positive, 107–108
removable appliances
  with buccal segment (posterior) crossbite,
      64
    bilateral crossbite, 68t
  with incisor absence (upper lateral), 12–13
  with incisor crossbite, 49
  with increased crowding (lowers - late
      presentation), 75–76
  with increased overbite, 56
  with severe crowding, 24
  slow tooth movement with, 91–92
  with unerupted upper permanent central
      incisor, 8
  with unerupted upper permanent palatal
      canines, 30
removal see extraction
replacement resorption with avulsed
    incisor, 128–129
replantation, avulsed central incisors, 128,
    129f
resin retained bridge (for replacement of
    upper lateral incisors), 13
resorption (root)
  central avulsed incisor, 128–129
  drifting upper incisors, 84
  lateral incisors, by ectopic canines, 35–36
  orthodontically-induced, 93
  prevention, 93
restorations (permanent teeth)
  in amelogenesis imperfecta, 151t
  incisor (central), with fractured crown,
      124
  molars, first
    diabetic patient, 158
    poor-quality teeth, 133
  with surface loss/wear, 145
restorations (primaries), 114
  incisors, upper, 102
  molars, 114
    first, 102
retention (primary teeth = delayed
    exfoliation), upper canines, 26–31
retention (technique)
  in bilateral crossbite, 69
  in crowding, 23–25
    and buccal upper canines, after first
        premolar extraction, 18
  following active tooth movement, 95
  in incisor crossbite, 49
  in incisor overbite, 56
  palatal upper canines, 30–31, 30t
  problems with retainers, 87–88
retraction, upper canines, 92–93

Ricketts' E-line, 205
root(s)
  fragment, first premolar, 92
  in incisor trauma, 123
    fracture, 84, 125
  resorption see resorption
  sensibility testing, incisors, 6
  shape anomalies, 149
root canal obliteration in dentinogenesis
    imperfecta, 153, 154f
root canal treatment/filling, incisor
  avulsed, 128
  discolouration following, treatment,
    136–137
  for orthodontic tooth movement, 8
rotations
  incisors
    increased overbite and, 56–57
    median diastema and, 1
  upper premolar, causes, 22

S

salivation and caries risk
  adolescent, 103
  infant, 96, 100, 101t
screw turning with palatal upper canines, 30
sedation/sedatives, 108–109, 117t
sensibility testing, incisor (root), 6, 94, 126
sensitivity with erosive loss, treatment,
    144–145
sex and cleft lip and palate, 96
shape
  abnormal, 146
  canines/incisors, 12
shell teeth, 154
size
  canines/incisors, 12
  discrepancies, 27–28
skeletal relationships/patterns
  absent upper lateral incisors, 12
  anterior open bite, 59t, 60
  buccal segment/posterior crossbite, 63t
    bilateral, 67t
  cephalometry, 204
  cleft lip and palate, 97
  increased overbite, 54, 55t
  increased overjet, 41–42, 42t
    effects of functional appliances, 44
  lingual crossbite, bilateral, 72t
  reverse overjet, 51, 51t
smile, attractive, 70
smoking and periodontal disease, 85
social factors, infant/early childhood
    caries, 101t
soft tissues
  cephalometric analysis, 205
  forces from, destabilizing orthodontic
    result, 94
  in increased overjet aetiology, 42t
  radiography for incisor fragment in lip,
    122
  trauma from increased overbite, 54–57
space
  closure (therapeutic), absent upper lateral
    incisors, 12
  creation (in natural development) for
    upper permanent incisors, 2
  creation (therapeutic)
    bucally-erupted upper canines, 80
    for replacement of absent upper lateral
      incisors, 12–13
    unerupted upper canines, 29–30

required to procline, with incisor
    crossbite, 48
speech
  with anterior open bite, 58–59
  with cleft lip and palate, 97
splints
  fractured permanent incisor root, 125–127
  TMJ pain and prominent chin, 80
springs, median diastema, 4
staining see discolouration
stainless steel crown, poor-quality first
    permanent molars, 133
stomach acid and its regurgitation, 143
stomatitis, palatal (red palate), with fixed
    appliances, 87–88
  see also gingivostomatitis
stress and TMJ pain, 77–78
study models
  in late lower incisor crowding, 75
  wax registration see wax registration
sucking see digit sucking
sugar-containing drinks and foods and
    infant/early childhood caries, 100
sugar-free chewing gum, adolescent, 106
supernumerary teeth, unerupted upper
    permanent central incisor due to, 6, 6b,
    8
surface (tooth), wear/loss/erosion,
    143–145
  increased overbite, 55
surgery
  cleft lip and palate, 97
  palatal upper canine exposure, 30, 30t
  in rapid palatal expansion (SARPE), with
    bilateral crossbite, 68t, 70
  TMJ pain and prominent chin, 80–81
swallowing pattern, anterior open bite, 58
sweet foods and caries, 100
swelling, orofacial
  dental abscess and, 116–118
  and fractured permanent incisor root,
    122
syndromes
  associated with genetic enamel defects,
    151
  associated with missing teeth, 146
systemic disease see medical conditions

T

talon cusp, 148–149
taurodontism, 149
  hypomature–hypoplastic amelogenesis
    imperfecta with, 151, 151t
teenagers see adolescence
tell-show-do technique of behaviour
    shaping, 107
temporary anchorage device (TAD), severe
    crowding, 23–24
temporomandibular joint pain and
    prominent chin, 77–82
tension zones in retraction of upper canines
    by tipping force, 91–92
tetracycline staining, 135
thrombosis, cavernous sinus, 116
thumb sucking see digit sucking
tipping movement, upper canine retraction
    by, 91
tongue
  brushing/scraping, 138
  and swallowing pattern with anterior
    open bite, 58–59
tooth mousse, adolescent, 106

toothbrushing
  advice, 138
    adolescent, 104
    infant/early childhood caries
      prevention, 101
  frequency, adolescent, 104
  gingival bleeding, 156–158
  overzealous, causing wear, 145
toothpaste see fluoride toothpaste
transpalatal arch, 23–24
transposition, canines, 32–34
trauma, 119–121
  dysmineralization of permanents
    following primary tooth trauma, 136
  incisors (upper), 119–121, 125–127
    permanent teeth, 122–130
    predisposing factors, 43
    primary teeth, 119–121
  soft tissue, with increased overbite, 54–57
  see also fracture
trisomy 21 (Down's syndrome), 146
tuberculated teeth, 149
Turner's tooth/hypoplasia, 21
Twin-Block appliance
  increased overbite, 56
  increased overjet, 44

U

ulceration, oral, 159–161
uncooperative child, 107–109
unerupted teeth (due to delay or failure)
  permanent dentition, 110–111
    upper canines, 20–31
    upper central incisor, 5–9
  primary dentition, 110

V

vacuum-formed retainers, 25
varicella–zoster virus, 160
veneers, composite, 136
  dentinogenesis imperfecta, 155
  fluorotic mottling, 141
vertical parallax for determining position
    of unerupted objects in anterior
    premaxilla, 7
viral infection, oral ulceration, 159–161
vital bleaching, fluorotic mottling, 140–142
vital pulpotomy, primary molar, 114
vitality
  of root-fractured incisors, maintenance, 127
  testing, traumatized anterior teeth, 123,
    125
voice control, 107
vomiting, recurrent, erosive loss, 143–144
VZV, 160

W

water, adolescent consumption, 104
wax registration
  for functional appliances
    increased overjet, 45
    reverse overjet, 52
  for study models
    late lower incisor crowding, 75
    posterior crossbite, 63
wear see surface
white patches or spots (incl.
    demineralization), 138
  with fixed appliance therapy, 18
  fluorosis, 139–142